SYMPTOMS AND EARLY WARNING SIGNS

SYMPTOMS AND EARLY WARNING SIGNS

A Comprehensive Guide to More Than 600 Medical Symptoms and What They Mean

Dr. Michael Apple, Dr. Roy Macgregor, and Dr. Jason Payne-James
Edited by Peter Curtis, M.D., and Carolyn Curtis, R.N.

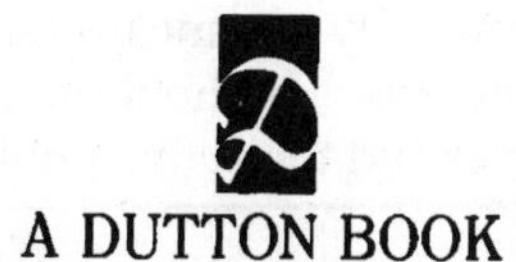

A DUTTON BOOK

DUTTON

Published by the Penguin Group
Penguin Books USA Inc., 375 Hudson Street, New York, New York 10014, USA
Penguin Books Ltd, 27 Wrights Lane, London W8 5TZ, England
Penguin Books Australia Ltd, Ringwood, Victoria, Australia
Penguin Books Canada Ltd, 10 Alcorn Avenue, Toronto, Ontario, Canada M4V 3B2
Penguin Books (NZ) Ltd, 182-190 Wairau Road, Auckland 10, New Zealand

Penguin Books Ltd, Registered Offices: Harmondsworth, Middlesex, England

Published by Dutton, an imprint of Dutton Signet, a division of Penguin Books USA Inc.

First Dutton Printing, January, 1994
10 9 8 7 6 5 4 3 2 1
First edition

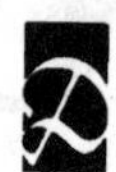

LIBRARY OF CONGRESS CATALOGING-IN-PUBLICATION DATA:

Apple, Michael.
Symptoms and early warning signs : a comprehensive guide to more than 600 medical symptoms and what they mean : Michael Apple, Roy Macgregor, and Jason Payne-James : edited by Peter Curtis and Carolyn Curtis.
p. cm.
ISBN 0–525–93732–3
1. Symptomatology—Popular works. I. Macgregor, Roy. II. Payne-James, Jason. III. Curtis, Peter, 1937- . IV. Curtis, Carolyn, R.N. V. Title.
RC69.A66 1994
616'.047—dc20 93–33383
CIP

The Editors

Dr Peter Curtis, MD co-editor, is Professor of Family Medicine at the University of North Carolina School of Medicine, where he has been teaching medicine for the past 19 years. He is also Director of the Institute for the Generalist Physician. He is board certified in Internal and Family Medicine and Obstetrics in the U.K. and in Family Medicine in the U.S.A. He has been practising medicine for 30 years and is particularly interested in musculoskeletal disease, women's health and medical education. He has published many scientific articles in medical journals and is a researcher in primary health care problems.

Carolyn Curtis, BA, RN co-editor, is a research associate in the School of Public Health at the University of North Carolina, where she co-ordinates and monitors clinical trials related to the investigation of heart disease. She has many years experience in women's health issues and has worked in a variety of fields emphasizing health care education. She has written and edited technical manuals for nurses and other health care professionals.

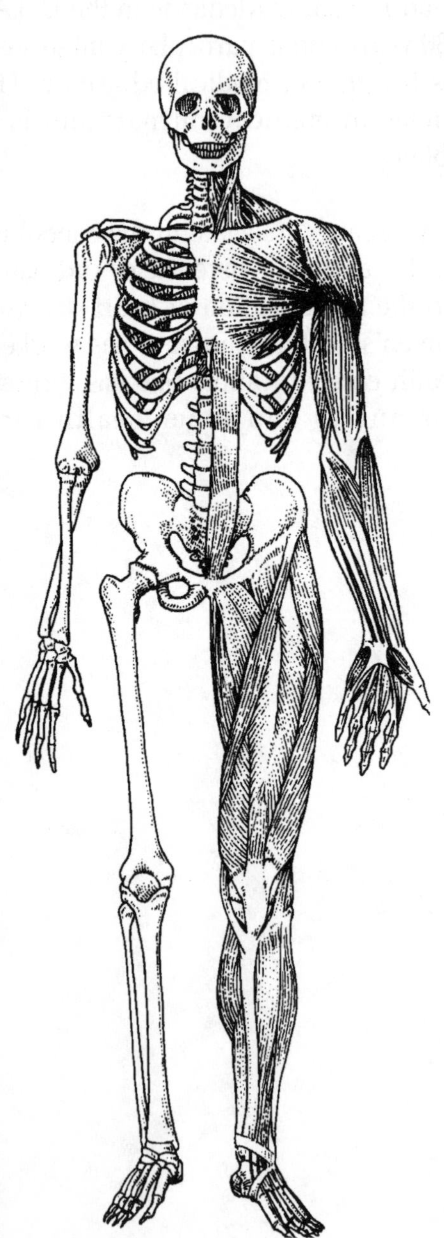

Contents

An explanation of how the contents are ordered is given on page 9. The book's main sections are:

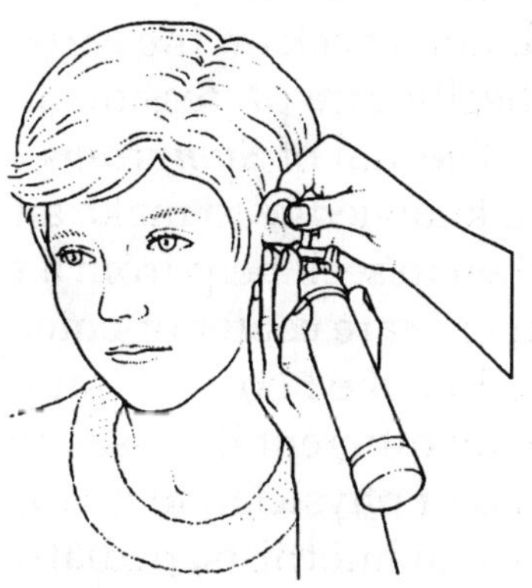

Introduction

This book is intended to help you understand your symptoms and check on the early signs of illness before getting help from a health care professional.

The aim of ***Symptoms and Early Warning Signs*** is to give you the knowledge to make an informed decision about whether and when to seek help from a nurse practitioner, pharmacist, physician, urgent care center or emergency room. As you will find out from reading the book, the same symptoms and signs can come from many different illnesses and diseases so you may not be sure what kind of physician to go to. Generalist clinicians, family physicians, general internists, pediatricians and family nurse practitioners treat a wide range of illnesses involving all body systems and they will refer you to a specialist if your problem is unusual, or not easily diagnosed, or for a special procedure or treatment such as surgery. If you choose to see a specialist for your symptoms, although he or she knows a great deal about a special area of medicine, it may not be possible to diagnose your problem without referring you to another specialist. This can be expensive and perhaps result in unnecessary and costly tests. Remember, whatever your symptoms or warning signs, many physicians' offices, clinics, health centers and some emergency rooms will offer advice over the telephone to help you decide what to do.

In ***Symptoms and Early Warning Signs,*** we have provided a picture of your signs and symptoms in the way that your physician thinks about them as she or he tries to make a diagnosis. Diagnoses are listed in order of probability: with the most commonly occurring diseases first, followed by the less likely and finally the rare causes of similar symptoms.

We hope that ***Symptoms and Early Warning Signs*** will give you the know-how to make important decisions about your health and help you separate the many minor health problems that we all encounter from the more serious illnesses that require more urgent attention.

Peter Curtis
Carolyn Curtis

The approach

For the first time ever in a popular medical guide, all the symptoms you are likely to experience are organized here in the same way that physicians think when they are trying to make a diagnosis.

Under each diagnosis the signs and symptoms are identified with a star. You do not have to experience all symptoms to make a diagnosis.

Throughout the book, diagnoses are divided into three categories:

■ **Probable**: the most likely causes of the symptom; the ones the physician would think of first. Physicians see these problems frequently.

■ **Possible:** If the probable causes have been excluded, these are the next most likely diagnoses. They may require special tests to confirm a diagnosis.

■ **Rare**: The frequency of these diagnoses is very variable. These diagnoses are *unlikely*, unless your own problem happens to match the listed signs and symptoms very closely. Remember, they are rare. Extensive testing may be required to confirm these diagnoses.

How to check your symptoms

1 Always start with your symptom or symptoms. (Often you will have a combination of symptoms rather than just one.) If it is easy to put a name to the symptom, such as headache or painful wrist, look for this in the index, which lists all the symptoms, and which will refer you straight to the relevant page number.

2 If your symptom is not quite so obvious, or easily defined, you need to decide if it can be isolated to a single part of the body — such as the knee, or abdomen — or whether it is a general, whole-body symptom, such as fever, or weight loss.

In the case of symptoms clearly occurring in one part of the body, or in one system of the body, for example the digestive system, turn straight to the relevant section and look through it. You will find that:

■ Each part of the body has its own section, clearly identified with a heading.

Using This Book

■ Symptoms are grouped like with like, so that, for instance, a common cold, shivers, chills and sweating all occur within the same few pages.

Simply look through the relevant section for the symptom, or combination of symptoms that fits your problem. If necessary follow the cross-referencing, which has been introduced to avoid too much unnecessary repetition.

3 If your symptom or symptoms cannot be isolated to a single part of the body, go to the "general" symptoms section, which comes last in the book.

Within this last section of the book, symptoms are again ordered like with like. To give additional help with symptom-finding in this section, the black bands down the sides of each page guide you to what is covered on these pages.

Medical terms

Certain terms are used so often in this book that explaining their meaning every time would be too space-consuming. They are:

Acute
Occurring now; a sudden appearance or sudden worsening.

Anxiety
Feelings of dread and concern.

Benign tumor
A lump which is not cancer.

Chronic
A disease or illness lasting usually more than six months.

Circulatory disease
Disease of the arteries or veins which carry blood around the body.

Cyanosis
Bluish skin coloration caused by lack of oxygen in the tissues.

Cyst
A sac within the body, usually fluid-filled; may also appear as a swelling in or on the body.

Follicle
Glandular structure under the skin from which a hair grows.

Immunosuppression
The immune system is the body's defence system against infection and other insults; if it is suppressed, by either illness or drugs, its normal function is limited or rendered less effective.

Indigestion, acidity
Both terms are used to describe discomfort after eating.

Lesion
A mark; a cut; a wound.

Malignant
Cancerous.

Nodule
A lump or swelling generally felt on the body's surface.

Non-specific
Usually describes a symptom which does not signify any disease in particular.

Palpable
Can be felt by hand.

Sepsis
Infection.

Systemic
Affecting all of the body's systems; widespread rather than local.

Tumor
A growth, often a lump, either benign or malignant.

Accents

Words spelt out in capitals do not carry accents in this book. They include Sjögren's disease; Ménière's disease and Guillain-Barré syndrome.

THE EYES, NOSE AND EARS

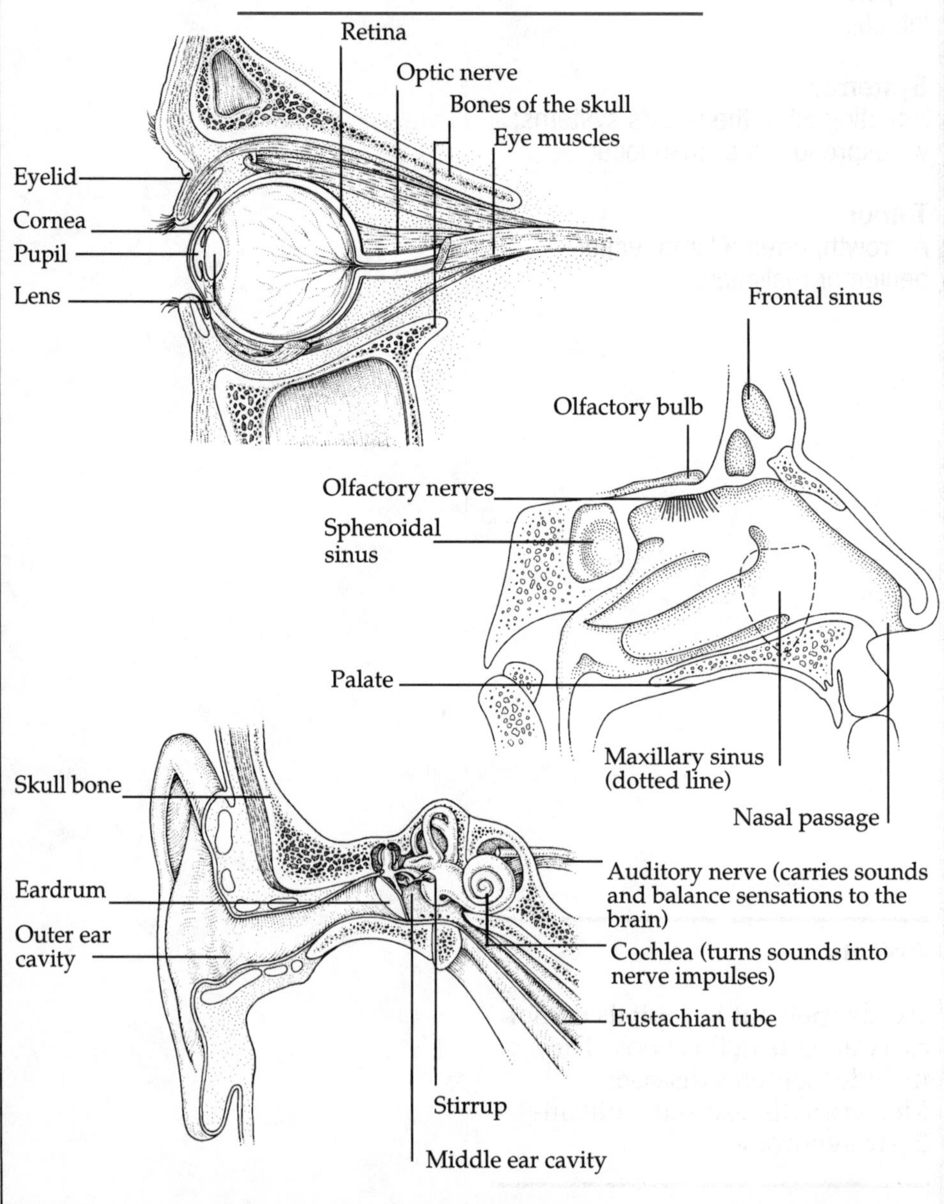

THE EYES INTRODUCTION

The eyes are delicate, highly sensitive, yet resilient structures. Light signals enter the eye through the lens which focuses the images on to the retina at the back of the eyeball. The optic nerve carries the visual impulse back to the brain where complex mechanisms translate the electrical and chemical messages into images of the world around us.

Eye problems are common in children and adults and if ignored may have serious consequences. The eyes can be affected by diseases in other parts of the body that seem to have no connection with the eyes. For instance, diabetes and high blood pressure can have serious effects on vision if not properly controlled. Report all but the most trivial eye symptoms to your physician, especially eye pain or blurred vision. Your physician will treat common problems and for anything more serious will refer you to an eye specialist (opthalmologist).

For a vision and glaucoma check, you may visit an optometrist who can prescribe eye-glasses and contact lenses, if they are required.

SKIN CHANGES AROUND THE EYE

Short-lived color change is likely, due to minor infection. Here are other possibilities to explain more long-lasting color changes.

PROBABLE

INJURY

POSSIBLE

ECZEMA

XANTHELASMA

SKIN CANCER

PROBABLE

■ INJURY

Any injury causing bruising of the forehead, or above the eye, may result in a blue/black eye, as the blood in the bruise tracks down the face to settle around the eye. A direct blow to the eye will cause the same symptoms.

* At first, redness and pain.
* Black eye appears after a few hours.
* Fades over seven to ten days.

POSSIBLE

■ ECZEMA
The skin of the eyelids and below the eyes is sensitive to many agents.
* Red, itchy skin.
* Dry and flaky.

People suffering from eczema elsewhere on the body can get this problem. Sometimes it is caused by an allergy to face make-up, nail varnish or soap. Often, an allergy test is needed to pinpoint the cause.

■ XANTHELASMA
* Yellowish, slightly raised nodules on the eyelids often close to the nose, in adults.
* Painless.
* Grow very slowly.
* Similar nodules may be found on elbows, hands, knees.

If you notice these, have a cholesterol check, since xanthelasma are often a sign of raised blood fats.

■ SKIN CANCER
Basal cell carcinoma or skin cancer is a slow-growing skin cancer often found on the lower lid and the side of the face including the ear. Common in older people.
* Begins as a slightly raised spot.
* Crusts as it grows.
* May bleed.

Cure can be virtually guaranteed if treated early.

RING AROUND CORNEA

PROBABLE
ARCUS SENILIS

POSSIBLE
IRON RING

RARE
COPPER RING

PROBABLE

■ ARCUS SENILIS
A white circle around part or all of the cornea, common in the over-60s. If seen in a younger person, it may be associated with raised blood cholesterol, which should be checked. Otherwise it is of no significance.

POSSIBLE

■ IRON RING
A brown ring may be left after a foreign body made of iron has been removed from the cornea.

RARE

■ COPPER RING
Also called Kayser-Fleischer ring. A brown or green ring associated with the rare condition of Wilson's

Disease, in which copper builds up in the body. A childhood disease, consisting of:
* Liver disease (swelling, easy bruising, jaundice).
* Tremor of the limbs.
* Dementia.
Early detection and treatment means a good prognosis.

RED AND PAINFUL EYE

Never ignore this symptom, which may be a sign of sight-threatening disease. Seek immediate medical attention.

PROBABLE
SEVERE CONJUNCTIVITIS

POSSIBLE
ACUTE IRITIS
ACUTE KERATITIS

RARE
ACUTE GLAUCOMA

PROBABLE

■ SEVERE CONJUNCTIVITIS
Conjunctivitis is inflammation of the white of the eye, giving rise to a mass of red blood vessels over the eyeball. It can be caused by contact with chemicals and fumes. Usually caused by a virus which is highly contagious, so tends to spread rapidly around a family.
* Initially, itching.
* Both eyes become red.
* The redness is greatest around the outer part of the eyeball.
* Bright light is mildly irritating.
* A yellow discharge.
* Crusted eyelids.
Antibiotic eyedrops are the widely used treatment. Sometimes the symptoms are confined to one eye only; in such cases a doctor will check-out other diseases.

POSSIBLE

■ ACUTE IRITIS
This is inflammation of the colored part of the eye, the iris, or associated structures. Iritis is not a final diagnosis in itself, since it can be caused by many diseases, in particular, arthritic disorders and connective tissue disorders.
* Usually only one eye is affected.
* Moderately painful and red.
* Redness is greatest around the colored iris.
* The pupil is smaller on the affected side.
* Vision is reduced, blurred.
* The pupil may appear irregular after repeated attacks.
Appropriate eye drops from the physician will reduce inflammation and dilate the pupil.

■ ACUTE KERATITIS
This is damage to the cornea caused by several types of infection or disease. The commonest problem is an ulcer on the cornea, or injury.
* Rapid onset of symptoms.

THE EYES

* One eye affected.
* No change in vision.
* Profuse watering; blinking.
* Light irritates the eye.

There are now highly effective anti-viral medications to counter the herpes virus which is the usual cause of this problem. Early treatment is needed.

RARE

■ ACUTE GLAUCOMA
The eyeball contains fluid which normally circulates via tiny channels. In glaucoma, pressure builds up in the eye, causing changes in vision. However, the changes usually happen so gradually that nothing is noticed until a late stage in the disease. For this reason, screening for glaucoma is important in anyone with a family history of the problem, and in anyone over the age of 60.

Sometimes, sudden, rapid rise in pressure can occur because of blockage in the channels, or perhaps if a medication constricts the pupils. This is acute glaucoma.

The early symptoms of glaucoma are:
* None at all.
* Possibly vague aching in the eyeball.
* Haloes around lights at night.
* Tunnel vision — *see page* 43.

Acute glaucoma is a medical emergency causing:
* Sudden, excruciating pain in the eye.
* Vomiting as a result of the pain.
* Redness around the iris.
* A hazy cornea.
* Vision severely reduced.

Urgent treatment is needed to reduce pressure within the eye and to save sight.

SLIGHTLY REDDENED EYE, OR RED EYE WITHOUT PAIN.

These are unlikely to signify any serious underlying cause, unless there is also blurred vision, or light hurts the eyes.

PROBABLE
CONJUNCTIVITIS
ALLERGY

POSSIBLE
SUBCONJUNCTIVAL HEMORRHAGE
FEVERISH ILLNESS

RARE
SCLERITIS/EPISCLERITIS
MENINGITIS

PROBABLE

■ CONJUNCTIVITIS
An infection of the conjunctiva, the thin membrane that covers the white of the eye.
* Eyes feel itchy and sore.
* Redness appears rapidly, due to many dilated blood vessels.
* The redness is least next to the

colored iris, greatest at the sides of the eyeballs.
* Yellow pus in the corners of the eyes.
* Eyelids may be crusted.

Conjunctivitis is usually a straightforward diagnosis, but if redness affects one eye only, other possibilities need to be considered. Antibiotic eyedrops are effective.

Contact lenses are frequently a cause of eye problems. Keeping extended wear lenses in your eyes for a long time means you are much more likely to have an eye infection or conjunctivitis.

Another common cause of infection is inadequate cleaning of lenses or the lens case.

■ ALLERGY

Recurrent, mildly red eyes raise the possibility of allergy. Common causes of allergies (allergens) are pollen, smoky atmosphere and air pollution. Sometimes, contact lenses, or the solutions used to clean them, are to blame.
* Mildly red, itchy eyes.
* May be seasonal, with sneezing and a runny nose.
* May be related to exposure to allergens as listed above.
* Discharge, if any, tends to be white and not yellow.
* Under-surface of eyelids may feel grainy.

Several effective anti-allergy medications can help, though for some this becomes a long-term problem.

POSSIBLE

■ SUBCONJUNCTIVAL HEMORRHAGE

This is blood under the conjunctiva of the eye. It may look alarming, but it is simply due to bleeding from a tiny blood vessel and will fade in a couple of weeks.
* Painless, so the condition is often pointed out by someone else.
* One eye has a bright red patch. on the white of the eye.
* Stops short at the iris.
* Fades away towards the sides of the eye.

In the elderly, it may call for a check on blood pressure. If, however, it occurs after a blow to the head, expert assessment is needed to check whether there is damage to the eye further back in its socket.

■ FEVERISH ILLNESS

Any such illness will give slightly red eyes; measles is well known for this effect.

RARE

■ SCLERITIS/EPISCLERITIS
* One part of the white of the eye is red.
* Prominent blood vessels are seen to cause the redness.
* Slight discomfort.
* Recurrent.

This condition is important since it tends to be associated with other diseases, especially joint problems. Should be seen by a physician.

The Eyes

■ MENINGITIS
A few red flecks suddenly appearing on the whites of the eyes may be the earliest signs of meningitis in a baby or child. There may also be:
* A high-pitched cry.
* Drowsiness.
* Photophobia.
* A bulging, soft spot (fontanelle) on the baby's scalp.
* A red rash elsewhere on the body.

This is a medical emergency: rush the baby or child to hospital.

ABNORMALLY SMALL PUPILS

The pupils are the openings through which light enters the eyes. Their size is controlled by nerves which make the pupils open and close. Those nerves are affected by changes within the brain.

It is normal for both pupils to be equal in size and for them to become smaller in bright light. The pupils of children and of the elderly tend to be smaller than those of adults. A young person, unconscious, and with pupils like pin points, arouses the immediate suspicion of a narcotic drug overdose.

PROBABLE
FAR-SIGHTEDNESS

POSSIBLE
MEDICATIONS
IRITIS

RARE
HORNER'S SYNDROME

PROBABLE

■ FAR-SIGHTEDNESS
Small pupils are normal in the far-sighted.
* Both pupils are small.
* The pupils react briskly to light and dark.

POSSIBLE

■ MEDICATIONS
Many medications, for example pilocarpine and timolol used to treat glaucoma (*page 45*), constrict the pupils by affecting the nerves controlling them. Small pupils may also be a side effect of the powerful narcotic painkillers such as morphine, dihydrocodeine and demerol or certain street drugs.

■ IRITIS
See page 36. Suggested by finding:
* Small, irregular pupil in one eye only.
* Pain in the same eye.
* Redness around the iris.

RARE

■ HORNER'S SYNDROME
A combination of:
* One abnormally small pupil.

* Drooping eyelid on that side.
* The eye bulging forward slightly.
* Decreased sweating on that side of the face.

Horner's syndrome reflects irritation of one of the nerves controlling the pupil somewhere along its route from the brain, down into the chest and up again to the eye. The irritation could be caused by a lung tumor; enlarged glands within the chest; multiple sclerosis; or brain disease. So although Horner's syndrome is uncommon, its significance is great, especially if there are associated symptoms such as:
* Chest pain.
* Coughing blood.
* Unsteady walking.
* Blurred vision, numb hands.

Seek medical attention.

WIDE PUPILS

PROBABLE
EMOTION
MEDICATIONS

POSSIBLE
THIRD NERVE PALSY
INJURY
COMA
ADIE'S PUPIL
BLINDNESS

RARE
IRRITATION OF NERVES TO EYE

PROBABLE

■ EMOTION
Both pupils will widen in response to emotional triggers such as fear, excitement and anxiety. Accompanying symptoms include:
* Rapid pulse.
* Thumping heart beat.
* Dry mouth.

■ MEDICATIONS
Commonly prescribed eye drops, such as atropine, are used to treat iritis and are intended to widen the pupil.

POSSIBLE

■ THIRD NERVE PALSY
See page 28. The third nerve is one of several nerves that control eye movements. If the nerve becomes paralyzed:
* The eye turns outwards.
* The eyelid droops.
* The pupil enlarges.

■ INJURY
A blow to the eye severe enough to damage its internal structure will upset movement of the pupil. This is not uncommon in sports such as baseball and raket ball.
* Probably bruising around the eye.
* Enlarged pupil, unreactive to light.
* Blurred vision is likely.

Emergency room treatment is required immediately.

THE EYES

■ COMA
A severe head injury or other serious disease affecting the brain, such as a stroke, may cause wide pupils.
* Deep unconsciousness.
* Breathing irregular and shallow.
* No response to painful stimulus.

At worst, wide pupils in both eyes which do not respond to light indicate brain death.

■ ADIE'S PUPIL
A harmless condition, generally in young women with:
* One wide pupil, which constricts in reaction to bright light, but more slowly than usual.
* Vision and health otherwise normal.

■ BLINDNESS
The pupil in a blind eye will be larger than the other eye because there is no reflex response to light.

RARE

■ IRRITATION OF NERVES TO EYE
The same process which produces Horner's Syndrome (*page 18*) can, in its early stages, irritate the nerve, causing a wide pupil. Associated symptoms which raise suspicion therefore include:
* Chest pain.
* Coughing blood.
* Unsteady walking.
* Blurred vision, numbness of hands.

Seek medical attention.

IRREGULAR PUPILS

Normal pupils are round or slightly oval. Minor irregularities are common. Major irregularities indicate disease.

PROBABLE
NORMAL VARIATION

POSSIBLE
IRITIS

RARE
MULTIPLE SCLEROSIS
SYPHILIS
BRAIN TUMOR

PROBABLE

■ NORMAL VARIATION
Minor irregularity is of no importance and may be hereditary, if there is also:
* No pain or visual disturbance.
* No change with passing of time.
* Otherwise good health.

POSSIBLE

■ IRITIS
See page 36. A small, irregular pupil is a particular feature of this painful condition, especially after repeated episodes.

RARE

■ MULTIPLE SCLEROSIS
A neurological disease usually beginning in early adult life.
* Sudden loss or blurring of vision in one eye.
* Numbness and weakness of different parts of the body.
* Tremor, unsteady gait.
Recent MRI technology has helped to make diagnosis easier.

■ SYPHILIS
A serious sexually transmitted disease affecting many parts of the body. Occurs more often now than in recent years. Some signs of syphilis are:
* Small, irregular pupils.
* Brief, severe limb pains.
* Unsteady gait.
* Loss of pain sensation in joints, leading to gross distortion of knees, ankles.
* Drooping eyelids on both sides.

■ BRAIN TUMOR
Might be possible if an irregular pupil is found together with:
* Severe and increasing headaches.
* Change of personality.
* Progressive weakness of one side of the body.

ENLARGED EYEBALL

PROBABLE
HYPERTHYROIDISM

RARE
TUMOR
THROMBOSIS
CONGENITAL GLAUCOMA

PROBABLE

■ HYPERTHYROIDISM
Also called Graves' Disease. The eyes may protrude giving a "bug-eyed" look. This responds effectively to medical treatment.
* Both eyeballs affected.
* Sweating, weight loss.
* Hyperactivity.
* Trembling of hands.

Though treatment controls the disease, the eyes may remain a little prominent.

RARE

■ TUMOR
* Progressive swelling of one eyeball. (Children or adults.)
* Cross-eyes, loss of vision, pain.

■ CONGENITAL GLAUCOMA
In children raised pressure inside the eye leads to:
* Bulging eyes.

■ THROMBOSIS
A risk in cases of meningitis and severe dehydration. Blood clots in structures behind the eyes rapidly causing:
* Painful protruding eyes.
* Restricted eye movements.
* Eyes that look swollen.

COLORED PATCHES ON EYEBALL

Doctors often check the eyes as a matter of routine because the eye may be an indicator of disease elsewhere in the body, for example jaundice or anemia.

The POSSIBLE and RARE causes of colored patches are really very infrequent.

PROBABLE
PTERYGIUM
PINGUECULA

POSSIBLE
SCLERITIS

RARE
GROWTHS

PROBABLE

■ PTERYGIUM
A wing-shaped sheath of blood vessels and tissue grows out along the white of the eye towards the cornea.
* Commonest in middle age.
* Small, triangular-shaped white tissue, blood vessels within.
* The broad base of the triangle is at the corner of the eye.

A pterygium usually causes only a cosmetic problem, or possibly slight irritation. It can be removed if it threatens to grow over the cornea.

■ PINGUECULA
The name comes from a word meaning "to do with grease". These yellowish discolorations are again little more than a cosmetic nuisance. Usually found in older people.
* Yellow, opaque raised lumps in the white of the eye.
* Triangular-shaped, with the broad base closest to the cornea.

POSSIBLE

■ SCLERITIS
In between episodes of inflammation, these groupings of blood vessels simply form a flat, discolored area to one side of the eyeball. *See page 17.*

RARE

■ GROWTHS
Any of the lumps, warts, cysts, moles and cancers that grow on skin anywhere in the body may appear on the white of the eye. Report any recently noticed spot to your physician. Remember, the appearance of any of these on the eye is very rare. Much more common are pterygium and pinguecula, above.

DISCHARGE FROM EYES

Eyes may discharge tears or pus, or a combination of both.

PROBABLE
CONJUNCTIVITIS
ALLERGY

POSSIBLE
BLOCKED TEAR DUCT
ECTROPION

RARE
GONORRHEA

PROBABLE

■ CONJUNCTIVITIS
* Red, itchy eyes develop over a day or so.
* Constant discharge of small amounts of yellow pus.
* Eyelids stick together in the mornings.

Minor infections are cleared by bathing the eyes with warm water. Severe infections, especially in children, need antibiotic drops. *See also page 16.*

■ ALLERGY
Likely if there is no seasonal tearing or itching. *See also page 17.*

POSSIBLE

■ BLOCKED TEAR DUCT
In babies, this is a common cause of eyes constantly tearing and of repeated episodes of conjunctivitis. The tear duct is too narrow for tears to drain normally into the nose.
* Usually only one eye is affected.
* Eye tears even when the baby is perfectly well.

Most babies grow out of this by their first birthday. If necessary, it is possible to dilate the tear duct surgically — a minor procedure.

■ ECTROPION
A lower eyelid turns outwards so that tears spill over; common in the elderly.

RARE

■ GONORRHEA
Though gonorrhea is a common sexually transmitted disease, routine antibiotic drops put in the baby's eyes at birth prevent infection.
* Profuse yellow pus surrounding the eyes and under the eyelids.
* Swollen eyelids, making it difficult to open the eyes.

Untreated, it causes blindness.

CONSTANT FLICKERING MOVEMENTS OF THE EYES

Medical term: nystagmus. It is not always an abnormality, as some people show a few beats of nystagmus if they look to the far left or right. Some people are born with a natural nystagmus. It is not a sign of disease in this case.

PROBABLE
VESTIBULITIS

POSSIBLE
UNCORRECTED POOR VISION
MULTIPLE SCLEROSIS
ALCOHOLISM

RARE
TUMORS
CONGENITAL BLINDNESS
ALBINISM

PROBABLE

■ VESTIBULITIS
A viral illness that upsets the organs of balance inside the ear.
* Abrupt dizziness.
* Nausea; on attempting to move.
* Eye flickering may be noticed by someone else.

Though alarming, it is a harmless condition that gradually fades away. Medication can improve the symptoms. *See also page 391*.

POSSIBLE

■ UNCORRECTED POOR VISION
An eye check-up is recommended if nystagmus is noticed in an otherwise well child.

■ ALCOHOLISM
Alcoholics with poor diets become deficient in vitamin B1, thiamine. The result is damage within the brain, causing:
* Nystagmus.
* Poor memory.
* Disorientation.
* Weak, tingling limbs.

■ MULTIPLE SCLEROSIS
Nystagmus is not an early sign of multiple sclerosis, but is found in more advanced cases.
* Muscular weakness.
* Shakiness.
* Stiff limbs.
* Blurred vision that comes and goes.

RARE

■ TUMORS
Nystagmus that has developed recently suggests that the individual should be checked for brain tumors, of which other features may be:
* Change of personality.
* Severe headaches.
* One-sided deafness.
* Ringing in the ear.
* Unsteadiness.

■ CONGENITAL BLINDNESS
The eyes of those born blind frequently show searching movements, that is, a constant slow shifting of the gaze.

■ ALBINISM
Some people lack the pigment in their bodies that protects skin and eyes from bright light. Their eyes continually move to escape the light.

CLOUDY CORNEA OR LENS

Disease in either of these structures causes a clouded, opaque appearance. Without the right equipment it may be difficult to decide whether the clouding is in the normally clear cornea, or whether it is in the deeper lens.

PROBABLE
CATARACT
INJURY

POSSIBLE
CONGENITAL

RARE
TRACHOMA
VITAMIN A DEFICIENCY
INFECTION
ACUTE GLAUCOMA
TUMOR

PROBABLE

■ CATARACT
The clouded appearance of a cataract causes:
* Circular, grey appearance over–lying the pupil.
* Gradually worsening, unclear vision.

Usually a disease of later life. Standard treatment is to replace the cataract with an artificial lens.

■ INJURY
Any serious injury or infection of the cornea will leave an opaque patch, which may obscure vision, depending on its position.

POSSIBLE

■ CONGENITAL
Several unusual inherited conditions can cause a cataract or lead to deterioration of the cornea during childhood. Diagnosis only established by a specialist examination.

RARE

■ TRACHOMA
Though rare in developed countries, this infection is one of the commonest worldwide causes of blindness.
* Swollen eyelids.
* Under surface of eyelids is granular.
* Gradual clouding of the cornea.

■ VITAMIN A DEFICIENCY
Associated with malnutrition. Worldwide, this is a serious and avoidable cause of blindness,

THE EYES

especially in children. Rare in developed countries.
* Hazy cornea with a thickened, coarse appearance.
* Night blindness.
* Colored whites of the eyes.

■ INFECTION
A hazard to vision confined mainly to undeveloped countries. Possible sources of infection are parasites, gonorrhea and syphilis; complications of each give rise to a clouded cornea.

■ ACUTE GLAUCOMA
The cornea is clouded and the eye is red and excrutiatingly painful. An emergency. (see page 45).

■ TUMOR
In children, the earliest sign of a tumor within the eye may be that the lens appears opaque.
* Often both eyes are affected.
* May be hereditary.
* Newly occurring cross-eyes is also cause for suspicion.

CATARACTS

A cataract is an opaque, clouded, patch within the lens of the eye. It cuts down the amount of light that can enter the eye and whatever light does enter is made hazy and blurred. An early cataract will not cause any symptoms and will only be spotted on examination of the eye; but a mature cataract is visible as a whitish haze on the lens. Between these two stages there will be variable symptoms.

Most cataracts are the result of

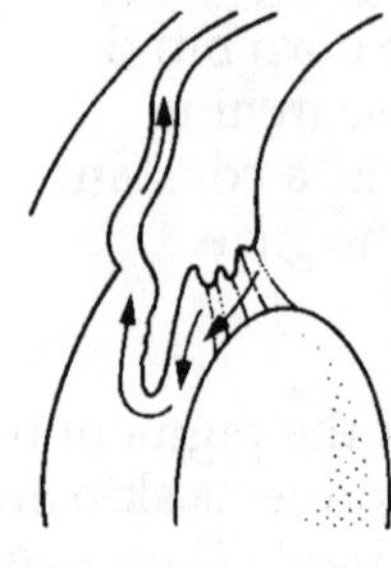

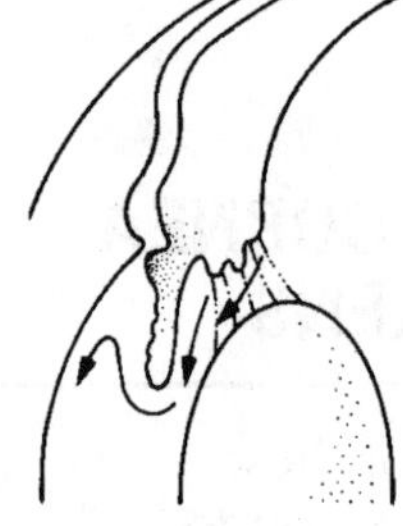

Left, a normal eye, fluid flowing freely for lubrication. Below left, drainage channel blocked by obstruction, causing the build-up characteristic of glaucoma.

aging. Occasionally they occur following injury or disease. On rare occasions, a child is born with a cataract because of infection during pregnancy.

PROBABLE
AGING
INJURY

POSSIBLE
DIABETES
STEROID USE

RARE
CONGENITAL RUBELLA
METABOLIC OR CONGENITAL DISEASE

THE EYES

PROBABLE

■ AGING
Most people over 60 will have some opacity of the lens, but if a cataract forms, it will be relatively obvious.
* No other general disease.
* Vision deteriorates slowly.
* Eyes are pain free.
Cataract surgery is an effective treatment for this common problem.

■ INJURY
Any but the most superficial injury to the cornea or lens leaves a permanent scar. This includes burns and infections, of which trachoma is the most common.
* The size of the opacity remains unchanged.
* Disturbance of vision depends on its size.

POSSIBLE

■ DIABETES
People suffering from this condition have an increased risk of developing cataracts in later life.

■ STEROIDS
Steroids, cortisone and prednisone, are invaluable medications used in the treatment of many diseases including severe asthma, joint diseases and inflammatory eye diseases such as iritis (*see page 36*). However, their long-term use can cause many side-effects, including early formation of cataracts. Do not use steroid eye drops without medical advice and monitoring. Otherwise, there is a risk of causing cataracts and of allowing infections to do severe damage to the cornea.

RARE

■ CONGENITAL RUBELLA
Rubella — German measles: infection during the first four months of pregnancy is likely to cause multiple abnormalities in the developing baby. These include:
* Cataracts.
* Mental retardation.
* Heart disease.
* Deafness.
These tragic consequences are avoided by routine vaccination of children and of mothers after pregnancy.

■ METABOLIC OR CONGENITAL DISEASE
Several unusual diseases may cause cataracts in children, usually in association with:
* Failure to grow normally.
* Developmental delay.

TWITCHING EYELID

This is often a sign of stress or fatigue.
* Brief, repeated twitching.
* Same lid is affected.
* Worse when tired or stressed.
* Rarely lasts for longer than a few days.

DROOPING EYELIDS

PROBABLE
ECTROPION

POSSIBLE
FACIAL NERVE PALSY
CONGENITAL

RARE
THIRD NERVE PALSY
MYASTHENIA GRAVIS
SYPHILIS

PROBABLE

■ ECTROPION
Sagging of the lower eyelids, very common in the elderly.
* The red under-surface of the lid is exposed.
* Tears spill out easily on to the cheek.
* Increased risk of conjunctivitis.
Really bad cases can be tightened up by a simple operation.

POSSIBLE

■ FACIAL NERVE PALSY
A paralysis of the facial nerve. Also called Bell's Palsy. Usually caused by a virus infection.
* One lower eyelid droops.
* Excessive tearing.
* Sometimes loss of taste.
* Occurs suddenly.
* The eye cannot be completely closed.
* The face sags on that side.
Recovery takes time and is usually complete. Medical treatment with steroids can speed recovery if given early. Should be seen quickly by a physician, to exclude stroke.

■ CONGENITAL
The probable diagnosis in a child with drooping upper eyelids.
* Normal eye movements.
* Normal muscular power.

RARE

■ THIRD NERVE PALSY
Refers to the third cranial nerve which is damaged (for example by pressure).
* Paralysis involves one eye only.
* Drooping upper lid.
* Eye turns outwards.
* Widened pupil.
Specialist investigation is needed to determine the underlying cause, which may be diabetes, a brain tumor, or an enlarged artery in the brain.

■ MYASTHENIA GRAVIS
A treatable disease causing rapid tiring of the muscles. Drooping eyelids are an early sign.
* Both upper eyelids are affected.
* Muscles elsewhere grow fatigued abnormally fast.

■ SYPHILIS
The late stage of syphilis, which may be 20 years after the first

infection, causes widespread nerve damage.
* Tingling feet.
* Brief shooting pains in the limbs.
* Unsteady movements.
* Pain sensation is reduced.
* Drooping eyelids on both sides.

EYELIDS INFLAMED OR ITCHY

Localized inflammation probably due to infection. More generalized itching is usually allergic.

PROBABLE
BLEPHARITIS
ALLERGY

POSSIBLE
INSECT BITES
PUBIC LICE

RARE
TRACHOMA

PROBABLE

■ BLEPHARITIS
Chronic inflammation of the margins of the eyelids along the roots of the lashes.
* Constant raw appearance.
* Crusting near the roots of the eyelashes.
* Flaking skin on eyelids.
* Intense irritation.

This common condition may be thought of as a type of dandruff affecting the eyelids. It is often associated with eczema. It helps to wash their eyelids nightly with a diluted solution of shampoo on a cotton bud. A physician can prescribe an antibiotic ointment.

■ ALLERGY
The upper eyelid is involved, causing a persistent mild irritation and desire to rub.
* Skin is slightly reddened.
* Dry, flaking skin all over upper eyelid.
* Often eczema elsewhere.

This is another minor but annoying problem, probably due to an allergic reaction. Possible triggers are hair spray, new eye make-up or nail varnish, but the cause often remains unclear even after allergy testing.

POSSIBLE

■ INSECT BITES
A common reason in the summer and autumn.
* Localized, raised red bump.
* Itchy for a few hours.

■ PUBIC LICE
Lice will happily make a home in any hairy area, including the eyelids.
* Tiny round insects seen adhering to root of eyelashes.
* May also inhabit the eyebrows.
* Will also be present in the pubic area.

See your physician for treatment.

The Eyes

RARE

■ TRACHOMA
A Third World infection causing
* Swollen eyelids.
* Grainy red under-surfaces of the eyelids.

One of the most common preventable causes of blindness.
See also page 25.

LUMPS ON EYELIDS

PROBABLE
STYE
INFECTED MEIBOMIAN CYST

POSSIBLE
MOLLUSCUM CONTAGIOSUM
SKIN CANCER

RARE
DACROCYSTITIS

PROBABLE

■ STYE
Infection at the root of a single eyelash.
* Often preceded by a day of mild discomfort.
* Swelling appears at root of hair.
* Pus appears.

Antibiotic drops help, as does removing the hair to allow drainage of pus.

■ INFECTED MEIBOMIAN CYST
The meibomian glands are helpful little structures which produce a greasy lubricant for the eyelashes. Infection reaches them via hair roots.

The important difference between this condition and a stye is that the lump is behind the root of the eyelash, on the flat part of the eyelid. It can be felt and seen as a small lump below the skin.
* Pain, redness inside an eyelid.
* Small, tender lump appears.

Treatment same as for a stye, although antibiotic pills may be required. Often an unsightly lump remains, which may need to be removed later.

POSSIBLE

■ MOLLUSCUM CONTAGIOSUM
A long name for a benign, wart-like condition, that appears in mini-epidemics among children.
* Small, rounded, slightly raised lumps.
* The center of the lump dips inwards.
* Other, similar lumps likely elsewhere on body.

Harmless, though cosmetically a nuisance; can be removed.

■ SKIN CANCER
Basal cell carcinoma or Rodent Ulcer is a slow-growing skin cancer commonest in the elderly and people who have much sun exposure.
* Begins as a small, pearly lump.
* Grows slowly.
* Center ulcerates and bleeds.

Considered curable, but needs

early medical attention.
See also page 14.

RARE

■ DACROCYSTITIS
Infection in the tear-producing glands, which are tucked away at the corners of the eyes.
* Pain, swelling near bridge of nose.
* Skin becomes red and tender.
* Pus discharges from eye.

A fairly serious condition that needs early treatment. *See also page 32.*

SWOLLEN EYELIDS

The loose skin of the eyelids easily swells to an alarming degree, but rarely for any serious reason.

PROBABLE
ALLERGY
STYE
BLEPHARITIS (CHRONIC)

RARE
ORBITAL CELLULITIS
NEPHROTIC SYNDROME

PROBABLE

■ ALLERGY
An allergic reaction of the skin of the eyelids to soap, hair spray or some other agent, though frequently the cause remains unknown. Usually both eyes are affected.
* Painless.
* Mild itching, flaking skin.
* Looks worse after sleep, because swelling worsens when a person lies flat.

■ STYE
A stye is a boil at the root of an eyelash. Large ones cause generalized swelling of the rest of the eyelid. *See also page 30.*
* Only one eye affected.
* Treatment as for a stye.

■ BLEPHARITIS (CHRONIC)
Prolonged inflammation of this kind, described on *page 29*, eventually makes the eyelids permanently swollen and roll-edged.

RARE

■ ORBITAL CELLULITIS
A spreading infection involving the skin of the eyelids and the surrounding parts of the face.
* Confined to one eye.
* May begin in a scratch or a stye.
* So much swelling that the eyelids cannot be opened.
* Red, tender eyelids.
* Raised temperature and chills.

Needs vigorous and immediate treatment with antibiotics (often intravenously) to prevent it spreading into the eye or elsewhere in the face.

■ NEPHROTIC SYNDROME
A kidney problem which has a variety of causes, as a result of which fluid builds up in several parts of the body. Can occur in

children and adults.
* Comes on slowly.
* Swelling of abdomen, ankles and face.
* Breathlessness.
Needs medical attention.

PAIN OR ACHING IN EYE AREA (even if slight)

PROBABLE
EYE STRAIN
NASAL CONGESTION
CONJUNCTIVITIS

POSSIBLE
GLAUCOMA
DACROCYSTITIS
FLU-LIKE ILLNESS
SINUSITIS

RARE
TUMOR

PROBABLE

■ EYE STRAIN
This familiar symptom arises after hours of close work, especially under poor or glaring light.
* Vision is normal.
* Aching in and around eyes.
* Relieved by a few hours' rest.
Recurrent eye strain means that you should have your vision checked, or consider adjustment to the lighting where you work.

■ NASAL CONGESTION
Along with a common cold there is often:
* Aching behind and around the eyeball.
* Blocked, runny nose.
* Mild headache.
These settle after a few days.

■ CONJUNCTIVITIS
Gives a prickling sensation, together with:
* Red eyes, worst around the margins.
* Mildly irritated by light.
* No loss of vision.
* Often a crusty deposit on the eyelashes.

POSSIBLE

■ GLAUCOMA
See page 45. This serious, but treatable condition frequently causes no other symptoms than a vague ache in and around the orbit.
It is easily detected with a simple eye check by an optician.

■ DACROCYSTITIS
An infection in the tear duct at the inner corner of the eye.
* Pain and swelling.
* A red lump appears.
* Eye runs with tears and pus.
Early treatment with antibiotics is advisable.

■ FLU-LIKE ILLNESS
Aching in the eyes is a frequent accompaniment to a feverish illness, including the common cold, or flu.
* Vision unaffected.

* Slight redness of eyes.
* Fever, aching muscles.

Within a few days, the underlying cause shows itself.

■ SINUSITIS
A very common cause of aching in and around the eyes.
* Usually develops after a common cold.
* Pain or pressure felt across the forehead or under the eyes.
* Worse on leaning forward and in the morning.

Sinusitis responds to steam inhalations, nose drops and antibiotics prescribed by your physician.

RARE

■ TUMOR
Needs to be considered in cases of persistent pain, especially with:
* Children
* Bulging eye.
* Changed vision.
* Newly occurring cross-eyes.

DRY EYES

* A constant feeling of irritation in the eyes.
* Frequent, mild conjunctivitis.

PROBABLE
AGING

POSSIBLE
DRY ATMOSPHERE

RARE
SJOGRENS' SYNDROME

PROBABLE

■ AGING
The eye's natural ability to lubricate itself with tears may decrease with age. "Artificial tears" in the form of eye drops are effective, but have to be used regularly.

Prolonged use of a VDU (visual display unit/computer screen) can cause uncomfortable or dry eyes. There is static electricity between the eyes and the screen. Dust is attracted to the eyes and can cause irritation. Tip: use an impregnated cloth to keep the area around your work-station as free from dust as possible.

POSSIBLE

■ DRY ATMOSPHERE
Many people complain of dry eyes during the winter, when heating systems are on and in the summer with air conditioning.

RARE

■ SJOGRENS' SYNDROME
A general term for a group of disorders in which the linings of the eyes and the salivary glands

dry out, leading to dry eyes and mouth. It may be associated with rheumatic diseases or with autoimmune diseases, causing:
* Joint pains.
* Swollen joints.
* Rashes.

Blood tests can usually pin down the underlying disease.

FEELING SOMETHING IN THE EYE

Considering how much dust flies around our city streets, it is remarkable how rarely anything gets into the eyes.
* A sudden, pricking feeling in one eye.
* Rapid blinking.
* Tears, sensitivity to light.
* Mild discomfort.
* The feeling that you must get something out of your eye.

PROBABLE
FOREIGN BODY
CONJUNCTIVITIS

POSSIBLE
INGROWING EYELASH
ALLERGY
STYE

RARE
CORNEAL ULCER

PROBABLE

■ FOREIGN BODY
Typically dust. Often a helper can see and remove the foreign body by washing the eye with water. But beware of a foreign body involving high-speed fragments, for example, while hammering concrete or drilling. Seek urgent care if symptoms continue for more than an hour or so, or if there are signs of infection.

■ CONJUNCTIVITIS
It is common, during the early stages of conjunctivitis before the redness is noticeable, to feel that something is lodged in the eye. Probably many cases of conjunctivitis do actually begin with a small foreign body, which then creates infection.

POSSIBLE

■ INGROWING EYELASH
A constant feeling of irritation in one part of the eye suggests that you should look carefully at the eyelids for this frequently overlooked cause.

■ ALLERGY
A recurrent feeling of irritation may be caused by allergy:
* Mild redness.
* Itching, rather than pain.

See also page 17.

■ STYE
An infection at the root of one of the eyelashes.

* Visible as a yellow swelling.
* The eye becomes red.
* Swelling of the eyelid is common.

Pulling out the eyelash allows drainage of the infection. Then gently apply a warm moist cloth or heating pad. Antibiotic ointment treatment may be necessary.

RARE

■ <u>CORNEAL ULCER</u>
A possibility if only one eye is inflamed. These uncommon infections begin with:
* Itching in one eye.
* Inability to look at light.
* Redness, mainly around the colored iris.

Another cause is damage by a foreign body.

A doctor will check for an ulcer using a fluorescent stain. The usual cause is the herpes virus. Vigorous treatment with anti-viral eye drops is necessary.

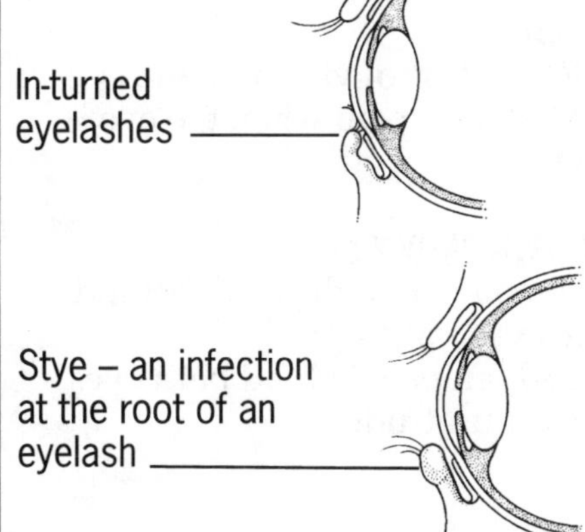

MODERATE TO SEVERE PAIN IN EYE

With the exception of an obvious foreign body, any such degree of eye pain needs expert assessment since neglect may permanently damage sight.

PROBABLE
FOREIGN BODY
ULCER OR ABRASION OF CORNEA

POSSIBLE
IRITIS
EPISCLERITIS
SHINGLES

RARE
ACUTE GLAUCOMA
RETROBULBAR NEURITIS
THROMBOSIS

PROBABLE

■ <u>FOREIGN BODY</u>
Dust, grit or in-growing eyelashes cause irritation out of all proportion to the size of the foreign body.
* One eye affected.
* Sudden onset, feeling something in the eye.
* Intense irritation and watering.
* Light irritates the eye.
* Vision unaffected, though may be blurred by tears.

THE EYES

The eye's own protective mechanisms sweep out the foreign body in most cases within an hour or so.

■ ULCER OR ABRASION OF CORNEA
An ulcer can quite easily occur on the delicate cornea, due to damage from a foreign body or from infection. The symptoms are:
* Intense discomfort in one eye.
* Builds up over a few hours.
* Light causes much discomfort.
* Redness around the iris (the colored part of the eye).

POSSIBLE

■ IRITIS
An inflammation of the iris; it may be associated with different types of joint disease.
* One eye affected.
* Redness, greatest around the colored iris.
* Inability to look at light.
* Blurred vision.
* Small pupil on affected side.

Treatment with eye drops, prescribed by a physician, is necessary to prevent permanent damage to the iris.

■ EPISCLERITIS
Irritation in one part of the eye:
* Redness in one obvious area of the white of the eye.
* Prominent blood vessels.
* Pain is moderate.
* Light irritates the eye.
* Vision is unaffected, apart from blurring due to tears.

■ SHINGLES
The medical name is Herpes Zoster. A disease caused by the chicken pox virus. But it is not highly infectious.
* At first, discomfort around one side of the face with no skin changes.
* After five to ten days, a rash appears.
* Crusting sores may develop over the forehead, eyelids, side of the nose and cheek.
* Severe pain.
* If spots appear on the tip of the nose, there is an increased chance of the eye being affected.

The main concern is ulceration of the cornea. There are now powerful anti-viral medications which need to be given early in the illness to reduce this possibility.

RARE

■ ACUTE GLAUCOMA
See page 45.

■ RETROBULBAR NEURITIS
Inflammation of the optic nerve, especially associated with multiple sclerosis.
* Rapid loss of vision in one eye.
* Moderate pain when the eye is moved.

■ THROMBOSIS
A blood clot in the skull behind the eyes, causing:
* Sudden pain behind both eyes.
* Eyes protrude.

EYES ABNORMALLY SENSITIVE TO LIGHT

Any existing irritation of the eyes will cause some discomfort in bright light. Persistent or severe sensitivity to light is called photophobia, and can be a symptom of:

PROBABLE
CONJUNCTIVITIS
ALLERGY

POSSIBLE
IRITIS
CORNEAL DAMAGE
MEASLES

RARE
MENINGITIS
ALBINISM

PROBABLE

■ CONJUNCTIVITIS
Mild redness around the outer parts of the whites of the eyes, plus:
* Sticky discharge.
* A mild, gritty feeling in eyes.
Antibiotic eye treatment is usually advisable. *See page 15.*

■ ALLERGY
Recurrent photophobia suggests an allergy, especially in someone with other signs of an allergic constitution, such as:
* Eczema.
* Runny nose: sneezing on exposure to pollens, animal hair.
* Itching eyes on exposure to dust or in specific environments.
* Vision is not affected, other than by the watering produced by the allergy.

Treatment is typically a combination of anti-histamine tablets and anti-allergic eye drops.

POSSIBLE

■ IRITIS
See page 36.

■ DAMAGED CORNEA
A picture similar to iritis, but with:
* Less severe pain.
* Redness around the cornea.
* History of abrasion or ulcer in the eye.

Needs appropriate treatment.

■ MEASLES
An increasing rarity in developed countries, where vaccination programs are leading to its eradication, measles can still be fatal to children in the Third World.

Sensitivity to light is common in the days before the rash appears.
* High fever for four days.
* Bloodshot eyes.
* Runny nose, cough.
* Blotchy red rash appears behind the ears and spreads over whole body.
* Temperature remains high for another three to four days.

Highly infectious.

The Eyes

RARE

■ MENINGITIS
Sensitivity to light is a significant symptom of meningitis, but there will usually be associated symptoms, including:
* Headache.
* Resistance and pain on attempting to bend the neck.
* Nausea and sometimes vomiting.
* Drowsiness, or confusion.
* In babies, a bulging, soft spot on top of the skull.

If you suspect meningitis, seek medical advice immediately.

■ ALBINISM
Due to lack of pigment, albinos have a special sensitivity to bright lights. Nystagmus (abnormal eye movements, *see CONSTANT FLICKERING MOVEMENTS OF THE EYES, page 24)* and cross-eyes are also common.

BLURRED VISION

Temporary blurring will result from any eye irritation causing tears to flow, for instance conjunctivitis. Persistent or recurrent blurring may result from the following:

PROBABLE
UNCORRECTED VISION

POSSIBLE
MACULAR DEGENERATION
CATARACT
EFFECTS OF MEDICATIONS

RARE
DIABETES

PROBABLE

■ UNCORRECTED VISION
The lens of the eye changes its shape to focus on near and far objects. Gradually, the power of the lens may change, also the strength of the muscles that move the lens.
* Gradual change.
* Can be corrected with eye-glasses.

Children are not usually aware of poor or changing vision, so eye checks are important in childhood.

POSSIBLE

■ MACULAR DEGENERATION
A process of deterioration of part of the retina of the eye in the elderly, causing loss of fine vision to a variable degree, not correctable with eye-glasses.
See page 45.

■ CATARACT
The interference with light caused by the cataract may be mis-interpreted as blurred vision. *See page 25.*

■ EFFECTS OF MEDICATIONS
Many medications affect the muscles in the eye, causing blurred vision. It is a question of relating the symptom to taking the medication. Common culprits include treatments to control bladder function, and depression.

RARE

■ DIABETES
Swings in the blood's sugar level can cause blurred vision.
* A temporary symptom which comes and goes.
* Undiagnosed diabetes usually causes thirst, frequent urination, tiredness and weight loss.

DISTORTION OF VISION

Objects look too small, or too large, and straight lines appear curved. Not a common symptom and, if persistent, needs expert assessment.

PROBABLE
UNKNOWN CAUSE

POSSIBLE
DETACHED RETINA

RARE
DISTORTION OF THE RETINA

PROBABLE

■ UNKNOWN CAUSE
The sensation of distortion of size or shape sometimes happens for just a brief moment. An object may suddenly seem to be distant.
* Vision otherwise unaffected.
* Recovers within moments.

POSSIBLE

■ DETACHED RETINA
Images falling on the crinkled, detaching retina seem distorted.
* Preceded by many floaters — *see page 42*
* The classic symptom is often described as a "curtain coming down to obscure the sight".
* Many flashing lights.

Seek medical help immediately, since early intervention can prevent loss of vision. *See page 47 for further details.*

RARE

■ DISTORTION OF THE RETINA
Just as distortion of a screen distorts the film projected on it, so distortion of the retina has the same effect on vision. This may be caused by tumors, bleeding or inflamation. Other symptoms, if any, include:
* Symptoms of retinal detachment, *above*.
* A bulging eye.
* Loss of vision.
* In children, a white appearance of the lens.

Seek medical help.

DOUBLE VISION

Movements of the eyes are delicately co-ordinated by an automatic process of the brain. Newborn babies have irregular, unco-ordinated eye movements and have to learn co-ordination. When things go wrong, we start seeing two of everything since the brain is no longer able to merge the vision from the two eyes into one image. Don't confuse this symptom with blurred vision, which raises quite different possibilities.

PROBABLE
USING EXTREMITIES OF GAZE
PARALYSIS OF EYE MUSCLES

POSSIBLE
MULTIPLE SCLEROSIS

RARE
DISPLACEMENT OF EYEBALL
MYASTHENIA GRAVIS
DISEASE OF ONE LENS

PROBABLE

■ USING EXTREMITIES OF GAZE
It is normal to experience double vision if the eyes are swivelled to the extreme left or right, up or down.

■ PARALYSIS OF EYE MUSCLES
The eye is moved by six muscles, each of which turns the eye in a particular direction. Paralysis of any of those muscles results in double vision because the affected muscle is unable to move the eye as well as the other eye can move. The pattern of weakness gives a clue as to which muscles are affected:
* The affected eye turning inwards or outwards.
* Eyelid may droop.
* Pupil on that side may be wider than on the unaffected side.

Many cases are unexplained. A head injury is a common cause and will be obvious. Other possibilities are meningitis, infections and nerve damage, but these give rise to more dramatic symptoms which overshadow the double vision, for instance:
* Severe headache.
* Confusion, drowsiness.
* The eye hurt by light.

POSSIBLE

■ MULTIPLE SCLEROSIS
A disease of the nervous system often beginning in early adult life. Double vision results from partial weakness of the eye muscles.
* Vision may also be blurred.
* Slight discomfort in the eye.
* Unsteadiness in walking.
* Shakiness or weakness in the arms or legs.
* Numbness of the limbs.
* Urinary control problems.

The double vision usually recedes over time.

RARE

■ DISPLACEMENT OF EYEBALL
Caused by something pushing the eye forwards and interfering with its movements. Bleeding behind the eye, or thrombosis, would be suggested by:
* Sudden onset.
* Pain in eye(s).
* Eye(s) suddenly bulging.

Graves' disease, associated with an overactive thyroid gland, or a tumor behind the eye, would produce:
* Slower onset of symptoms.
* Gradual bulging of one or both eyes.
* Sweating, rapid pulse and weight loss.

■ MYASTHENIA GRAVIS
An unusual disease in which muscles anywhere in the body tire rapidly. Eye symptoms are an early feature.
* Eyelids droop.
* Double vision may occur in any direction of gaze.
* Both eyes are affected.

The diagnosis is confirmed by the individual's response to certain injected medications.

■ DISEASE OF ONE LENS
The apparently impossible symptom of double vision affecting one eye may, in fact, though rarely, be due to disease in one lens which splits the image like a prism.

FLASHING LIGHTS

Caused by individual light receptors firing off in the retina.

PROBABLE
NORMAL

POSSIBLE
MIGRAINE

RARE
DETACHED RETINA

PROBABLE

■ NORMAL
Flashing lights are frequently experienced after a blow to the head or after suddenly getting up from a squatting position, when blood flow to the brain is briefly disturbed.
* Both eyes affected.
* You feel light-headed, briefly.
* Return to normal within seconds.

POSSIBLE

■ MIGRAINE
Flashing lights shimmering in one section of the field of vision are a typical warning of the onset of migraine.

* Usually both eyes are affected.
* Nausea.
* Headache.

See also page 113.

RARE

■ DETACHED RETINA

See page 47.

* One eye affected.
* A shower of flashes.
* Numerous floaters.

These symptoms need urgent medical attention

FLOATERS - FLOATING SPOTS BEFORE THE EYES

The interior of the eye consists of a liquid, in which it is normal for clumps of cells to float around, hence the term "floaters". An alternative medical term is muscae volitantes, meaning "flying flies".

PROBABLE
NORMAL

POSSIBLE
SEVERE NEAR-SIGHTEDNESS

RARE
DETACHED RETINA
DAMAGE TO RETINA

PROBABLE

■ NORMAL

A floater is probably harmless if:
* There are only one or two.
* Vision is otherwise normal.
* The eye is painless.

POSSIBLE

■ SEVERE NEAR-SIGHTEDNESS

This can cause the release of more than usual numbers of floaters.

RARE

■ DETACHED RETINA

See page 47. Before complete detachment, warning signs include:
* Large numbers of floaters.
* Showers of flashing lights.

If you have these symptoms, you need urgent medical attention.

■ DAMAGE TO RETINA

Inflammation or bleeding within the eye causes:
* Many floaters in one eye.
* Blurring of vision.
* Pain.
* Redness.

Treatment depends on the cause.

SEEING HALOES (RINGS) AROUND LIGHTS

This happens if the cornea becomes waterlogged, as in glaucoma, or if something within the lens is scattering light.

PROBABLE
GLAUCOMA

POSSIBLE
CATARACT

PROBABLE

■ GLAUCOMA
See page 45.
* Haloes, seen especially at night.
* Tunnel vision.

Untreated, glaucoma progressively destroys sight, producing few symptoms until the disease is well advanced. So it is important to have your eyes checked if a close relative suffers from glaucoma. People over 60 should be checked regularly.

POSSIBLE

■ CATARACT
See page 25. The haziness in the lens acts like a prism: it scatters light so that objects appear to be surrounded by haloes and rainbows.

TUNNEL VISION

Loss of the outer field of vision: you seem to look at the world through a tube. The brain is so adaptable that the problem can progress unnoticed for quite some time.

PROBABLE
GLAUCOMA

POSSIBLE
RETINITIS PIGMENTOSA
MIGRAINE

RARE
BRAIN TUMOR
SYPHILIS

PROBABLE

■ GLAUCOMA
Suggested by the combination of:
* Tunnel vision.
* At night, bright lights appear to be surrounded by haloes.
* Sometimes, aching in eyes.

See page 45.

POSSIBLE

■ RETINITIS PIGMENTOSA
See page 46.

THE EYES

■ MIGRAINE
* Symptoms develop over a few minutes.
* Visual field appears to shrink.
* Followed by severe headache, nausea.
* Vision recovers.
Can often be prevented or helped by medical treatment.

RARE

■ BRAIN TUMOR
Can cause tunnel vision by increasing the pressure inside the brain, or by a direct destruction of the parts of the brain required to interpret vision. There are likely to be other symptoms such as:
* Severe chronic headache, typically on waking at night.
* Persistent nausea.
* Change of personality.
* Altered awareness.

■ SYPHILIS
Years after infection, the widespread damage caused by this disease also causes a multitude of symptoms including:
* Severe shooting pains in limbs.
* Unsteady gait.
* Drooping eyelids.
* Loss of pain sensation in limbs, leading to grossly deformed joints.
* Some degree of mental disturbance.

BLINDNESS

Many causes of blindness cannot be treated. It is, therefore, important to know which causes of blindness are treatable, or controllable. People with high blood pressure, diabetes or a family history of glaucoma should take special care of their eyes and watch out for warning signs, including flashing lights, pains in the eyes and pain in the temples.

BLINDNESS, GRADUAL

Gradual, permanent loss of vision.

PROBABLE
CATARACT
MACULAR DEGENERATION
DIABETIC EYE DISEASE
GLAUCOMA

POSSIBLE
HIGH BLOOD PRESSURE
CHOROIDITIS
RETINITIS PIGMENTOSA

RARE
TRACHOMA

PROBABLE

■ CATARACT
A white patch seen in the lens of the eye and nearly always due to the aging process.
* Very gradual loss of clear vision.
* The awareness of light is not lost, only clarity.

Cataract surgery is a very successful form of treatment. *See page 25.*

■ MACULAR DEGENERATION

The retina of the eye is made up of a sandwich of light-sensitive receptors. The macula is a small area of the retina where these receptors are most concentrated and where the sharpest vision is achieved.

"Degeneration" means, literally, decrease in function — part of the natural process of aging. This is the commonest cause of worsening eyesight in the elderly. Disease in the macula has a serious effect on vision, but does not cause total loss of sight. Unfortunately, little can be done to halt established degeneration, but sometimes it is possible to seal blood vessels with a laser.

* Gradual, painless loss of vision.
* Central vision deteriorates.
* Vision, especially close vision, is blurred and not improved with eye-glasses.
* Outer vision is unaffected.
* Objects may look distorted or small.

There is never complete loss of vision, because the outer parts of the retina are spared.

■ DIABETIC EYE DISEASE

One long-term effect of diabetes is degeneration of blood vessels within the retina. This causes loss of vision that can be gradual or sudden, depending on the pattern of degeneration. Diabetics, therefore, need annual eye checks by an opthalmologist. It is possible to treat blood vessels which appear diseased with a laser beam.

■ GLAUCOMA

Raised pressure inside the eye, a common condition, which should be screened for in the elderly and earlier in those with a family history of glaucoma. The features of blindness caused by this insidious disease are:

* Painless.
* Peripheral vision is lost, giving rise to tunnel vision.
* Occasionally, aching in eyes.
* At night, bright lights appear to be surrounded by a halo.

POSSIBLE

■ HIGH BLOOD PRESSURE

This may increase the likelihood of macular degeneration (*see this page*) and should be treated. Mild to moderate high blood pressure has no symptoms. Very high blood pressure over a long period may cause:

* Severe headaches.
* Symptoms due to strain on the heart such as breathlessness, ankle swelling, palpitations or chest pain.

■ CHOROIDITIS

The choroid is one of the layers in the sandwich that makes up the retina. Inflammation in the choroid results in a gradual, but permanent, loss of vision corresponding to the site of damage. The reason for most cases of choroiditis is unknown, although there is a proven association with toxoplasmosis, an infection that causes an illness similar to glandular fever.

Syphilis used to be a more common cause.

* You may recall an episode of disturbed vision in one eye.
* You then become aware of an area of blindness in that eye.
* Only one eye affected.
* The area is fixed, and neither grows nor shrinks.

■ RETINITIS PIGMENTOSA
A degenerative condition affecting the retina and so called because of the dark pigment that is visible over the retina through an opthalmoscope. This tends to be an inherited condition and nothing can be done to stop it.
* Symptoms begin in adolescence.
* Gradual loss of the peripheral field of vision, leading eventually to tunnel vision.
* Night blindness.

RARE

■ TRACHOMA
Worldwide, trachoma is a common cause of blindness, but it is rare in the developed world. The infection causes:
* Extremely sore, puffy eyes.
* Running eyes.
* Scarring of the cornea, resulting in partial or total blindness.

SUDDEN BLINDNESS

Unusual, but when it does occur, it has a serious underlying cause.

PROBABLE
BLOCKAGE OF CENTRAL RETINAL ARTERY
BLOCKAGE OF CENTRAL RETINAL VEIN
DETACHED RETINA
AMAUROSIS FUGAX – MINI-STROKE
STROKE

POSSIBLE
TEMPORAL ARTERITIS
MIGRAINE
OPTIC NEURITIS
VITREOUS HEMORRHAGE
ACUTE GLAUCOMA

RARE
METHYL ALCOHOL POISONING
INJURY
HYSTERIA

PROBABLE

■ BLOCKAGE OF CENTRAL RETINAL ARTERY
This artery supplies blood to the back of the eye. Blockage may occur because of a tiny blood clot or because the artery constricts to the point where it cuts off blood flow:

* Sudden, total blindness.
* No pain.
* One eye affected.

If the blockage is a result of spasm of the artery, there is a chance of vision returning after an hour or so. Otherwise, there is no treatment. It is important to search for causes that may threaten the sight of the other eye, for example, a source of blood clots in the heart, or temporal arteritis (*see below*).

■ BLOCKAGE OF THE CENTRAL RETINAL VEIN

This vessel carries blood away from the eye. Blockage is usually caused by pressure from a diseased retinal artery, which lies very close to the vein.
* The elderly, and those with diabetes or high blood pressure, are at increased risk.
* Loss of vision is rapid, but not instant, as in arterial blockage.
* Usually, light can still be seen.

Sometimes partial vision returns, though this can take a few weeks.

■ DETACHED RETINA

The retina is not firmly attached to the back of the eye, but is held in place by the pressure of fluid within the eye. The retina can rip, allowing fluid to leak behind it and to peel it off the back of the eye. A blow to the head may also dislodge the retina, or, rarely, a tumor growing at the back of the eye.
* Most common in the very near-sighted.
* Multiple flashing lights may be a warning of detachment.
* A shadow appears to fall over the field of vision. Sometimes described as a curtain descending over the field of vision.

With early treatment, the retina can often be anchored back into place.

■ AMAUROSIS FUGAX — MINI-STROKE

This is, in fact, a blockage of the central retinal artery; however, the blood clot rapidly dislodges.
* Sudden, painless loss of vision in one eye.
* Vision returns after a few minutes.

Your doctor must search for the site where the blood clots originate. It is usually in the carotid artery, which runs up the neck.

■ STROKE

A stroke is caused by blockage of blood flow within the brain. If the blockage involves the part of the brain that processes the information from the eyes, the result is full or partial blindness.
* Sudden, painless onset.
* Vision is usually lost in both eyes at once.
* Sudden paralysis of one side of the body.
* In severe strokes, unconsciousness follows.

The exact nature of the loss of vision can give a clue as to where in the brain damage has occurred.

See also BLIND SPOTS, page 49.

THE EYES

POSSIBLE

■ TEMPORAL ARTERITIS
This cause of blindness should be better known because it is treatable. It is often associated with a condition known as polymyalgia rheumatica *(see also page 272)* and occurs in the elderly.
* Gradual development of a vague weakness and malaise.
* Muscular tenderness, especially around shoulders and neck.
* Tenderness over the temples: a very significant symptom.

The disease responds dramatically to steroid (cortisone) medication, which can save sight if the problem is recognized in time.

■ MIGRAINE
Visual disturbances, including temporary blindness, are common in migraine. Commonest in, but not confined to, the young and middle-aged.
* Shimmering lights in the eyes.
* Nausea, vomiting.
* One-sided blindness.
* Possibly slurred speech, loss of use of one hand.
* As symptoms fade, a severe headache begins.

The first time this happens, it may seem like a stroke. Many doctors recommend further tests, since occasionally there is a cause for the migraine within the brain.

■ OPTIC NEURITIS
Inflammation of the optic nerve, usually in a young adult.
* Sudden loss of vision in one eye.
* Usually, the loss is confined to the central field of vision, so the individual can still see "at the edges of vision".
* The eye may ache.

Recovery after a few days. Optic neuritis can be a warning sign of multiple sclerosis. Other underlying causes may be syphilis, diabetes, and lack of B vitamins.

■ VITREOUS HEMORRHAGE
Bleeding into the fluid within the eyeball. Associated with diabetes, and with general arterial disease.
* Mild cases give rise to multiple floaters — *see page 42.*
* Otherwise painless partial loss of vision in one eye.

The problem is confirmed by looking at the interior of the eye with an opthalmoscope. There is rarely any treatment. The outcome depends on the size of the bleed and any underlying disease.

■ ACUTE GLAUCOMA
See page 45. Suggested by the sudden onset of:
* Excruciating pain in one eye.
* Red eye.
* Glazed appearance of the eye.

Requires emergency treatment.

RARE

■ METHYL ALCOHOL
Drinkers of methanol are at risk of sudden blindness in one or both eyes.

■ INJURY
A head injury can cause sudden blindness by damaging the part of the brain involved in vision, or by causing retinal detachment — see above.

■ HYSTERIA
Blindness of psychological origin is suspected if the back of the eye appears normal and if electrical tests show that visual stimuli are reaching the brain. The individual has usually exhibited other odd physical symptoms, such as:
* Unexplained paralysis.
* Loss of speech.
* Abnormal gait.
* Does not show the expected emotional reaction to blindness, which for most people is a devastating event.

There is often previous psychotic history.

BLIND SPOTS

You may become aware of an area of your field of vision where the vision is poor or absent altogether. Wherever you look, that patch remains fixed in relation to the rest of your visual field. This is known as a scotoma. A scotoma that suddenly appears will be obvious, but you may be unaware of a slowly enlarging scotoma until it is quite large. You are aware only of some blurring of vision.

Scotomas in both eyes are due to damage to the optic nerves somewhere in the brain. A scotoma in one eye is nearly always due to a cause within that eye.

A scotoma should not be confused with the blind spot which every one has: an area of low vision which might possibly be noticed if one eye is covered and an object slowly moved to the side. There is a point at which the object briefly disappears from vision. This corresponds with the part of the retina where the optic nerve leaves the eye and where, therefore, there are no visual receptors.

PROBABLE
MACULAR DEGENERATION
STROKE
INJURY

POSSIBLE
PITUITARY TUMOR

RARE
POISONING
CAROTID ANEURYSM
HEREDITARY

PROBABLE

■ MACULAR DEGENERATION
Age-related deterioration of the eye causing a fixed area of poor or absent vision. *See page 45.*
* One eye affected more than the other.
* A loss of vision in the center of the field.
* The area of loss may increase very slowly.

■ STROKE
A stroke affecting the back of the brain causes:
* Loss of part of the field of vision.

THE EYES

* Both eyes are affected.
* Other features of a stroke, such as paralysis, confusion.

See also page 47.

■ INJURY
A blow to the head severe enough to damage the eye or the brain may cause loss of vision.
* Usually both eyes are affected.

POSSIBLE

■ PITUITARY TUMOR
The pituitary gland is a structure in the brain which lies close to the nerves coming from the eyes. Any tumor in the gland presses on those nerves, producing a characteristic blind spot.
* Painless.
* Loss of the outer field of vision.
* Both eyes affected.
* Mild headache.

There may be other symptoms as a result of abnormal hormone production: for example, excessive height, absent menstruation, breasts constantly leaking milk.

RARE

■ POISONING
Tobacco, ethyl alcohol and lead are some of the many poisons that may affect the optic nerve.
* Gradual loss of the central field of vision.
* Vision is generally dimmed.
* Loss of vision may be abrupt after an alcoholic binge.

Recovery depends on how long-standing the damage is.

■ CAROTID ANEURYSM
A swollen carotid artery within the brain, which presses on the optic nerve.
* A blind area in the outer field of vision.
* Affects one eye at first.
* Gradually involves both eyes.

■ HEREDITARY
Rare, inherited conditions might be a possibility in young adults who develop a scotoma.

NIGHT BLINDNESS

PROBABLE
RETINITIS PIGMENTOSA

POSSIBLE
SEVERE NEAR-SIGHTEDNESS
CONGENITAL

RARE
VITAMIN A DEFICIENCY

PROBABLE

■ RETINITIS PIGMENTOSA
See page 46. Suspected in a young adult with:
* Night blindness.
* Tunnel vision.

POSSIBLE

■ SEVERE NEAR-SIGHTEDNESS
* Difficulty seeing when the light is poor.
* Blurred vision, helped by glasses.

■ CONGENITAL
Occasionally, poor night vision is present from birth.

RARE

■ VITAMIN A DEFICIENCY
Vitamin A is required for vision, and is the basis for the idea that eating carrots, a rich source of Vitamin A, will help night vision. People with no vitamin A deficiency cannot improve their night vision. But a lack of this vitamin is a major cause of blindness in the Third World.
* Night blindness is an early symptom.
* The eyes appear leathery, the lenses clouded.

High doses of Vitamin A given early can save sight.

COLOR BLINDNESS

A condition affecting about one in 12 males and about one in 200 females. In the commonest form, red–green vision is partly or completely absent; less commonly, blue–green vision is affected. Total absence of any color vision is very rare. So adaptable is the brain that it is possible to reach adult life without any suspicion of a problem. The individual appears to distinguish colors by noting subtle differences in brightness and greyness; context also helps — for example the lowest traffic light is green because that is what everyone else calls it.

Normal color vision is needed in certain occupations — typically pilots and truck drivers — where it is essential to see color absolutely correctly.

Occasionally, someone with previously normal color vision finds it deteriorating for one of the following reasons:

PROBABLE
CATARACT
DAMAGE TO THE RETINA

POSSIBLE
MALNUTRITION

RARE
TOXIC MEDICATIONS

PROBABLE

■ CATARACT
This common problem, typically experienced as haziness in the lens, does not really destroy color vision but makes colors less easy to distinguish. *See page 25.*

■ DAMAGE TO RETINA
Many retinal diseases can affect color vision by damaging the receptors responsible for seeing

color. Other symptoms, considered fully elsewhere in this section, can include:
* Gradual loss of vision.
* Sudden loss of vision.
* Blind spots.

It is not possible to be more specific without medical assessment of the eye, optic nerve and the parts of the brain responsible for vision.

POSSIBLE

■ MALNUTRITION
Lack of vitamins and protein needed for the visual receptors can cause color vision to deteriorate. It is a possibility among the very poor, alcoholics, people with wasting diseases or mental illness.

There is likely to be also:
* Night blindness. *See page 50.*
* In children, failure to grow.
* Hair loss, loss of skin color.
* Swollen ankles.

RARE

■ TOXIC DRUGS
This includes massive over-use of tobacco and alcohol.

Overdosage of digoxin, used in heart disease, can make the world look yellow or green.

CROSS-EYES

Cross-eyes (or strabismus) are the result of the eyes being out of alignment: they appear to point in different directions. Often cross-eyes are suspected as an impression rather than definitely seen: you may have the feeling on looking at someone that their eyes are not quite in line. If that someone is a child, please do not ignore your impression, for cross-eyes is an important symptom that should never be ignored.

Forget the old story of children growing out of cross-eyes; it does not happen. What does happen is that the child experiences double vision and gradually its brain learns to ignore the vision from one eye in an effort to overcome the defect. If unrecognized, this leads to permanently damaged vision in one eye. Symptoms which suggest cross-eyes are:
* Obvious misalignment of one or both eyes.
* Head held in an unusual posture, to compensate.
* Cross-eyes noticed if child is tired.

The assessment and treatment of cross-eyes is complex. In most cases the cause is either muscle imbalance or different strengths of the lens of each eye. Both causes are treated by surgery or by eye-glasses.

THE EYES

PROBABLE
MUSCLE IMBALANCE OR INEQUALITIES OF VISION

POSSIBLE
PROMINENT SKIN FOLDS

RARE
NERVE PALSIES
TUMORS OF EYE OR SOCKET

PROBABLE

■ MUSCLE IMBALANCE OR INEQUALITIES OF VISION
If the head is held at an unusual angle, it suggests the likelihood of muscle imbalance underlying the cross-eyes. You may also notice that one eye cannot turn beyond a certain point. Otherwise it is likely that one eye is far-sighted or, less commonly, near-sighted compared to the other. A physician must evaluate all the possibilities.

POSSIBLE

■ PROMINENT SKIN FOLDS
In children, the folds of skin by the bridge of the nose may be unusually wide, giving the impression that the eyes turn in. Even if this happens to be the case, the child should still be checked.

RARE

■ NERVE PALSIES
It has been mentioned (*see PARALYSIS OF THE EYE MUSCLES page 40*) that six muscles control movements of the eyes. Each muscle can become paralyzed for a variety of reasons. Nerve damage is probably the cause if there is:
* Sudden onset of previously unnoticed cross-eyes.
* A drooping eyelid.
* Changes in size of the pupil; *see page 19.*

Nerve paralysis has a variety of causes, which need further evaluation.

■ TUMORS OF EYE OR SOCKET
These can occur at all ages, producing cross-eyes by pressure on one eyeball. So don't ignore newly occurring cross-eyes, especially in children.
* The eye bulges more and more.
* There is a pain behind the eye.
* The pupil may appear white if the tumor is inside the eye.

The Nose

DEFORMED NOSE

PROBABLE
INJURY

POSSIBLE
RHINOPHYMA

RARE
NASAL SEPTAL NECROSIS
LEPROSY
MALIGNANT TUMOR

PROBABLE

■ INJURY
Typically, the nose is flattened or made crooked (you may hear doctors describe the latter as deviated septum). This is likely to be caused by fracture of the nose bone, swelling and bleeding.

It is normal to wait for a week to allow swelling to go down before deciding whether the nose needs straightening by surgery.
* Nasal bone fracture.
* Flattening of the nose.
* Deviation of the nose.
* Swelling.
* Bleeding.

POSSIBLE

■ RHINOPHYMA
Also known as "potato nose" or "bottle-nose". Caused by overactivity of the sebaceous glands of the nose. It takes some years to develop.
* Large, bulbous nose.
* Purplish-red in color.
* Irregular "pitted" surface: the pits mark the entrances to the glands.
Can be treated by cosmetic surgery.

RARE

■ NASAL SEPTAL NECROSIS
A blow to the nose may not break the nasal bones, but instead damage the nasal septum (a thin layer of cartilage separating the nostrils). Pressure from a blood clot under its mucous membrane covering causes:
* Headache.
* Local pain at the tip of the nose.
* Apparent widening of the tip of the nose.
* Loss of sensation over the skin of the nose.
* Destruction of the nasal septum over a number of weeks, causing the nose to dip at the bridge.

■ LEPROSY
Causes collapse of the nose due to septal ulceration.

This is one of several obvious symptoms which will be apparent.

■ CANCER OF THE NOSE
Any irregular sore on the nose that enlarges over months or years, that bleeds, ulcerates or is painful could be malignant. Enlargement of local lymph nodes suggests malignancy.

RED NOSE

PROBABLE
STAPHYLOCOCCAL INFECTION

POSSIBLE
ACNE ROSACEA
ERYSIPELAS
RHINOPHYMA

PROBABLE

■ STAPHYLOCOCCAL INFECTION
An infection of the skin follicles in a part of the nose.
* Local swelling.
* Local redness
* Local pain.
* Local heat.

May need antibiotics.

POSSIBLE

■ ACNE ROSACEA
A rash caused by over-activity of the sebaceous glands.
* Associated with facial flushing.
* Redness from small blood vessels.
* Rash covers nose, forehead, face and chin.
* Small pustules may be evident.
* May persist for years.

Treatment is available to control symptoms.

■ ERYSIPELAS
A bacterial skin infection.
* Associated with a break in the skin.
* Often near eye, nose or mouth.
* Fever.
* Feel sick.
* Hot, reddened swelling all over affected area.
* Painful.
* Blisters may appear.

Antibiotics will treat this effectively if given at an early stage.

■ RHINOPHYMA
See page 54.

RUNNY NOSE

PROBABLE
COMMON COLD
VASOMOTOR RHINITIS
ALLERGIC RHINITIS

POSSIBLE
SINUSITIS
FOREIGN BODY
NASAL POLYP
DRUG WITHDRAWAL

RARE
CANCER OF THE NOSE

THE NOSE

PROBABLE

■ COMMON COLD
See page 454. There are many different types of common cold virus. As you get over each new one, you develop a natural immunity to it. Children often have a "perpetual runny nose". This is because they are being exposed to new viruses in day care and at school. The elderly rarely get colds for they have built up immunity to many of the viruses.

■ VASOMOTOR RHINITIS
See also page 129. Some individuals suffer from hypersensitivity of the nasal lining. This leads to an excess of the usually small amounts of "normal" nasal discharge. Some medications taken as nasal sprays may help this condition. It is similar to allergic rhinitis.

■ ALLERGIC RHINITIS
See also page 129. Many allergens (molds, dust, pollen etc) can cause a running nose. Locally applied steroid nasal sprays and antihistamines can be effective in preventing the reaction.

POSSIBLE

■ SINUSITIS
See page 130. Nasal discharge will often be yellow or green, sometimes thick. There may be an associated headache. Antibiotic treatment is usually needed.

■ FOREIGN BODIES
See page 58. A small object in a nostril. Discharge is foul-smelling and on one side only.
Antibiotics may help after removal.

■ NASAL POLYP
Polyps are benign, fleshy growths inside the nose. They may be associated with allergies. As well as obstructing the nasal passages they can cause an increase in the volume of secretions, which will appear as a runny nose. May also be a cause of bad breath.
Treatment is either steroid nasal spray or surgical removal of the polyps.

■ DRUG WITHDRAWAL
A clear, runny discharge is a common symptom when withdrawing from hard drugs such as cocaine. Other signs include:
* Running eyes.
* Sweating.
* "Goose flesh".
* Yawning.
* Stomach cramps.
* Diarrhea.

RARE

■ CANCER OF THE NOSE
See page 59. Any tumor of the nose or in the spaces around the nose may cause a nasal discharge. Recurrent nosebleeds or bloody streaks in the discharge may occur.

NOSEBLEEDS

Also known as epistaxis. A particularly common problem in children, although most adults have episodes of bleeding from the nose at some time. There are many causes, some due to local disease and some indicative of systemic, or "whole body", disease. Most nosebleeds can be treated by continuous, firm pressure across the fleshy part of the nose just below the bridge. Pressure should be maintained for as long as 15 minutes in severe cases. Sit forward with the head supported and breathe through your mouth. Local application of ice may also help. Only in rare cases is medical or surgical intervention required. But see your doctor or urgent care facility about any heavy or prolonged bleeding.

PROBABLE
MINOR INFECTION
NOSE-PICKING
INJURY
COMMON COLD

POSSIBLE
FOREIGN BODY
CHRONIC SINUSITIS
MEDICATION-INDUCED
BENIGN TUMORS, INCLUDING NASAL POLYPS

RARE
HEREDITARY HEMORRHAGIC TELANGIECTASIA
DISORDERS OF BLOOD CLOTTING
HIGH BLOOD PRESSURE
CANCER OF THE NOSE

PROBABLE

■ MINOR INFECTION
The commonest cause of nosebleeds is a minor nasal infection. This brings blood vessels very close to the surface on the inside of the nose. The slightest irritation or injury will then start a nosebleed. Antibiotic ointment used inside the nose for a few days will give improvement.

■ NOSE-PICKING
Probably the commonest cause in children. The finger, or the fingernail, damages an area of the lining known as Little's area, at the entrance to the nose.
* Occasionally, profuse bleeding.
* Often occurs at night.
* Almost always cures itself after applying pressure.
* May be repeated.

■ INJURY
If the nose is clearly deformed or misaligned as a result of an injury, see a physician. There could be an underlying fracture.

■ COMMON COLD
Nosebleeds are a surprisingly frequent symptom of common colds because of inflammation of the lining.

The Nose

Repeated nose-blowing to clear mucus may also bring on bleeding.

POSSIBLE

■ FOREIGN BODY
A toddler or young child pushes a bead or some other small object into a nostril, which remains unrecognized for days, weeks or months. Inflammation develops, causing:
* Discharge from one nostril; it may be
* Purulent — yellow-green.
* Possibly bloodstained and foul smelling.

Must be removed under medical supervision.

■ CHRONIC SINUSITIS
The linings of the bony sinuses become chronically infected.
* Profuse discharge back into throat, rather than out through the nostrils.
* Blockage of the nose.
* Head pain, particularly in the forehead or under the eyes.
* Loss of sense of smell and sometimes taste.
* Nosebleeds, often from excessive nose-blowing.

■ MEDICATION-INDUCED
A number of medications, typically coumadin, which thins the blood, and some medications used to treat arthritis may cause nosebleeds.

If nosebleeds occur while you are taking coumadin, see your physician immediately to check your dose.

The sinuses

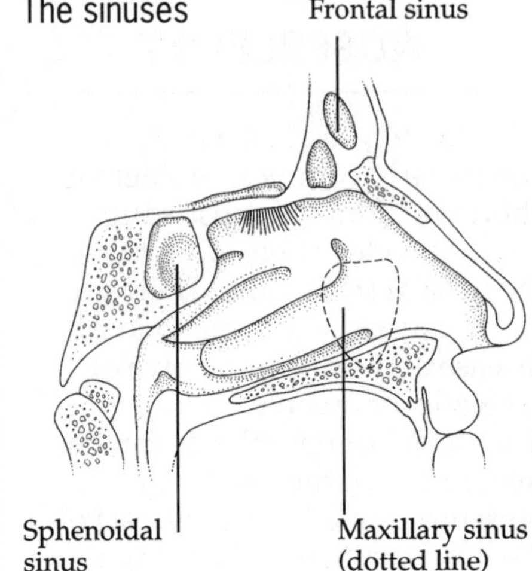

■ BENIGN TUMORS, INCLUDING NASAL POLYPS
These can bleed from time to time, particularly after nose-picking or blowing.
* Obstruction of the nose.
* Associated sinusitis.
* Discharge of mucus.
* Loss of sense of smell.

RARE

■ HEREDITARY HEMORRHAGIC TELANGIECTASIA
See page 87.

■ DISORDERS OF BLOOD CLOTTING
The commonest are Factor 8 deficiency (true haemophilia) Christmas disease and von Willebrand's disease. Common symptoms include:
* Persistent bleeding after minor cuts and abrasions.
* Frequent, easy bruising.

* Bleeding after extraction of teeth.
* Bleeding into joints, causing severe pain.
* Spontaneous nosebleeds.

Specific blood tests will determine whether there is any abnormality of clotting. It is particularly important to know if you have a clotting problem before dental treatment. If in doubt, check with a physician.

■ HIGH BLOOD PRESSURE

An otherwise healthy person who suddenly gets recurring nosebleeds must have blood pressure checks and tests of clotting ability. More likely in people past middle age.

■ CANCER OF THE NOSE

There are several potential symptoms:

* Blockage of the nose.
* Discharge from the nose.
* Pain in the teeth.
* Loosening of the teeth.
* Ill-fitting dentures.
* Associated sinusitis.
* Nose-bleeds.
* Bulging eyes.
* Visual disturbance.
* Sensory changes in face, nose and mouth.
* The skin may be involved.
* Lymph nodes may enlarge.

It is *very* rare for anyone to present nosebleeds to their physician as a symptom of cancer of the nose.

The naso-pharynx

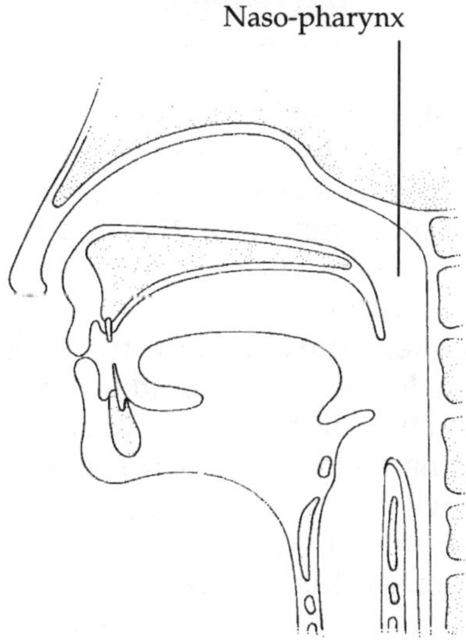

NASAL-SOUNDING SPEECH

Any disease or injury that blocks the nose or distorts the naso-pharynx will alter the quality of the sound produced. Commonest of the causes are the common cold; septal deviation *(page 61)* ; "adenoids" *(page 60)*; and injury. Less common, but worth considering, are: cleft palate *(page 88)*; a foreign body *(page 58)*; chronic sinusitis *(page 58)*; and benign tumors, including polyps *(page 58)*.

The Nose

SNORING

A common problem, rarely reported to physicians by snorers.

It happens when the tongue and other soft structures at the back of the mouth obstruct air flow causing vibration. Most common in drinkers, the obese, the over-40s and males, and those with nasal obstruction or misshapen noses. Sleeping on the side, rather than the back, will probably help.

Exceptionally severe, persistent snoring justifies surgery. A modern operation known as a uvuloplasty, which reshapes the soft palate at the back of the mouth, can transform the lives of severe snorers and their partners.

There are a number of tricks which may prevent snoring such as sewing a tennis ball in the back of the pyjama jacket. This wakes you when you roll on to your back. Also try adjusting pillow height and changing the ventilation in your bedroom.

■ SLEEP APNEA

Occurs when soft structures at the back of the mouth close-down and prevent breathing. Breathing starts again with loud snorting and snoring. This may occur many times during the night. Commonest in overweight men with a history of snoring. Leads to daytime sleepiness. Medication or surgery can often help.

BREATHING THROUGH THE MOUTH: A BLOCKED NOSE

The effects of a blocked nose depend somewhat on the cause, but may include:

* Pain in the nose.
* Discharge from the nose.
* No sense of smell.
* Breathing through the mouth.
* Snoring.
* Dry mouth.
* Bad breath.

For details, see the sections concerning those symptoms. Causes of obstruction include:

PROBABLE

"ADENOIDS"
SEPTAL DEVIATION
INJURY
COMMON COLD
VASOMOTOR RHINITIS
ALLERGIC RHINITIS

POSSIBLE

FOREIGN BODY
CHRONIC SINUSITIS
BENIGN TUMORS, INCLUDING NASAL POLYPS

PROBABLE

■ "ADENOIDS"

Perhaps the commonest reason for "mouth breathing". The adenoids are lymph tissue lying at the back

of the nose and pharynx near the soft palate. They are commonly the site of acute or chronic infection. **Acute infection gives:**
* Pain behind nose.
* Congestion.
* Nasal obstruction (due to enlargement of the adenoids).
* Enlarged neck lymph nodes.

Chronic infection gives:
* Enlarged adenoids.
* Chronic congestion.
* Persistent cough.
* Breathing through the mouth.
* Ear infection, possibly leading to impaired hearing.

Both types of "adenoiditis" cause alteration in the quality of speech.As the adenoids perform no vital function, removing them is a common operation in childhood.

However, current understanding is that adenoids and the tonsils shrink naturally as a child reaches his or her tenth birthday. An operation can be avoided if symptoms are not too troublesome.

■ SEPTAL DEVIATION
The septum is the thin layer of cartilage separating the two sides of the nose. "Deviation" may occur during birth (one to two per cent of babies have permanently deviated septa). It may also occur as the result of injury at a later age. The result is obstruction of one or other of the nostrils, either partially or completely. *See DEFORMED NOSE, page 54.*

■ INJURY AND COMMON COLD
See page 54; and page 454.

■ VASOMOTOR RHINITIS and ALLERGIC RHINITIS
See page 129.

POSSIBLE

■ FOREIGN BODY, CHRONIC SINUSITIS AND BENIGN TUMORS INCLUDING NASAL POLYPS: *see page 58.*

PAINFUL NOSE

This is such a general symptom that analyzing it in its own right is not helpful. There will always be some other associated factor(s). Is there nasal discharge or bleeding? Is the speech affected? Is the nose mis-shapen? Does the nose itch? Has the sense of smell gone? These are all covered in detail in neighboring pages and will give proper insight into "pain in the nose".

TINGLING NOSE; SNEEZING

Look for an outside cause first: is it the smell of a houseplant, or an animal? Or a chemical? Or chili powder or pepper? Some people sneeze in bright sunlight. There are many different causes, a large number unique to individuals. Failing these, consider vasomotor rhinitis, or allergic rhinitis, *page 129.*

THE NOSE

NO SENSE OF SMELL

Any progressive loss of the sense of smell suggests an underlying medical problem and needs proper medical attention.

PROBABLE
SMOKING
COMMON COLD
VASOMOTOR RHINITIS
ALLERGIC RHINITIS

POSSIBLE
OBSTRUCTIVE LESIONS OF NOSE
BREATHING THROUGH THE MOUTH
SINUSITIS

RARE
HEAD INJURY
MENINGIOMA
FRONTAL LOBE TUMOR

PROBABLE

These diagnoses are either self-evident or covered in detail elsewhere: *see pages 454 and 129.* With a common cold, the loss of smell is passing; vasomotor rhinitis and allergic rhinitis cause intermittent loss of smell, which may become long-term.

POSSIBLE

■ OBSTRUCTIVE LESIONS OF THE NOSE
See BREATHING THROUGH THE MOUTH etc, page 60.

■ BREATHING THROUGH THE MOUTH
See page 60.

■ SINUSITIS
See NOSEBLEEDS page 57 and MUCUS IN THE THROAT, page 129.
Acute sinusitis may lead to temporary loss and chronic sinusitis to long-term loss of smell.

RARE

■ HEAD INJURY
A blow to the head may cut the nerves in the roof of the nose. If the nose is pushed in, or the forehead struck, there is a bony movement or fracture which can cut the nerve responsible for sensing smell.
Permanent loss.

■ MENINGIOMA
A tumor of the protective sheath covering the brain. It can press on the olfactory nerve, causing progressive loss of smell and other symptoms, such as headache.

■ FRONTAL LOBE TUMOR
This can cause pressure on brain tissue involved in sensing smell, and it can damage the pathways conducting sense of smell. Loss is progressive and other symptoms will be apparent.

THE EAR

There is much more to the ear than you see, since most of it is hidden inside the head. The visible outer ear is cartilage, covered with skin, and it is subject to any of the problems that affect skin elsewhere: bruising, infections and eczema.

Hidden from view, at the end of the outer canal, is the eardrum, which guards the middle ear, a beautifully intricate structure that turns sound waves into the electrical impulses for transmission to the brain.

The inner ear contains the fluid-filled semi-circular canals which give you your sense of balance and orientation. There are also passages connecting the middle ear to the back of the throat: they allow equalization of air pressure on both sides of the eardrum, without which you experience pressure or "popping" in the ears. Skin, nerves, bones, fluid: little wonder that there are many minor diseases which can afflict the ear, and a few serious ones.

BLEEDING EAR

Blood from the ear, usually mixed with pus, is a common symptom, not often due to a serious cause.

PROBABLE
MIDDLE EAR INFECTION

POSSIBLE
BOIL
POLYP
INJURY

RARE
CANCER

PROBABLE

■ MIDDLE EAR INFECTION
This problem is common in childhood, occasional in adults and usually accompanies a common cold. The eardrum becomes red and bulges. If the drum bursts, pus and blood ooze from the ear for a few days.
* Pain in the ear for a day or two.
* Then, suddenly, a smelly, bloodstained discharge.
* The pain goes.
* The discharge lessens over a few days.

The eardrum nearly always heals, but your doctor will want to watch progress and will usually treat you with antibiotics.

POSSIBLE

■ BOIL
Just like a pimple elsewhere, a boil in the canal of the ear may burst, discharging a few specks of blood.
* An extremely tender spot, just inside the ear canal.
* Bursts after a day or two.
* Symptoms then rapidly vanish.

The Ears

■ POLYP
These fleshy lumps can form deep inside the ear if there is recurrent infection. They are painless, but may ooze or bleed and can be seen through an otoscope, an instrument for looking inside the ear.

■ INJURY
A severe blow to the head may rupture the eardrum and cause bleeding.

RARE

■ CANCER
Growths within the ear canal or within the inner ear are unusual.
* Intense, persistent pain in the ear.
* Constant discharge of pus mixed with blood.
* Partial paralysis of one side of the face.
* Dizziness or ringing noises.

BOIL IN THE EAR

PROBABLE
BOIL

POSSIBLE
HERPES SIMPLEX
SHINGLES

PROBABLE

■ BOIL
Boils form at the root of the tiny hairs lining the ear canal. They cause pain out of all proportion to their tiny size because the skin of the ear canal is unable to stretch much without intense pain.
* Localized, throbbing pain.
* You may be able to feel a tender lump.
* Reaches a peak after a day or two.
* Discharges small amounts of blood and pus for a couple of days.

Will usually clear by itself, but antibiotic drops help. A heating pad may speed the process.

POSSIBLE

■ HERPES SIMPLEX
A cold sore in the ear canal will give symptoms similar to a boil, but:
* The pain is more prolonged and recurrent.
* The sore is filled with clear fluid, rather than pus.

■ SHINGLES
See page 69.

LUMPS AND BUMPS ON THE EAR

PROBABLE
HEALING BOIL
CAULIFLOWER EAR

POSSIBLE
AURICULAR APPENDAGE
WART

RARE
GOUT
TUMORS

PROBABLE

■ HEALING BOIL
* Initially, pain and redness from the boil.
* May discharge pus.
* Becomes smaller over a few days.
* Firm lump left at the site.
Usually the lump disappears, but this can take months.

■ CAULIFLOWER EAR
This is the permanently enlarged, fleshy, misshapen ear left after injury. It results from permanent scarring of the cartilage that makes up the external ear and is an occupational hazard of boxers.

POSSIBLE

■ AURICULAR APPENDAGE
A small, painless outgrowth between the ear canal and the cheek. It is present from birth, harmless and removable.

■ WART
Can occur on the ear as on other parts of the skin.
* Appears rapidly, then stops growing at about 1/4 inch in length.
* The surface is rough, with black spots.
Removable. See physician or pharmacist.

RARE

■ GOUT
A disorder of body chemistry causing the appearance of crystals of uric acid in many parts of the body, especially the joints.
* Firm, irregular lumps called tophi in the outer ear.
* These become extremely painful.
* Acute pain, redness and swelling in other joints, especially the big toe.

■ TUMORS
A slow-growing skin cancer can occur on the ear. Common in farmers and others who work outside in the sun.
* Begins as a small, crusted spot.
* Develops a rolled edge.
* May bleed.
* Does not heal.
* Gradually enlarges.
This is a slow form of cancer, treated by freezing, surgery, special medications or radiotherapy.

DISCHARGING EAR

PROBABLE
EAR INFECTION
OTITIS EXTERNA

POSSIBLE
CHRONIC OTITIS MEDIA

RARE
CHOLESTEATOMA
POLYP
RUPTURE OF EARDRUM

THE EARS

PROBABLE

■ EAR INFECTION
See page 63.
Produces pain, pus and blood for a few days.

■ OTITIS EXTERNA
Inflammation/irritation of the lining of the ear canal. Commonly known as Swimmer's Ear.
Aggravating factors include swimming-pool chemicals, poking in the ear with pencils or earbuds, dandruff from the hair and even medicated ear drops. Frequently, bacteria or fungi invade the ear lining creating a mixture of infection and inflammation which is difficult to cure.
* Intensely itching ear canals.
* Persistent, thin, watery discharge.
* Discharge thicker if infection occurs.
Treatment is with anti-fungal, anti-inflammatory ear drops and often needs to continue for many weeks.

POSSIBLE

■ CHRONIC OTITIS MEDIA
Literally, chronic infection of the middle ear, often with pus discharging through a hole in the eardrum. There is usually a history of repeated ear infection.
* Yellowish discharge.
* Quantity varies from day to day.
Treatment involves eradicating infection, getting air into the ear and, eventually, repairing the hole in the eardrum.

RARE

■ CHOLESTEATOMA
This is a mass of abnormal cells which forms usually as a result of recurrent ear infections. The cells destroy surrounding tissues, so causing symptoms of:
* Deafness.
* Discharge.
* Dizziness.
Treatment consists of surgically removing the cholesteatoma and often reconstructing the middle ear. This is a complex operation.

■ POLYP
A fleshy, non-cancerous growth arising from a cholesteatoma and causing discharge, sometimes bloodstained.

■ RUPTURE OF EAR DRUM
Caused by injury or infection and resulting in:
* Deafness, which may be partial or total.
* Ringing in ears.
* Bloody discharge.
An injury serious enough to fracture the skull near the ear may lead to a leakage of brain fluid from the ear. This serious injury causes the above symptoms plus:
* Painless, persistent leakage of clear fluid.
This needs urgent medical attention.

EARACHE

Pain in the ear is usually caused by a relatively minor problem within the ear. It can, however, be a symptom of disease elsewhere.

PROBABLE
INFECTION
EUSTACHIAN CONGESTION
WAX
BOIL

POSSIBLE
THROAT INFECTION
TEETH PROBLEMS
MASTOIDITIS
PERICHONDRITIS

RARE
SKIN CANCER
NEURALGIA
SHINGLES
CANCER OF EAR
CANCER OF TONSIL
CANCER OF TONGUE

PROBABLE

■ EAR INFECTION
See page 63.

Pain, pus and discharge arising over a few hours or days. A routine symptom in children with common colds.

■ EUSTACHIAN CONGESTION
This condition may be described by your physicianas Eustachian tube blockage.

If fluid builds up inside the middle ear, it muffles hearing. This condition is common for a few days or weeks after a common cold. Chronic congestion is also familiar to those who suffer from hay fever or sinusitis. It is particularly important to identify in childhood since it can cause deafness severe enough to interfere with speech development and to hinder progress in school.
* Hearing is muffled.
* A feeling of pressure inside the ear.
* Yawning relieves pressure temporarily.
* In children, delay in learning to speak.

Adults rarely need any treatment other than decongestants; children suffering deafness may need surgery to drain the fluid through ear tubes.

The Eustachian tube is a ventilation canal which goes from the back of the throat to the middle ear. Air passes through the tube to equalize the pressure on either side of the eardrum. This is why swallowing relieves popping ears. The tube is narrowest in childhood and it is then that most problems occur.

■ WAX
A block of hard wax in the ear canal may eventually become painful and give rise to muffled hearing. People vary a lot in how

THE EARS

much ear wax they produce and often recognize for themselves when their ears need washing out. This cannot be done at home. See your physician.

The ear is a self-cleaning organ. It is rarely necessary to have ears washed-out. Small hairs move the wax to the outer ear where it can be wiped away.

Avoid cleaning your ears with cotton buds — it causes more problems than it cures. Ear wash-outs once started, tend to need repeating. This is thought to be due to damage to the hairs in the ear canal. Always try simple earwax softening drops first, to allow the ear to clear naturally.

■ BOIL

See page 64. A pimple in the ear canal, causing a remarkable amount of pain for such a small problem.

POSSIBLE

■ THROAT INFECTION

A throat infection (including tonsilitis) may seem obvious and recognizable, but often the throat symptoms are overshadowed by earache. Especially common in young children.
* Sore throat.
* Pain on swallowing.
* If tonsilitis, white patches may be present on tonsils.

■ TEETH PROBLEMS

The large molar teeth, if decayed, may cause earache. In children, the back teeth coming in can cause a combination of symptoms easily taken for an ear infection:
* Feverish, unhappy child.
* Rubbing ear.
* Dribbling.

■ MASTOIDITIS

The mastoid bone is the bony swelling just behind the ears and it was once common for ear infection to spread into that area. With the routine use of antibiotics, this is now unlikely.
* Pain behind the ear.
* Tender, red swelling of the mastoid bone.
* Fever and discomfort.
* Heavy yellow discharge from the ear.

The condition urgently needs surgical drainage of the mastoid bone.

■ PERICHONDRITIS

Occasionally, the outer ear, which is made up of cartilage, becomes inflamed, typically after an injury, or in cold weather.
* Throbbing pain over part of the outer ear.
* Skin is reddened.

Symptoms settle over a few days, occasionally needing antibiotic treatment.

RARE

■ SKIN CANCER

Can occur anywhere on the ear or in the ear canal.
* Starts by looking like a small sore that does not heal.
* Grows very slowly.

* May bleed and cause pain.
Cured by medical treatment given at an early stage.

■ NEURALGIA (NERVE PAIN)
An unpleasant condition caused by irritation of the fifth cranial nerve which supplies feeling to much of the face and the ear. The cause is unknown. Commonest in the late middle-aged and elderly.
* Sudden, severe shooting pains across ear, face, nose.
* Pains set off by eating, cold weather or other triggers.
There are several effective medications for this miserable, though harmless illness.

■ SHINGLES
An unusual form of form of shingles which can be a puzzling cause of ear pain.
* Pain in one side of throat and the ear on that side.
* Hearing may seem hyper–sensitive.
* Loss of taste on that side of the tongue.
* Rash may appear on the ear lobes.
* Small, crusting spots appear on throat and ear after a week or two.

■ CANCER OF THE EAR
Cancer of the ear canal or inner ear is unusual.
* Sometimes painful.
* Bloody discharge.
* Blocked hearing.

■ CANCER OF THE TONGUE
It is important to check the back of the tongue in cases of persistent earache where there appears to be no cause within the ear itself.
* A persistent, shallow ulcer on the back of the tongue.
* Commonest in smokers.
* Gradually enlarges, with pain and bleeding.

■ CANCER OF TONSIL
Another unusual cancer, most common in old age.
* One tonsil is enlarged.
* Earache.
* Pain on swallowing.

EAR FEELS "FULL"

A familiar sensation, variously described as fullness, cotton wool between the ears, pressure in the ears, fuzziness in the head. The basic features are slight deafness and muffled hearing due to some physical obstruction to hearing. The causes are often obvious and readily treatable.

PROBABLE
EUSTACHIAN CONGESTION
WAX
INFECTION

POSSIBLE
HAY FEVER

RARE
CHRONIC OTITIS EXTERNA

THE EARS

PROBABLE

■ EUSTACHIAN CONGESTION
See EARACHE, page 67. Caused by build-up of fluid within the inner ear after a common cold; treatment, if needed, consists of decongestants and steam inhalations.

■ WAX
Probably the commonest cause of a slight feeling of fullness, often accompanied by dizziness, discomfort, mild earache *(see page 67)*.

Simple earwax softening drops often allow the ear to clear naturally. Ear wash-out may be needed.

■ INFECTION
Rather than causing the painful picture described elsewhere (*see, for example, EARACHE, page 67*, infections sometimes run a less obvious course with:
* Vague mild discomfort.
* Fluctuating, mild deafness.
* Feeling of pressure in ear.

The diagnosis has to be made by viewing the eardrum.

POSSIBLE

■ HAY FEVER
Causes fullness as a result of swelling of the lining of the nose and ears.
* Seasonal sneezing, sore eyes.
* Persistent runny nose during the pollen season.
* Often associated with eczema, asthma.

Treatments include anti-histamine tablets and nose sprays. Excessive use of nose sprays is damaging to the nasal lining.

RARE

■ CHRONIC OTITIS EXTERNA
Severe cases give rise to chronic swelling of the ear canal, which also becomes blocked with debris. Regular cleansing is needed under medical supervision. *See page 66*

DEAFNESS OR HEARING DIFFICULTIES IN ADULTS

Adult deafness or loss of hearing is, to a large extent, a normal part of the aging process. The hearing loss can gradually worsen, unnoticed, until it interferes with work or social relationships, at which point it is suddenly seen as a "new" problem. Special attention should always be given to sudden deafness, deafness affecting one ear only or when it is associated with pain, dizziness (vertigo), or ringing in the ears (tinnitus).

PROBABLE
WAX
CHRONIC OTITIS MEDIA
OTOSCLEROSIS
PRESBYACUSIS

POSSIBLE
MENIERE'S DISEASE
ACOUSTIC TRAUMA
ARTERIOSCLEROSIS

RARE

INFECTION
ACOUSTIC NEUROMA
SKULL FRACTURE
MEDICATIONS
PAGET'S DISEASE

PROBABLE

■ WAX
An extremely common cause for a mild degree of hearing loss.
* Often causes sudden, partial hearing loss.
* "Blocked" feeling in ears.

■ CHRONIC OTITIS MEDIA
Long-term infection within the ear leads to:
* Deafness.
* Persistent discharge of pus-like material.
* Sometimes pain and vertigo.

Treatment is meticulous cleansing of the ear in a specialist clinic. The sudden appearance of pain and vertigo calls for urgent specialist assessment. Normally, continuous cleansing of the ear will allow healing. Occasionally, when the infection has cleared, skin grafting to the ear drum is necessary to allow complete healing.

■ OTOSCLEROSIS
A condition causing increasing stiffness of one of the bones that transmits sound waves from the eardrum.
* Often runs in families.
* Commonest in women, and gets worse in pregnancy.
* Progressive deafness, starting in early adulthood.
* Ringing in the ears — tinnitus — is common.

Surgery can help, but usually a hearing aid is the simplest treatment.

■ PRESBYACUSIS
This is the hearing loss that comes with age, caused by degeneration of the pathway that turns sound waves into electrical impulses for transmission to the brain.
* Typically noticed in late 60s.
* Both ears affected.
* Pain-free.

POSSIBLE

■ MENIERE'S DISEASE
Suggested by repeated attacks of deafness along with vertigo and ringing in the ears — tinnitus.

■ ACOUSTIC TRAUMA
Repeated loud noise damages hearing. Rock concert deafness may be temporary; but prolonged and repeated exposure to loud noise will result in some loss of hearing. Ringing in the ears is common after hearing loud noises. Workers exposed to loud noise should wear ear protection and have regular hearing checks.

Prolonged use of a "walkman" at high volume damages ears. The direct delivery of high volume sound, has been shown significantly to affect young people's hearing. If others around you can hear it — it is too loud.

The Ears

■ ARTERIOSCLEROSIS
Poor blood flow to the arteries supplying blood to the ear can cause a range of symptoms, usually confined to the elderly.
* Fluctuating deafness, dizziness, ringing in the ears.
* Symptoms may vary, depending on the position of the neck.
There is no specific treatment.

RARE

■ INFECTION
Deafness is a rare and unpredictable complication of certain infectious illnesses, especially measles and mumps. It is also a possible consequence of menin–gitis and syphilis. In babies it may the result of rubella infection during pregnancy.

Children who have recurrent ear infections may have decreased hearing. *See also HEARING DIFFICULTIES IN CHILDREN, this page.*

■ ACOUSTIC NEUROMA
A slow-growing tumor on the nerve of hearing. Though rare, it is suspected on the basis of the following suggestive symptoms:
* One-sided progressive deafness.
* One-sided tinnitus.
* Vertigo.
* Later numbness of face, unsteadiness.

A brain scan allows for quite precise localization, improving the chances of successful removal by surgery.

■ SKULL FRACTURE
Could damage the nerve of hearing and disrupts the delicate bones that transmit sounds, causing sudden loss of hearing.

■ MEDICATIONS
The nerve of hearing is sensitive to several medications. The commonest among adults is aspirin, taken in large doses.
* Tinnitus is an early warning sign.
* Dizziness.

■ PAGET'S DISEASE
Occurs in later life.
* Bones become tender.
* Bowing of the legs.
* Enlargement of the head.
* Gradual deafness.

The deafness is caused by pressure on the nerve of hearing by enlarged bone. This disease is frequently unrecognized until characteristic signs are noticed on an X-ray.

DEAFNESS OR HEARING DIFFICULTIES IN CHILDREN

Hearing problems in childhood are difficult to detect. In a baby, suspect a hearing problem if there is no startled reaction to sudden, loud noises, or if he or she does not turn to a sound. Later, delay in starting to speak should arouse suspicion. Later again school performance may deteriorate for no obvious cause; once more, consider the possibility of loss of hearing. You cannot be too careful.

THE EARS

PROBABLE
WAX
SEROUS OTITIS MEDIA

POSSIBLE
CONGENITAL

RARE
CONGENITAL RUBELLA
INFECTIONS
NEO-NATAL JAUNDICE
MEDICATIONS
HYPOTHYROIDISM

PROBABLE

■ WAX
Simple to detect, and simple to remedy with drops to soften the earwax. The wax will usually clear naturally. May need wash-out of the ears.

■ SEROUS OTITIS MEDIA
A common reason for hearing loss in children who have regular ear infections leading to a build-up of fluid within the middle ear. The condition is also known as glue ear because the fluid can be thick and sticky. The condition may cure itself, but frequently other treatment is needed. Symptoms are:
* Deafness, which may be partial or total.
* Occasional pain in ear.

Certain typical changes in the appearance of the eardrum will alert a physician to the problem. Ear tubes may be inserted.

POSSIBLE

■ CONGENITAL
Always to be considered in children born deaf, in whom there may have been a failure of development of the organs of hearing. Sometimes deafness runs in the family; sometimes the mother has been exposed to medications or infection in pregnancy which damage the ear (*see below*)

In most cases of congenital deafness, however, no cause can be found. There are many syndromes in which deafness is one of several other abnormalities, but this is a matter for specialist assessment.

RARE

■ CONGENITAL RUBELLA – GERMAN MEASLES
A rarity since vaccination has become generally available. Rubella contracted in the first four months of pregnancy can damage the developing child. As well as deafness, it can cause:
* Poor development of the brain and mental retardation.
* Cataracts.
* Heart defects.

This tragic outcome is becoming much less frequent as state immunization programs against Rubella improve. Check on your Rubella immunity before you get pregnant.

THE EARS

■ INFECTION
Deafness is an unusual and unpredictable complication ofcertain infectious illnesses, such as measles and mumps, both of which are increasingly rare, thanks to immunization. It may also be a consequence of meningitis.

■ NEONATAL JAUNDICE
Severe jaundice in the days after birth can cause brain damage, including deafness. Hence the vigorous treatment given to babies who develop severe jaundice.

■ MEDICATIONS
The nerve of hearing is sensitive to several medications, the commonest of which is aspirin taken in high doses. Another is gentamicin, now reserved for life-threatening
disease such as meningitis, where the risk of damage to hearing is outweighed by the risk to life.
* Tinnitus (ringing in the ears) is an early warning sign.
* Dizziness.
If a potentially harmful drug has to be used, blood levels will be monitored to avoid damage.

■ CONGENITAL HYPOTHYROIDISM
A child with an under-active thyroid gland will have:
* Coarse features.
* A gruff cry.
* Enlarged tongue.
In many countries there are screening blood tests to detect this curable illness as early as possible in new-born babies.

ITCHING EAR

PROBABLE
OTITIS EXTERNA

POSSIBLE
FUNGAL INFECTION

PROBABLE

■ OTITIS EXTERNA
A form of eczema or inflammation affecting the skin of the ear canal, often called Swimmer's Ear. Common in adult life, typically in those with eczema elsewhere.
* Intense itching.
* Skin of ear canal and ear itself is flaking, crusting, swollen.
* Ear feels wet, with a thin, clear discharge.
The outer ear canal can become sensitised to chemicals. Common among these are chlorine in swimming pools, hair spray and antibiotics in drops sometimes used to treat otitis externa.

POSSIBLE

■ FUNGAL INFECTION
Organisms known as fungi can invade skin which is alreadybroken down by otitis externa.
* Symptoms of otitis externa.
* Black spores may be visible in the discharge.
Diagnosed by a special test. Treated with anti-fungal drops.

NOISES IN THE EAR

Noises other than ringing in the ear are very common and usually not serious. They nearly always get better within a week or two. Many cases remain unexplained, the symptoms improving as mysteriously as they came. If noises occur in a particular location, check for a cause as simple as the hum from central heating, power lines or similar noise source. *See also RINGING IN THE EAR, page 76.*

PROBABLE
EUSTACHIAN CONGESTION
ACUTE MIDDLE EAR INFECTION

POSSIBLE
ATHEROSCLEROSIS

RARE
HEART MURMUR
ANEMIA

PROBABLE

■ EUSTACHIAN CONGESTION
Blockage caused by fluid building up inside the ear, often experienced with a common cold.
* Muffled hearing.
* Popping or crackling inside the ears.
* Slight discomfort from a feeling of pressure in the ears.
* Swallowing gives temporary relief.

■ ACUTE MIDDLE EAR INFECTION
Causes noises for similar reasons as does congestion (*see above*).
* Rapid onset of pain.
* Temporary deafness.
* Crackling inside ears.

Antibiotics are usually given for this condition.

POSSIBLE

■ ATHEROSCLEROSIS
In the elderly, narrow or twisted arteries in the neck can cause a whooshing noise in the ears. Needs evaluation by a physician.

RARE

■ HEART MURMUR
The sound arising from a diseased valve in the heart may be heard inside the head when there is no competing noise.
* A whooshing noise.
* In time with heart beat.

Needs to be assessed by a doctor.

■ ANEMIA
If extreme, anemia is said to cause noises in the ear. This symptom is likely to be over–shadowed by other features of anemia such as:
* Pale skin.
* Tiredness or exhaustion.
* Sore tongue.

* Dizziness on standing.
A blood test will quickly confirm the diagnosis.

SORENESS BEHIND THE EAR

Immediately behind the ear is a bone known as the mastoid, felt as a prominent swelling. Pain and swelling in this area is always to be taken seriously.

PROBABLE
ACUTE EAR INFECTION

POSSIBLE
MASTOIDITIS

PROBABLE

■ ACUTE EAR INFECTION
Although the infection is confined to the middle ear, occasionally there is a mild degree of soreness over the mastoid bone. Middle ear infections are usually treated with an antibiotic, which should prevent further spread.

POSSIBLE

■ MASTOIDITIS
Though now uncommon, this was once a serious complication of ear infections, since infection can spread from the mastoid region into the brain.
* Begins with an ear infection.

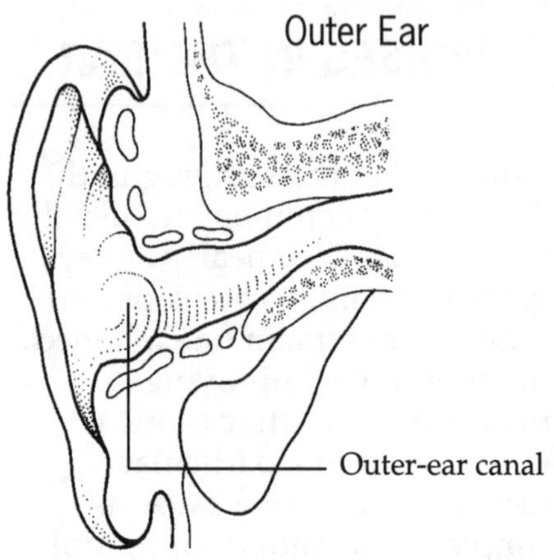

* Redness, swelling over mastoid bone.
* Yellow/green discharge from ear.
* Fever, pain, malaise.
Urgent surgical and antibiotic treatment is needed.

RINGING IN THE EAR — TINNITUS

This problem may be very persistent. It is usually described as a ringing noise, but sometimes it is lower-pitched than that, more of a hum. As an occasional symptom it is quite common, gets better quickly and is no more than a nuisance. Brief episodes of tinnitus may be caused by a blow to the head, wax in the ears, a foreign body, infection or sudden changes in air pressure.

Chronic tinnitus is another matter. Therapy varies from medications to devices that mask the sound, but there is no real cure. Persistent symptoms may be due to the following:

PROBABLE
OTOSCLEROSIS
MENIERE'S DISEASE
PRESBYACUSIS

POSSIBLE
ARTERIOSCLEROSIS
MEDICATIONS
PSYCHOLOGICAL

RARE
PAGET'S DISEASE

PROBABLE

■ OTOSCLEROSIS
This is a common cause of deafness. *See page 71.* Tinnitus tends to be the earliest symptom of the condition, which is due to increasing stiffness of one of the bones that transmit sound.

■ MENIERE'S DISEASE
The classic symptoms of this disease are varying combinations of:
* Tinnitus.
* Vertigo.
* Deafness.

■ PRESBYACUSIS
Hearing loss as part of the aging process is frequently accompanied by tinnitus. *See page 71.*

POSSIBLE

■ ARTERIOSCLEROSIS
The blood supply to the brain and ear arrives via major arteries in the neck which, with age, can become narrowed. This is thought to be responsible for tinnitus in the elderly associated with:
* Dizziness on standing up.
* Dizziness caused by head movements, especially looking up.
* Deafness.

It helps to take your time when getting up and to avoid sudden, extreme movements of the neck.

■ MEDICATIONS
Common medications which can cause tinnitus include aspirin, quinine and streptomycin.

■ PSYCHOLOGICAL
Occasionally, tinnitus or other noises in the ears are actually hallucinations in someone suffering from serious mental disease. Suspicion aroused by reports of:
* Bizarre noises.
* Voices commenting on the individual's activities.

The individual may also appear:
* Unusually suspicious.
* Moody to an exaggerated degree.

This situation needs sensitive, expert assessment.

THE EARS

RARE

■ PAGET'S DISEASE
A disease of bone which can press on the nerve of hearing, resulting in:
* Deafness.
* Tinnitus.

See also page 72.

VERTIGO

Vertigo means a sense of spinning. Dizziness is a mild form of the same symptom. This is frequently caused by disorders of the ear, although the connection may not be obvious since there may be no other signs of ear trouble such as pain, discharge or tinnitus. For that reason, vertigo/dizziness is covered in detail elsewhere in this book. *See THE BRAIN AND NERVOUS SYSTEM.* The following conditions are, however, relevant to the ear.

PROBABLE
CONGESTION
VESTIBULITIS
MENIERE'S DISEASE

POSSIBLE
CHRONIC OTITIS MEDIA
OTOSCLEROSIS
WAX

RARE
ACOUSTIC NEUROMA

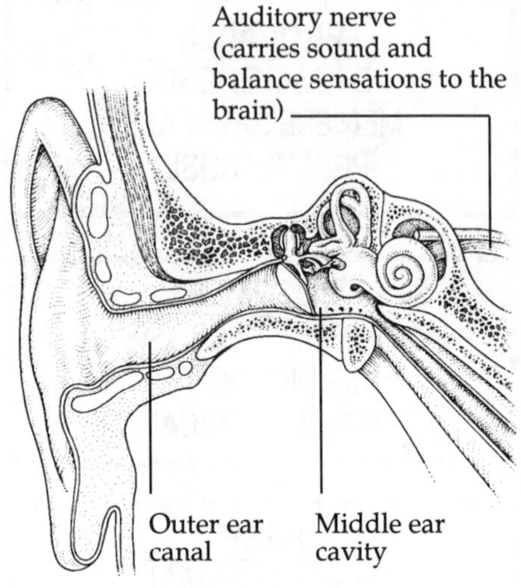

PROBABLE

■ CONGESTION
The congestion which accompanies a cold often also causes mild dizziness for a few days.
* Nasal congestion.
* Slight pressure in ears.
* Mild deafness and ringing in the ears — tinnitus.

■ VESTIBULITIS
A common, alarming, but harmless condition, often occurring in mini-epidemics. It is a viral infection of the balance organ in the middle ear. The nerve endings that normally transmit messages telling us how we are balanced become inflamed and send off inaccurate and confusing messages. This causes acute loss of balance and intense vertigo, with the room spinning round.
* Abrupt, disabling vertigo: you may even find it impossible to

Ear syringing

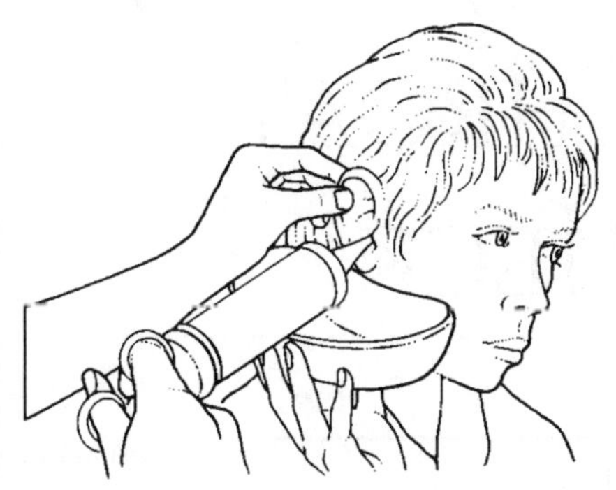

Ear examination

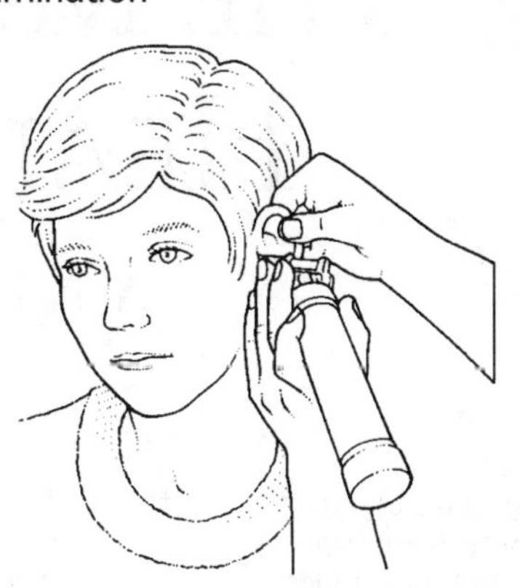

stand up.
* Usually noticed on attempting to get up in the morning.
* Nausea or vomiting are common.
* Vertigo returns each time you move your head.

This is very disabling but be reassured that the symptoms will fade usually over several days. Medication can help the symptoms significantly. Minor recurrences are possible for several months afterwards.

■ MENIERE'S DISEASE
Vertigo can be an early symptom of this condition. Later there is:
* Ringing in the ears — tinnitus.
* Deafness.

POSSIBLE

■ CHRONIC OTITIS MEDIA
See page 71. Persistent yellow or green discharge from one ear, together with:
* Discomfort.
* Deafness.

Needs specialized treatment to clean the ear and to eradicate infection.

■ OTOSCLEROSIS
A cause of deafness in middle life, but as early features there can be:
* Tinnitus.
* Vertigo.

■ WAX
If there is mild dizziness, with no other symptoms except that the ears are full of hard wax, it is reasonable for a physician to exclude wax as a cause of vertigo. The wax should be softened with drops and if necessary washed-out.

RARE

■ ACOUSTIC NEUROMA
See page 72. This growth on the nerve of hearing is suspected if, as well as vertigo, there is progressive:
* One-sided deafness.
* One-sided vertigo.
* One-sided tinnitus.
* Sometimes ear pain.

The Mouth, Face, Head, Throat and Neck

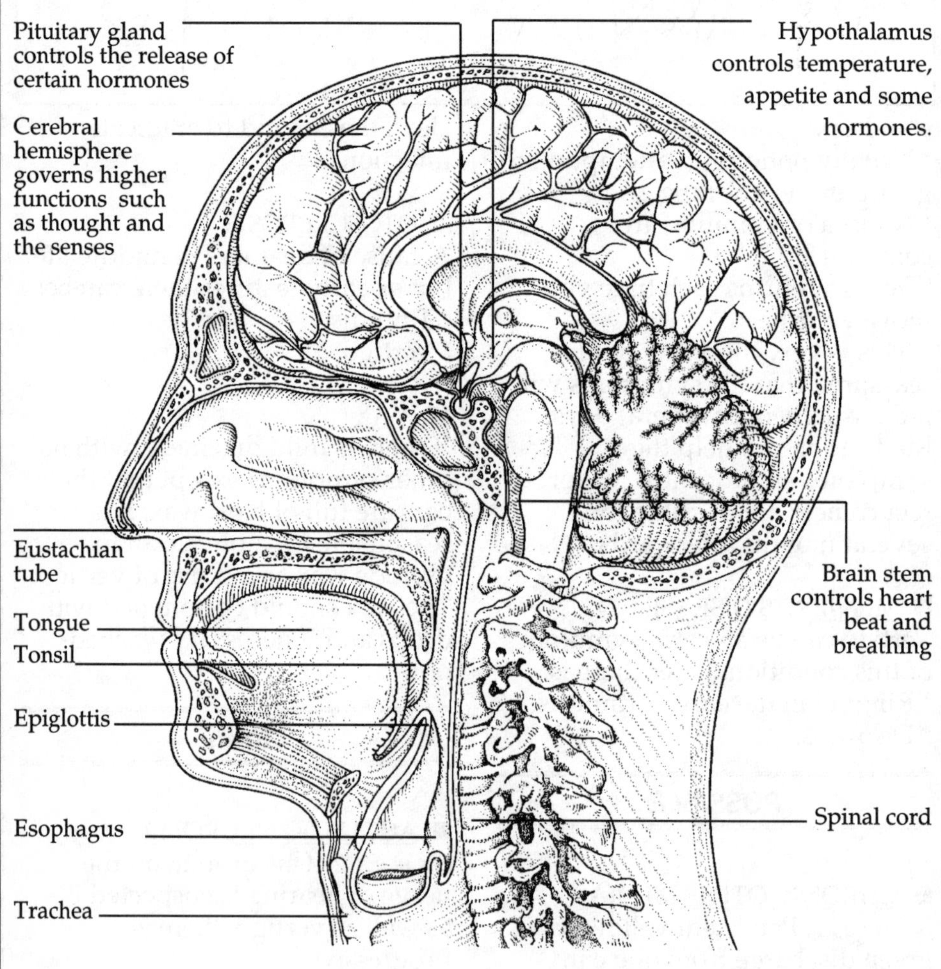

BLUISH-PURPLE LIPS

A sign of cyanosis, covered in detail on *page 424.* It can be caused by low body temperature. But long-term cyanosis suggests that blood oxygen levels are low. Similar discoloration may be noticed in the ear lobes, all the mucus membranes, the tongue and anywhere that blood flows close to the surface of the skin, such as the beds of the fingernails. In general, cyanosis suggests either heart or lung disease.

PROBABLE
LOW TEMPERATURE
CHRONIC BRONCHITIS
EMPHYSEMA
PULMONARY EDEMA

POSSIBLE
SHOCK
PNEUMONIA

RARE
PULMONARY EMBOLUS
CONGENITAL HEART DISEASE
AIRWAYS OBSTRUCTED BY A FOREIGN BODY
LARYNGEAL EDEMA
FIBROSING ALVEOLITIS
PNEUMOCONIOSIS
EXTRINSIC ALLERGIC ALVEOLITIS

PROBABLE

■ LOW TEMPERATURE
It may occur with low temperature in the elderly. Consider hypothermia if there are other symptoms, such as:
* Confusion.
* Slowness of thought.
* Decreased movement
* Cold skin.

The individual should be warmed gradually: layers of blankets are best. Hot drinks, such as tea, may be given. Avoid alcohol, which increases heat loss. In all cases, seek medical help urgently — hypothermia must be dealt with in hospital.

■ CHRONIC BRONCHITIS (COPD)
See page 222.

■ EMPHYSEMA (COPD)
Described in detail on *page 222.*
* Shortness of breath which gets progressively worse.
* The chest becomes expanded, as though permanently inhaling.
* May accompany chronic bronchitis.
* Respiratory infections.
* Cyanosis.
* Respiratory failure.

■ PULMONARY EDEMA
Retention of fluid in the lungs as a result of failure of the heart to pump effectively. Heart failure may have occurred because of either poor blood supply to the heart, or because of structural abnormality such as disease of the heart's valves. Symptoms can come on very quickly and include:

MOUTH

* Shortness of breath on effort.
* Shortness of breath when lying down flat.
* Night-time shortness of breath.
* Frothy sputum, sometimes pink with blood.
* Cyanosis.
* Fast or irregular heart rate.
* Swelling of ankles.

Needs urgent medical treatment.

POSSIBLE

■ SHOCK

Covered in detail on *page 408.* Cyanosis is just one of several noticeable signs. May be an emergency.

■ PNEUMONIA

See page 214.

Some types of pneumonia may still be fatal, particularly in the very young or the elderly: see a physician without delay.

RARE

■ PULMONARY EMBOLUS

Covered in detail on *page 218.* Bluish lips are just one of several more dramatic features, such as sudden shortness of breath, chest pain, bloody sputum and collapse.

■ CONGENITAL HEART DISEASE

Cyanosis is a typical and obvious feature of new-born babies with heart abnormalities. Fallot's tetralogy and transposition of the great arteries are probably the most well known. Heart defects may also accompany abnormalities such as Down's Syndrome, or those caused by the mother having Rubella during pregnancy. In addition to cyanosis:
* Shortness of breath.
* Swelling of finger tips.
* Swelling of toe ends.
* Polycythemia: excess hemoglobin to compensate for poor oxygenation.
* Weakness.
* Poor growth.

■ AIRWAYS OBSTRUCTED BY A FOREIGN BODY

Any object that obstructs the free passage of air in an out of the lungs may result in cyanosis. The sudden onset of blueness, choking in someone eating, or in a child, might be caused by inhalation of a foreign body, perhaps a peanut, or a piece of a toy. This is a life-threatening emergency. *See HEIMLICH'S MANEUVER, page 204.*

■ LARYNGEAL EDEMA

An infection (typically diphtheria, epiglottitis) or a severe allergic reaction may cause swelling of the soft tissues of the larynx (voice box area), preventing air getting into the lungs.
* Difficulty in getting breath.
* Blue lips.
* Stridor: a harsh and frightening noise heard as air is forced past a blockage in the upper airways.
* Distress.

Laryngeal edema is an emergency: get help quickly.

■ FIBROSING ALVEOLITIS (COPD)

Tends to develop in middle age and progresses gradually.
* Increasing shortness of breath.
* Dry cough.

* Swollen finger ends.
* Cyanosis.

■ PNEUMOCONIOSIS (COPD)
A term used for a number of occupationally related lung diseases, typically associated with work in dusty environments.
* Gradual onset.
* Increasing shortness of breath on exertion, and then at rest.
* Intermittent cough.
* Chronic bronchitis.
* Cyanosis.
* Respiratory failure.
* Heart failure.

■ EXTRINSIC ALLERGIC ALVEOLITIS (COPD)
A disease that develops because of recurrent allergic reactions to dusts from animals or plants. Quite common in farm workers.
* Recurrent brief attacks, up to a couple of days, of shortness of breath, fever and cough, when exposed to the dust.

After repeated exposure over the years a chronic condition develops, with:
* Shortness of breath.
* Finger and toe swelling.
* Cyanosis.
* Respiratory failure.
* Heart failure.

COPD – Chronic Obstructive Pulmonary Disease – is the term often used by physicians to refer to various lung diseases that produce the same effects: breathlessness, limited physical activity and, if severe, heart strain and cyanosis.

CRACKING AT CORNERS OF MOUTH

On its own this symptom is normally of no great significance.

PROBABLE
CHILDHOOD CRACKING
AGE

POSSIBLE
WEAKNESS OF MOUTH MUSCLES

RARE
VITAMIN C DEFICIENCY
ZINC DEFICIENCY
VITAMIN B2 DEFICIENCY

PROBABLE

■ CHILDHOOD CRACKING
If the corners of your child's mouth are constantly wet, they will be at increased risk of cracking. Children who suck their thumbs may develop inflammation at the corner(s) of the mouth. This may also occur in older children, with no very obvious cause.
* Redness.
* Cracking.
* Pain.
* Improves on its own.
* May develop on one side only.

Mouth

■ AGE
As individuals age, they can develop a crease running downwards from the angle of the mouth, along which saliva flows, causing skin irritation and:
* Redness.
* Cracking.
* Pain.
* May be on one or both sides. Clears up of its own accord.

POSSIBLE

■ WEAKNESS OF MOUTH MUSCLES
Anyone who has suffered brain injury (stroke, accident) or who has facial weakness or swallowing problems may dribble saliva out of the mouth.
* Redness.
* Cracking.
* Pain.
* Clears up on its own.
* May be on one side only (after stroke) or on both sides if there is a swallowing problem.

RARE

■ VITAMIN C AND ZINC DEFICIENCY: *see pages 426 and 86 respectively*. Vitamin B2 is a water-soluble vitamin present in many foods. Deficiency is likely to be a feature only of severe, general malnutrition. It does occur in the elderly. Smooth, sore red tongue is a symptom, *page 125*.

HARE LIP

Common term for cleft lip. *See CLEFT LIP AND PALATE, page 88.*

SORES ON LIP AND INSIDE MOUTH

Sore, inflamed lips are common in adults and children: the lips look red and are often cracked. The usual cause is regular exposure to heat and cold. The skin of the lips loses its natural oil, becoming dry and uncomfortable or "chapped".

Other common causes are lip-licking and lip-chewing. The first is typical of children with colds who develop running noses and continually lick or wipe their upper lips, causing inflammation. The second is a comfort habit adopted at times of stress.

The lips and the surrounding skin are possible sites of sores or lesions for many diseases. Some are local and some general; some are permanent and some temporary, some need treatment and some don't. The following list cannot be exhaustive, but it does highlight examples of all these types.

PROBABLE
APHTHOUS ULCER
HERPES SIMPLEX
MUCOCELE OR RETENTION CYST
INJURY
BURN
IMPETIGO

POSSIBLE
CANDIDIASIS
LEUKOPLAKIA
CHICKEN POX
MEASLES
STOMATITIS

RARE
ZINC DEFICIENCY
HEREDITARY HEMORRHAGIC TELANGIECTASIA
CHANCRE
DERMATITIS
BEHCET'S SYNDROME
ERYTHEMA MULTIFORME
CANCER
LICHEN PLANUS
MEDICATIONS

PROBABLE

■ APHTHOUS ULCER (CANKER SORE)

May develop after injury, when the individual is stressed (physically or mentally) or often for no clear reason.
* Very painful.
* After 24 hours mucus membrane breaks down to form an ulcer.
* Often a greyish/white appearance.
* Ulcer is normally about 3-4 mm in diameter and oval shaped.
* Pain can make eating, talking or brushing teeth difficult.
* May be multiple.
* Tend to be on inner aspect of lips.
* Healing occurs between five days and two weeks.

Treatment is available.

■ HERPES SIMPLEX

Also known as a cold sore or fever blister. A virus which infects the skin.
* Often caused by upper respiratory tract infection when the individual is stressed.
* Also brought on by weather extremes (heat or cold).
* Initially a slightly irritating itchy patch on the lip or skin.
* Little fluid filled vesicles develop.
* These become crusted and a scab develops.
* The disease runs its course in ten to 14 days, but can return from time to time.

If severe, and recognized at an early stage, can be helped by anti-viral medication.

■ MUCOCELE OR RETENTION CYST

Blockage of one of the small glands on the inner aspect of the lips causes:
* Sudden appearance of a lump, a few millimetres in diameter.
* Painless.
* Translucent/bluish colour.
* Suddenly empties.
* Rarely lasts for more than a few days.

■ INJURY

Injury from a sharp object such as a fork, ballpoint pen or from biting the lip or cheek can produce a small sore. It will heal on its own.

MOUTH

■ BURN

In this location usually caused by food hot from the oven, such as pizza. May be the result of a cigarette burn while under the influence of alcohol. Will heal in a few days.

■ IMPETIGO

A highly infectious skin infection, which can occur anywhere, but commonly on the face and lips and other exposed parts. Commonest in children.

* Starts with redness.
* Fluid filled sacs develop on the skin surface.
* These burst and crusting occurs.
* May spread over a large area of the face.
* Asymmetrical: does not spread evenly over both sides of face.

Needs antibiotic treatment.

POSSIBLE

■ CANDIDIASIS

A "thrush" infection of the lips and inner cheeks may occur in the elderly, people with dentures, with diets deficient in vitamins or iron, and in AIDS patients. Treatment is anti-fungal creams or lozenges.

* Redness.
* Soreness.
* Slight swelling.
* Occasional cracking and bleeding.
* White plaques or patches may be seen.

■ LEUKOPLAKIA

* White patches on the tongue or lining of the mouth.
* Cannot be scraped off.
* Occasionally disappear leaving a red base.
* Localized hardening under the patch may occur.

It is associated with smoking, heavy liquor intake, spices, infection, sharp teeth, and syphilis.

Leukoplakia may also be an early warning sign of cancer, so long-standing firm white patches on the tongue or in the mouth must not be ignored.

■ CHICKEN POX/MEASLES

These very infectious diseases produce blisters inside the mouth and a rash on the skin.

* Fever.
* Skin rash.
* Feel sick.

■ STOMATITIS

Painful mouth ulcers on the gums, lips and cheeks caused by a virus, usually in children.

* Painful mouth.
* Difficulty swallowing.
* Excessive saliva.

Needs medical attention for relief.

RARE

■ ZINC DEFICIENCY

Any elderly person on a poor diet or with malabsorption or malnutrition problems who develops intermittent sores on, or around, the mouth may be zinc-deficient. A blood test may be needed to confirm this, and zinc supplements can be given.

■ CANCER
Any long-standing ulcer or growth on the lip, particularly in elderly smokers with poor oral hygiene, may be cancerous.
* Persistent ulcer or irregular lump.
* Persistent painless, but enlarged lymph nodes, usually in the neck area.
* Bleeding from lesion.
* Loss of weight.
* Feeling unwell.

■ HEREDITARY HEMORRHAGIC TELANGIECTASIA
Also known as Osler-Weber-Rendu Disease. Hereditary.
* Small red lesions on lips and in mouth that disappear when pressed on.
* Similar lesions throughout gastro-intestinal tract.
* The gastro-intestinal lesions may cause internal bleeding.
* Rarely seen before the age of 40.

■ CHANCRE
The first sign of infection with syphilis. May occur on the lips or in the mouth after oral sex.
* Appears three to four weeks after contact.
* Initially, a hardened, elevated solitary lesion.
* Becomes a shallow ulcer.
* Painless.
* Does not bleed.
* Raised, red edges.
* Local, painless lymph node enlargement in face and neck area.

If suspected must be seen and treated by a physician.

■ DERMATITIS
Any area of skin may develop sensitivity to some irritant. Habitual sucking or chewing of pens or application of some lipsticks or lip balms are examples of agents to which some may react.
* Redness.
* Itching.
* Soreness.
* Sometime crusting and weeping.
* Normal lips when the irritant is not being used

■ BEHCET'S SYNDROME
Commonest in men from the teens to the early thirties.
* Painful ulceration of the mouth.
* Genital ulceration a few weeks after the oral lesions.
* Eye inflammation (uveitis) with the genital ulceration.

The condition comes and goes. Treatment is aimed at relieving the symptoms.

■ ERYTHEMA MULTIFORME
Associated with reaction to medications or infection. Commonest in young males.
* Extensive painful ulcers inside the mouth.
* Gum inflammation.
* Crusting, bloodstained lesions on lips.

Treatment is via identifying and removing or treating the cause.

■ LICHEN PLANUS
In the over-30s.
* Multiple, fine white lines on lips. tongue and the cheek.
* Tiny white spots in the same region.
* Sometimes ulcers between the spots and lines.
* Occasionally fluid-filled sacs develop, then burst, causing painful ulcers.

Mouth

■ MEDICATIONS
A number of medications, such as arsenic, bismuth, lead and mercury, will cause pigmentation of the mouth and lips, in addition to their other symptoms and signs. In the absence of other definite causes for mouth pigmentation, accidental or deliberate taking of such drugs should be considered.

CHAPPED LIPS

Essentially the same as *SORE LIPS, page 84*.

CLEFT LIP AND PALATE

These terms cover a fairly wide range of abnormalities that occur during development in the womb. They are quite common. During development of the fetus, areas of tissue fail to "join", and the resulting gap is seen at birth, sometimes on one side, or in severe cases as a cleft lip and palate on both sides beneath the nose.
* Distortion of the nostril on the affected side.
* In more than half the cases, there is also a defect in the roof of the mouth.
* Food may go up into the nose.
* Speech problems, typically nasal speech, will develop if left untreated.

The trend at present is to repair these deformities by plastic surgery as soon as reasonable after birth so that breast feeding and speech development are affected as little as possible.

SKIN AROUND MOUTH LOOKS PALE

This is a very specific symptom, otherwise known as circumoral pallor, associated with scarlet fever. It should not be confused with more general pallor of skin, mucus membranes and nails associated with anemia or blood loss. *See pages 417-24.* The symptoms of scarlet fever are:
* Tonsilitis and pharyngitis.
* Red rash, predominantly on trunk.
* Sore and coated tongue.
* Circumoral pallor.
* Otitis media may develop; *see page 66.*

Caused by streptococcus bacteria. Treated with antibiotics.

BLEEDING GUMS

This is almost always due to over-vigorous brushing of the teeth, and can be a normal daily occurrence for some people. If bleeding is persistent, or the gums are painful, some degree of *GUM DISEASE* (also known as gingivitis or periodontal disease) may be present; *see page 90.* This may settle without treatment but if there is infection, antibiotics may be necessary. The care of a dental hygienist may be beneficial. A very rare cause of bleeding gums is caused by Vitamin C deficiency.

FOUL-SMELLING BREATH

Halitosis. Most often bad breath is attributable to poor oral hygiene. There are, however, other causes, related to a variety of abnormalities of the mouth, the sinuses, and the lungs, as well as disease elsewhere in the body.

PROBABLE
POOR ORAL HYGIENE
FOOD OR DRINK
SMOKING
DENTAL CARIES
MOUTH BREATHING
MOUTH OR THROAT INFECTION
GUM DISEASE
DENTURES
POST NASAL DRIP

POSSIBLE
SINUSITIS
CONGESTION
CHRONIC LUNG CONDITIONS
PYORRHEA ALVEOLARIS
DIABETIC KETOACIDOSIS

RARE
VINCENT'S ANGINA
CANCERS OF THE MOUTH, UPPER RESPIRATORY TRACT AND LARYNX
KIDNEY FAILURE – UREMIA
LIVER FAILURE
MEDICATIONS AND POISONING

PROBABLE

■ POOR ORAL HYGIENE
The surest way to develop bad breath is to fail to clean your teeth. Even regular tooth brushing may not be enough to prevent the accumulation of food debris between teeth which decays causing odor and plaque. Dental flossing cleans between the teeth and helps prevent bad breath.
* Staining between teeth.
* Irregular color to teeth.
* Breath worse in the morning, on waking.

In addition to brushing and flossing your teeth, regular descaling by a dentist or an oral hygienist can help prevent bad breath and gum disease.

■ FOOD AND DRINK
* Individual has recently eaten spiced foods or drunk alcohol.
* No other evidence of disease in mouth or elsewhere.
* Not present if diet is confined to non-spicy food, or if alcoholic drink is stopped.

■ SMOKING
* Bad breath.
* Stained teeth.

■ DENTAL CARIES
Caries means tooth decay. The enamel covering of the tooth is damaged by bacteria. Regular brushing and avoidance of sugary foods may help, as may fluoride treatments and toothpaste — ask your dentist's advice.
* "Sensitive teeth".

MOUTH

* Painful tooth or teeth.
* Bad breath.
* Pain is worse with very hot or cold food and drink.

■ MOUTH BREATHING

Any condition which makes you breath through your mouth rather than your nose may result in halitosis because of drying up of the salivary secretions which act as a rinsing agent. Nasal polyps, a broken nose, hay fever or even snoring may cause halitosis.

■ MOUTH OR THROAT INFECTION

Any mouth or throat infection may cause bad breath; all may be associated with:
* Pain.
* Fever.
* Feeling unwell.
* Bad breath.
* Unpleasant taste in the mouth.

■ GUM DISEASE

Disease of the gums and tooth sockets, with inflammation of the gums (also known as gingivitis). Caused mainly by poor oral hygiene.
* Bleeding gums particularly after brushing teeth.
* Sensitive gums.
* Bad breath.
* Often occurs with dental caries.

■ DENTURES

If not cleaned regularly and adequately, food debris or saliva may accumulate on dentures, giving off an offensive smell, even when in the mouth.

The sinuses

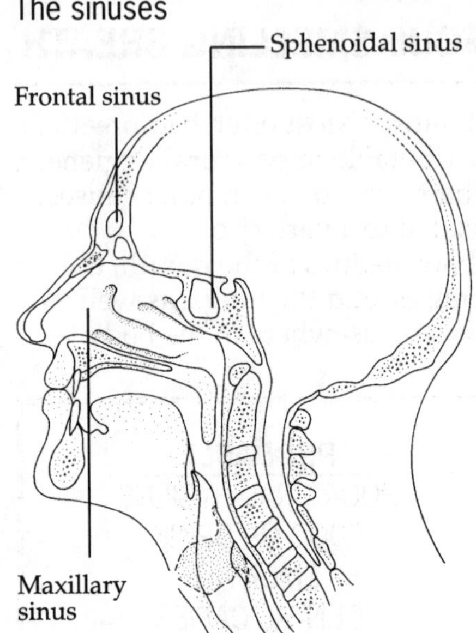

■ POST NASAL DRIP

* May be present for some weeks after flu/colds or sinusitis.
* Mucus drips back into throat causing reflex coughing.
* Worse at night.
* General health otherwise good.
* Bad breath may be present.

See also MUCUS IN THE THROAT, page 129.

POSSIBLE

■ SINUSITIS

Infection of any of the sinuses may cause:
* Persistent nasal discharge (out through the nose or back into the throat).
* May be green or yellow mucus.
* Possibly headache or pain in cheeks or eyes.
* Occasionally fever.
* Congestion.
* Feeling unwell.
* Bad breath.

■ CONGESTION
It often results in bad breath, either because of accompanying infection in the mouth or nose, or because a blocked nose is making you breathe through your mouth.

■ CHRONIC LUNG CONDITIONS
See also FOUL-SMELLING BREATH AND COUGH, page 92.

Any lung condition that causes persistent production of mucus, or where the lung has a long-standing focus of infection may cause bad breath. Patients with chronic bronchitis, tuberculosis, cystic fibrosis, bronchiectasis, emphysema and other diseases may complain of bad breath. The main symptoms of the underlying disease usually include:
* Purulent (green/yellow) mucus.
* Cough.
* Fever.
* Feeling unwell.
* Breathlessness or reduced breathing capacity.

■ PYORRHEA ALVEOLARIS
A disease of gums and tooth sockets, actually a severe, advanced form of gum disease (*see above*).
* Gum margins recede.
* Teeth loosen.
* Pus caused by infection of the tooth socket leaks out between gums and teeth.
* Pain.
* Bad breath.

■ DIABETIC KETOACIDOSIS
Diabetics whose blood sugar is not properly controlled can develop an excess of sugar (ketoacidosis). This is characterized by a sweetish smell on the breath (some describe it as sickly).

RARE

■ VINCENT'S ANGINA
This is a bacterial disease of the tonsils which spreads to the gums. Associated with poor hygiene.
* Fever.
* Sore throat.
* Infected gums.
* Enlarged lymph nodes in the neck.
* Often only one tonsil is affected, with ulceration, and a membrane which may spread to soft and hard palate.

Highly infectious. Responds rapidly to antibiotics.

■ CANCER OF THE MOUTH, UPPER RESPIRATORY TRACT AND LARYNX
Bad breath may be an accompaniment to any site of cancer in the mouth, upper respiratory tract and larynx, particularly if the tumor has become infected and ulcerated. Thus persistent bad breath, in addition to some or any of the following, particularly in elderly smokers, needs close evaluation:
* Persistent, painless enlarged lymph nodes.
* Other lumps developing in mouth/tongue or palate.
* Change in voice.
* Loss of weight.
* Feeling unwell.
* Persistent pain in mouth or neck.
* Dentures not fitting.
* Anemia.

Mouth

■ KIDNEY FAILURE
Uremia is present. Urea is a waste product produced by the kidneys normally excreted in the urine.
* Browny/yellow appearance of skin.
* Bruising.
* Fast rate of breathing.
* Swollen ankles.
* Heart failure.
* Breath smells of urine/ammonia.
* Altered sensation in limbs.

■ LIVER FAILURE
This may occur as a result of a number of diseases that damage liver tissue, such as hepatitis or cirrhosis. It may cause many symptoms, including:
* Jaundice.
* Fatigue.
* Mental deterioration.
* Reddened palms ("liver" palms).
* The appearance of tiny blood vessels in the skin — "vascular spiders".
* Fever.
* Breath smells of feces.

■ MEDICATIONS AND POISONING
Some medications have characteristic smells, excreted in air exhaled from the lungs. Examples are paraldehyde, now rarely used, and disulfiram, a drug prescribed for alcoholics.

FOUL-SMELLING BREATH AND COUGH

PROBABLE
CHRONIC BRONCHITIS

POSSIBLE
LUNG CANCER
BRONCHIECTASIS
CYSTIC FIBROSIS
PULMONARY TUBERCULOSIS
(TB OF THE LUNG)

RARE
LUNG ABSCESS

PROBABLE

■ CHRONIC BRONCHITIS
Covered in detail on *page 212*.
Usually there is:
* Smoker's cough, especially in the early morning.
* Cough in winter.
* Wheezing.
* Sputum varying from white to yellow/green.
* Increasing breathlessness over the years.
* Cyanosis.
* Bad breath.

POSSIBLE

LUNG CANCER
Covered in detail on *page 223*.
Associated symptoms which may be noticeable include:
* Dry cough.
* Bloody sputum.
* Hoarse voice.
* Shortness of breath.
* Chest pain.
* Infection in the lung.

* Feeling weak.
* Weight loss.
* Blockage of neck veins.
* Bad breath.

■ BRONCHIECTASIS
The air passages are damaged, preventing oxygen entering the circulation efficiently. Features include:
* History of repeated chest infections.
* Lots of yellow/green sputum with or without blood.
* Fever.
* Looking unwell.
* Weight loss.
* Feeling sick.
* Severe halitosis.

■ CYSTIC FIBROSIS
See page 223.

Later in infancy, symptoms may include slow growth, offensive diarrhea and/or respiratory infections, which may be associated with bad breath.

■ PULMONARY (LUNG) TUBERCULOSIS
Most frequent in malnourished, immunosuppressed or elderly patients. Features may include:
* Feeling unwell.
* Fatigue.
* Weight loss.
* Cough with sputum — sometimes bloody.
* Chest pain.
* Shortness of breath
* Bad breath.

New resistant strains are developing.

RARE

■ LUNG ABSCESS
A collection of pus lying within the lung tissue. It may be caused by inhaling infected material, as a complication of pneumonia, or by rare causes such as spread of a liver abscess into the chest. In general, features include:
* A pre-existing infection.
* Fever.
* Shivering.
* Sweats.
* Feeling sick.
* Pleurisy (pain in the chest on breathing in and out).
* Foul sputum.
* Bad breath.

BREATH SMELLS OF URINE

Covered in detail under *KIDNEY FAILURE* in *FOUL-SMELLING BREATH, page 92.*

BREATH SMELLS SWEET

See *DIABETIC KETOACIDOSIS* and *LIVER FAILURE*, covered in detail under *FOUL-SMELLING BREATH, page 92.*

ABNORMAL TEETH

Including discoloration and deformity. These following diseases and predisposing factors are worth considering:

Mouth

■ AGE
Teeth tend to become discoloured with age. Periodontal disease such as gingivitis causes gum loss, making the teeth appear longer than normal: hence the expression "long in the tooth".

■ SMOKING
Yellowy-brown staining, even with regular brushing. It also hastens the age-related color changes of teeth.

■ BETEL-NUT CHEWING
Brownish-red discoloration of all teeth, seen in some Asian men and women who chew betel nuts.

■ TETRACYCLINE STAINING
Permanent brown transverse staining of teeth may be caused by administering an antibiotic, called tetracycline to young children or by the mother taking it during pregnancy.

■ TRANSVERSE RIDGES
Transverse ridges on teeth may be seen in people who had Vitamin C or D deficiencies while the surface enamel of their teeth was forming.

■ CHONDRO-ECTODERMAL DYSPLASIA
A congenital disorder. Features include:
* Short stature.
* Short fingers.
* Small teeth.
* Dry skin.
* Scanty hair.

Upper and lower teeth are rooted in the bones of the maxilla and mandible

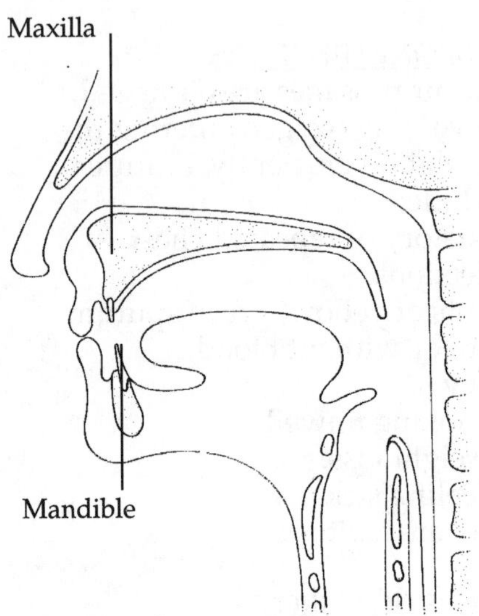

GRINDING THE TEETH

This is a symptom of more concern to the partner or parent of the affected person. It is observed commonly at night and may be associated with snoring. The noise is caused by movement of the upper and lower teeth against each other. The symptom often disappears spontaneously. Only rarely does it cause permanent tooth damage. If the symptom persists the advice of a dentist should be sought.

"Made-to-measure" molds which fit over the teeth can be worn at night to protect the teeth and to prevent grinding.

There is an association between tooth grinding and migraine: some people have both conditions.

DAMAGED TOOTH

If possible, the broken fragment(s) should be kept, and taken with you to a dentist. If the entire tooth and root has been displaced, it may be possible to reimplant it. This should be done as soon as possible. A heavily bleeding tooth socket can be stopped by biting down on a wet tea bag. If there is a possibility that the jaw is fractured, get professional help quickly. The cosmetic problems of a broken or chipped tooth are less important than underlying bone damage if the injury is severe. The bones may need to be realigned. *(See UPPER AND LOWER TEETH NOT CLOSING etc, page 100).*

TEETHING PAIN

The first baby teeth, normally the lower central incisors, appear at the age of six to ten months. Teeth continue to appear until about 30 months. Most infants will have episodes of crying, fever and salivation which may be attributed to teeth coming in.

Fever is not a usual symptom in a teething child: if your child has a fever, it is probably not due to teething. Pain and discomfort are the major symptoms, leading to irritability and crying. It is reasonable to use infant tylenol to soothe a teething child.

It is always important to exclude other obvious sites of infection such as ears or throat.

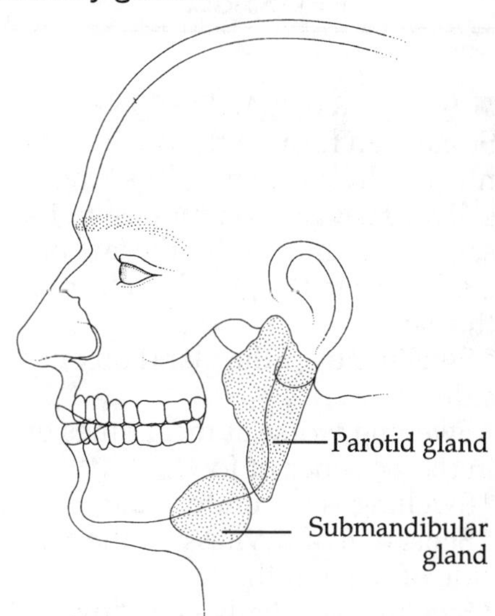

DRY MOUTH

The PROBABLE causes are, dehydration, mouth breathing and fear or anxiety. The first two are covered on *pages 483 and 60, the last on page 377.* Remove the cause, and a normal "wet" mouth returns. If a dry mouth persists, then it might indicate underlying disease.

Anesthetics, antihistamines, sinus medications and anti-depressants can also cause a dry mouth.

POSSIBLE

SALIVARY GLAND STONE

RARE

SJOGREN'S SYNDROME

MOUTH

POSSIBLE

■ SALIVARY GLAND STONE

Stones can form in the ducts of the major salivary glands, blocking saliva. They are commonest in the salivary glands under the jaw but also occur in the glands in front of the ear.

* Swelling over the gland on one side.
* Swelling worse at meal times or in the presence of food.
* Swelling is uncomfortable.
* Sensation of dryness on the same side of the mouth.
* Swelling suddenly goes down — you may note saliva trickling into mouth.

Sometimes the stones are passed, sometimes they need surgery to relieve an abscess or remove the stone.

RARE

■ SJOGREN'S SYNDROME

Probably an auto-immune disease, commonest in middle-aged women.

* Dry eyes, causing a painful, gritty feeling.
* Dry mouth, with bad breath.
* Salivary gland swelling.

Other connective tissue disorders may be associated, for example rheumatoid arthritis.

GENERALLY INFECTED MOUTH

Severe generalized infection of the oral cavity, including tongue, roof of mouth and gums, is a medical emergency. It is rare, and happens if oral hygiene is extremely poor.

RARE
VINCENT'S ANGINA AND VINCENT'S ACUTE ULCERATIVE GINGIVITIS
CANCRUM ORIS

RARE

■ VINCENT'S ANGINA AND VINCENT'S ACUTE ULCERATIVE GINGIVITIS

These are bacterial diseases of the mouth which may originate in the gums between the teeth, or the tonsils and spread rapidly to adjacent tissues.

Vincent's angina:

* Fever.
* Local pain.
* Sore throat.
* Enlarged neck lymph nodes.
* Often only one tonsil affected which is ulcerated, with a membrane present.
* The membrane may spread to soft and hard palate.
* Excessive salivation may occur.
* Highly infectious.

Responds rapidly to appropriate antibiotics.

Vincent's acute ulcerative gingivitis: in addition to the preceding symptoms,

* Deep gum ulcers.

■ CANCRUM ORIS
A severe form of the conditions described above which occur in poorly nourished children. Even with treatment, severe scarring of the cheek can result, also limitation of jaw movement.

DIFFICULT TO OPEN MOUTH

This is usually the result of a disease affecting structures involved in opening the mouth, causing a combination of either pain or swelling. Pain makes it difficult to open the jaw rather than it being a mechanical problem. It is, however, rarely a primary symptom. The diseases are listed here in order of **frequency**, not in order of how often they cause difficulty in opening the mouth.

PROBABLE
APHTHOUS ULCER
DENTAL CARIES
DENTAL INFECTION
UPPER RESPIRATORY TRACT INFECTION
TONSILITIS
MUMPS

POSSIBLE
INFECTIOUS MONONUCLEOSIS
PERITONSILLAR ABSCESS
IMPACTION OF WISDOM TOOTH
ARTHRITIS IN TEMPOROMANDIBULAR JOINT

RARE
TETANUS
STRYCHNINE POISONING

PROBABLE

■ APHTHOUS ULCER
See page 85.

■ DENTAL CARIES
See page 89.

■ DENTAL INFECTION
See page 138.

■ UPPER RESPIRATORY TRACT INFECTION
See page 138.

■ TONSILITIS
See page 138.

■ MUMPS
* Inflammation of the parotid glands in front of the ear.
* Both glands affected and markedly swollen.
* Swelling makes opening the jaw uncomfortable.
* Occasionally, pancreas and testes are affected (after puberty).

POSSIBLE

■ INFECTIOUS MONONUCLEOSIS
See page 139.

■ PERITONSILLAR ABSCESS
See page 139.

■ IMPACTED WISDOM TOOTH
Emerging wisdom teeth,

especially if obstructed by existing teeth, may cause such pain and discomfort at the back of the mouth that it is difficult to open your mouth. Dental opinion should be sought.

■ ARTHRITIS IN TEMPOROMANDIBULAR JOINT
This joint is where the jaw hinges with the skull. Arthritis can develop with age, or after injury.
* Pain localized just in front of the ear.
* Pain may extend across side of face.
* Pain worse on chewing or moving jaw.
* A grinding sensation over the joint may be noted.
* At first, only on one side.
* May eventually affect both sides.

RARE

■ TETANUS
A disease caught by soil penetrating a trivial skin wound and contaminating it with the organism *Clostridium tetani.* It can be fatal.
* Local muscular weakness near the wound.
* Muscular spasms develop.
* Inability to open the mouth, called trismus or "lockjaw".
* The spasms and trismus give rise to a grinning appearance, "risus sardonicus".
* Fever.

Keeping your tetanus immunization up to date is essential. After the teen years, choose a birthday as the date for your shot, and have a tetanus shot every tenth year; for example, at 20, 30, 40 years old, and so on.

Temporomandibular joint

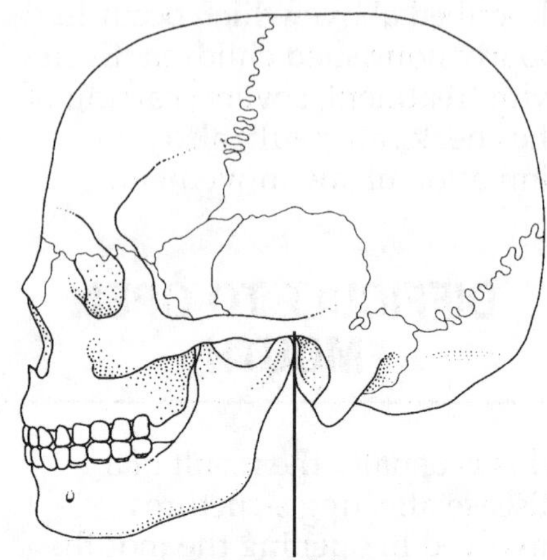

Region of the temporomandibular joint

■ STRYCHNINE POISONING
The symptoms of strychnine poisoning are similar to those of tetanus (*see this page*) but without a history of wound contamination.

TOO MUCH SALIVA

In the absence of any other problems, this is rare. Any condition that causes painful swallowing or a sore throat may lead to an apparent excess of saliva, as the pain prevents the usual frequency of clearing of the saliva from mouth to stomach.

However, there are some conditions in which excessive saliva is a notable feature.

MOUTH

PROBABLE
SMOKING
NAUSEA AND VOMITING
TONSILITIS
PHARYNGITIS

POSSIBLE
INFECTIOUS MONONUCLEOSIS
BRAIN INJURY
NEUROLOGICAL DISEASE
PERITONSILLAR ABSCESS

RARE
CANCER OF THE ESOPHAGUS

PROBABLE

■ SMOKING
Many smokers, especially pipe and cigar smokers, notice that they salivate excessively when smoking, an effect of nicotine.

■ NAUSEA AND VOMITING
Prior to vomiting, the mouth often appears to fill with salty saliva.

■ TONSILITIS
See page 138. Excessive saliva is a typical feature.

■ PHARYNGITIS
See page 124. There may be an apparent excess of saliva because of pain on swallowing.

POSSIBLE

■ INFECTIOUS MONONUCLEOSIS
See page 139.

■ BRAIN INJURY
See page 380.

■ NEUROLOGICAL DISEASE
See multiple sclerosis, Parkinson's disease, motor neurone disease, pseudobulbar and bulbar palsy, under PROBLEMS WITH SWALLOWING PLUS WEIGHT LOSS, page 122.

■ PERITONSILLAR ABSCESS
See ENLARGED LYMPH GLANDS IN NECK, page 137.

RARE

■ CANCER OF THE ESOPHAGUS
See page 121.

IMPACTED TOOTH

Meaning a tooth that cannot come in because it is blocked or prevented from emerging by other teeth. This applies most frequently in adult life to the wisdom teeth. The impacted tooth may be covered by a flap of gum that can become infected and painful. Extraction of the tooth is the usual — and effective — treatment. General or local anaesthetic may be used.

LOOSE TEETH

See DENTAL CARIES, page 89; GUM DISEASE page 90; PYORRHEA ALVEOLARIS , page 91. These are associated with, or lead to, loose teeth, decaying teeth and toothache.

UPPER AND LOWER TEETH NOT CLOSING PROPERLY

Medical term, malocclusion. Teeth should snap shut directly opposite each other. Most people have some degree of malocclusion, typically protruding front teeth — overbite. Some people have irregular teeth. Dentists can correct deformities to improve function and cosmetic appearance.

Damage to the jaw bones, into which the teeth are bedded, can also give malocclusion. If bone damage is suspected, specialized treatment is essential. Deformity will give rise to pain around the face and ear — *see DIFFICULT TO OPEN MOUTH, page 97.*

Arthritis may develop.

SENSITIVE TEETH

Most people suffer from sensitive teeth at some time, frequently caused by injury, leading to receding gums. This exposes the nerve fibres around the tooth, producing sometimes extreme sensitivity to heat and cold. When a tooth is damaged or infected, the nerves will be exposed and unusually sensitive.

See DENTAL CARIES, page 89; GUM DISEASE page 90; PYORRHEA ALVEOLARIS, page 91. Special toothpastes for sensitive teeth coat the nerves and reduce sensitivity. They should be used only after a dentist has excluded gum disease, dental caries or infection.

DECAYING TEETH

See DENTAL CARIES, page 89; GUM DISEASE page 90; PYORRHEA ALVEOLARIS , page 91.

TOOTHACHE

See DENTAL CARIES, page 89; GUM DISEASE page 90; PYORRHEA ALVEOLARIS , page 91.

THE FACE — INTRODUCTION

Many symptoms of the face can also appear elsewhere on the body. This section concentrates on conditions most likely to be localized to the face.

SWOLLEN OR PUFFY FACE

Generalized swelling or puffiness of the face, as distinct from, say, swelling in the neck, is rather uncommon. Considered here is true, overall facial swelling or puffiness.

For causes of local swelling, see the sections on skin, and on the neck.

PROBABLE
INSECT BITE
DENTAL ABSCESS
POISON IVY

POSSIBLE
ANGIONEUROTIC OEDEMA
ERYSIPELAS
CHRONIC CORTISONE THERAPY
NEPHROTIC SYNDROME
HYPOTHYROIDISM
GLOMERULONEPHRITIS

RARE
ACROMEGALY
HYPERADRENALISM

PROBABLE

■ INSECT BITE
* Sudden onset of swelling localized to site of bite.
* Often very itchy.
* Subsides after a day or so.
* Occasionally becomes infected, with swelling becoming red and hot, and fever developing.

■ DENTAL ABSCESS
* Painful swelling above or below lower or upper jaw.
* Whole cheek may be swollen.
* No obvious dental pain or decay (caries).
* Swelling worsens over two to three days.

A visit to your dentist plus a course of antibiotics should provide rapid relief. Dental treatment may subsequently be required.

■ POISON IVY
After exposure in the yard or woods, itching, blisters and swelling may affect the face.
* Patch or line of blisters.
* Crusting.
* Swelling around eyes.
* Spreads on body.

Helped by cortisone cream, if mild. Wash all clothes and bed linens. Severe episode needs medical attention.

The Face

POSSIBLE

■ ANGIONEUROTIC OEDEMA
Also known as giant urticaria. Normally caused by insect bite or allergy to a food or medication, but often the cause is not identifiable. Symptoms may include:
* Swelling of lips and eyes.
* Marked itching.
* Wheezing.
* Breathlessness.
Needs urgent medical attention.

■ ERYSIPELAS
An infection of the skin and underlying tissues. Often, germs get in through a cut or graze.
* Red, shiny, hot skin.
* Painful.
* Fever
* Feeling unwell.
Needs antibiotic treatment.

■ CHRONIC CORTISONE THERAPY
Long term cortisone therapy is used for some diseases such as rheumatoid arthritis and severe skin diseases. It can cause:
* Moon face.
* Thinning of bone.
* Weight gain.
* Thinning and reddening of the skin.
* Raised blood pressure.
* Increased likelihood of infections.

■ NEPHROTIC SYNDROME
See page 430.

■ HYPOTHYROIDISM
Weight gain and other changes associated with this condition may give the appearance of a puffy face, although there is no true swelling.
See page 460.

■ GLOMERULONEPHRITIS
One of the conditions described by *NEPHRITIS, page 429.*

RARE

■ ACROMEGALY
Enlargement of the jaw is one of the symptoms of acromegaly and might be mistaken for facial swelling. *See page 275.*

■ HYPERADRENALISM
See page 273.

FACIAL NODULES OR BUMPS

A possible cause is gout, covered in detail on *page 278*. Also possible are skin papilloma, *page 251* and pigmented mole, *page 244*. A very rare cause is leprosy, *page 319*.

FACIAL BLISTERS OR ULCERATIONS

PROBABLE
COLD SORE
POISON IVY
IMPETIGO

POSSIBLE
ECZEMA
SHINGLES

RARE
SKIN CANCER
PEMPHIGUS VULGARIS
DERMATITIS HERPETIFORMIS
PEMPHIGOID
ERYTHEMA MULTIFORME
STEVENS-JOHNSON SYNDROME

PROBABLE

■ COLD SORE (CANKER SORE)
Common, and caused by a herpes virus. They often develop when someone is or has been unwell, or subjected to extremes of weather, either hot or cold, or windy.
* Initially, irritation noted on skin around mouth.
* Becomes progressively more painful.
* Skin reddens and little vesicles (fluid-filled blisters) appear.
* Vesicles burst and crusts form.
* Clears up in about two weeks.

A similar type of infection may occur in the genital region.

■ POISON IVY
After exposure in the yard or woods, itching, blisters and swelling may affect the face.
* Patch or line of blisters.
* Crusting.
* Swelling around eyes.
* Spreads on body.

Helped by cortisone cream, if mild. Wash all clothes and bed linens. Severe episode needs medical attention.

■ IMPETIGO
A bacterial infection of the skin. Very contagious. May occur in children and adults.
* Blisters may develop wherever the infection starts.
* Blisters burst, forming dark scabs.
* Large areas can be infected if untreated.

At some stages, impetigo can be difficult to distinguish from a cold sore.

Antibiotics are required.

POSSIBLE

■ ECZEMA
Sometimes called dermatitis. On the face, cosmetics are a common cause. Symptoms include:
* Redness (where the cosmetics were applied).
* Red, raised spots.
* Small blisters which weep.
* Crusting and scaling.

It is not uncommon for patches of eczema to appear eventually all over the body.

■ SHINGLES
An infection caused by the virus that also causes chicken pox.
* Red, blistering rash.
* Can be very painful (often preceding the rash).
* May be extensive (typically covering one side of the face).
* Localized to one side of the body's center line.
* Crusting of the blisters.
* Heals in about two weeks, but in

rare cases pain may persist for months or years.

If the eye is affected, seek medical help urgently.

RARE

■ SKIN CANCER
A small cancerous sore, which virtually never spreads to distant parts of the body. Often appears in the elderly around nose, eyes, ears or mouth.
* Starts as a small pink lump.
* After some weeks or months become ulcerated.
* Gradually, if undiagnosed and untreated, it invades underlying tissues, for example the bones of the nose.

Once diagnosed, treatment is effective.

■ PEMPHIGUS VULGARIS
See page 240.

■ DERMATITIS HERPETIFORMIS
See page 240.

■ PEMPHIGOID
See page 240.

■ ERYTHEMA MULTIFORME and STEVENS-JOHNSON SYNDROME
The second is a severe form of the first and both are reactions to infection or medications.

Symptoms include:
* Red rash of different shapes which may be present all over the body.
* Raised red lesions and blisters may occur.
* Each episode may last two to three weeks.

Stevens-Johnson syndrome may also include:
* Fever.
* Feeling sick.
* Lung inflammation.
* Kidney damage.

REDDENED FACE

The probable causes are blushing, heat and alcohol, all of which can make the blood vessels in the skin widen so that they carry more blood than usual. In each case, the redness may well extend across not only face and head but neck and upper trunk.

POSSIBLE
ACNE ROSACEA
EPILEPSY
MENOPAUSE
SYSTEMIC LUPUS ERYTHEMATOSIS

RARE
MITRAL VALVE DISEASE
CARCINOID SYNDROME
PHEOCHROMOCYTOMA

POSSIBLE

■ ACNE ROSACEA
Most common in the middle-aged and elderly.
* Facial reddening.
* Some inflamed pustules.
* Skin is shiny.
* May become permanent.

Food, alcohol or emotion can exacerbate the reddening.

■ EPILEPSY
Epileptics may be aware of facial flushing just before a seizure, and observers will often notice it afterwards.

■ MENOPAUSE
"Flashes" are commonly experienced by women as they approach the "change of life". Symptoms can continue for years.

■ SYSTEMIC LUPUS ERYTHEMATOSUS
See page 448.

RARE

■ MITRAL VALVE DISEASE
* Shortness of breath.
* Lung congestion.
* Coughing blood.
* Bronchitis.
* Heart failure.
* Facial flush, very marked below the eyes.

■ CARCINOID SYNDROME
A tumor that may occur in many parts of the body. Most of its symptoms are caused by chemicals it secretes, and may include:
* Facial flushing, extending over body.
* Diarrhea, abdominal pain.
* Enlarged liver.
* Wheezy chest.
* Heart problems.

■ PHEOCHROMOCYTOMA
Another tumor whose symptoms are caused by the chemicals it secretes. It is very rare.
* High blood pressure.
* Diarrhea.
* Nausea.
* Abdominal pain.
* Facial flushing.

ADENOIDAL FACE

A term used for individuals who tend to mouth-breathe because their enlarged adenoids prevent them from breathing through their nose. Their voice may also be affected and is often described as "adenoidal". Symptoms may include:
* Breathing through the mouth.
* Snoring.
* Open mouth — the jaw hangs down.
* Nasal speech.
* Dark around eyes.

EXPRESSIONLESS FACE

Parkinson's disease is the classic reason for an expressionless, immobile face. However, a number of conditions can give rise to a similar appearance as a result of damage to the part of the brain that controls facial, and other, movement.

PROBABLE
PARKINSON'S DISEASE
DEPRESSION

The Face

POSSIBLE
MEDICATIONS
SCLERODERMA

RARE
HEPATOLENTICULAR DEGENERATION

PROBABLE

■ PARKINSON'S DISEASE
A slowly progressive disease of the middle-aged and elderly.
* Tremor.
* Rigidity and some muscle pain.
* Slow movement.
* Immobile, mask-like face.
* Difficulty in writing.
* Occasional swallowing disorders.
* Salivation.

Can be controlled with medication.

■ DEPRESSION
A depressed person may progressively lose the expression from his or her face. A dull, saddened, flat face is characteristic of depression. *See also page 389.*

POSSIBLE

■ MEDICATIONS
Medications that may cause some of the same symptoms as Parkinson's disease include phenothiazines and butyrophenones. Both these groups of medications are commonly used as tranquillizers.

■ SCLERODERMA
A multi-system disease, usually afflicting women, which is likely to have already been diagnosed; *see page 124.*
* Stiffness of hands leading to rigidity.
* Smooth, hard, shiny skin.
* Difficulty in opening mouth.
* Immobile face with loss of expression.
* Gastric tract, heart and kidneys may become involved.

RARE

■ HEPATOLENTICULAR DEGENERATION
Wilson's disease. An inherited disorder, usually showing itself during the teens.
* Parkinson's disease symptoms, plus:
* Liver damage leading to jaundice in some cases.
* Yellow-brown rings on the eyes.

PART OF THE FACE PARALYZED

Excluded here is immobility of the entire face, covered under *EXPRESSIONLESS FACE, page 105.*

PROBABLE
FACIAL PARALYSIS
STROKE

POSSIBLE
INJURY
POLIOMYELITIS

RARE
TUMORS
HERPES
GUILLAIN BARRE SYNDROME
MOTOR NEURONE DISEASE

PROBABLE

■ FACIAL PARALYSIS (BELL'S PALSY)

The cause is unknown, but the facial nerve is damaged on one side. The affected individual may note the symptoms on waking up one morning, or after having been out in cold weather:
* May be a dull ache on the affected side.
* Cannot close eye.
* Mouth drawn to the side, away from the damaged nerve
* Saliva may dribble from the affected side.
* Cannot smile properly or bare the teeth.
* Occasionally, taste sensation to one side of the tongue is affected.
* With luck, recovery commences within seven to ten days, but may take several weeks.

If you suspect Bell's palsy, see a doctor as soon as possible. Some doctors believe that high doses of steroids, given early enough, may improve the chances of recovery.

■ STROKE

Any stroke may damage part of the brain that controls the nerve that makes the facial muscles work. Different types of stroke may affect the face in slightly different ways so that a number of symptoms can be present to a greater or lesser degree. These include:
* Difficulty or inability to wrinkle the forehead.
* Difficulty or inability to blink or close the eye.
* Difficulty or inability to smile symmetrically.
* Difficulty or inability to bare the teeth.
* Difficulty or inability to whistle.
* Saliva may leak out of the affected side of the mouth.
* The body will be affected on the same side as the face: for example, weakened left hand and face paralyzed on left side.

Paralysis of the face is unlikely to occur in the absence of other symptoms — which may help to determine the diagnosis.

THE FACE

POSSIBLE

■ INJURY
All or part of the facial nerve, which controls movement of the facial muscles, may be damaged — sometimes permanently. The symptoms are the same as for facial palsy (*see above*). Knife wounds to the face or motor vehicle accidents may be a cause.

■ POLIOMYELITIS
"Polio" can also affect the facial nerve, with similar results to *FACIAL PALSY, page 107*.

RARE

■ TUMORS
Primary or secondary cancerous tumors developing in the part of the brain that controls facial movement or that involve or press on the facial nerve, may cause a mixture of symptoms similar to those of *STROKE* or *FACIAL PALSY, page 107*.

■ HERPES
A herpes infection of the mouth, palate or ear can damage the nerve supply to the face causing symptoms similar to FACIAL PALSY, *page 107*.

■ GUILLAIN-BARRE SYNDROME
A disease of the nervous system with many different symptoms, ranging from mild to severe. Most cases recover, but this may take many months.
* Altered sensation in the arms and legs.
* Weakened legs or arms.
* Shoulder and back pain.
* Facial palsies.
* Muscles of respiration may be so weakened that assisted breathing by machine is required.
* Swallowing may be affected and tube-feeding may be needed while recovery progresses.

■ MOTOR NEURONE DISEASE
See page 123.

FACIAL PAIN

Covered here are causes of pain that have no *visible* symptoms, so, for example, shingles is excluded.

PROBABLE
DENTAL DISEASE
REFERRED PAIN

POSSIBLE
MIGRAINE
POST HERPETIC NEURALGIA
TRIGEMINAL NEURALGIA

RARE
CANCER
PAGET'S DISEASE
PSYCHOGENIC FACIAL PAIN

PROBABLE

■ DENTAL DISEASE
Check teeth and gums first if local

face pain develops with no obvious cause. Is it an abscess? If in doubt, always check with your dentist.

■ REFERRED PAIN
Because the body's "wiring" — its nervous system — is interconnected, pain arising in one place can travel or "be referred" to another. If the teeth and gums appear normal, then pain in the face may arise from elsewhere in the head, for instance the facial sinuses.

POSSIBLE

■ MIGRAINE
See page 113, for full details. Facial pain can be felt as part of a migraine attack.
* The pain will usually be severe and piercing.
* Only one side of the face will be affected.

■ POST-HERPETIC NEURALGIA
Persistent burning pain at the site of a previous attack of shingles; *see page 239*.
* Usually in elderly patients.
* Pain is so severe that suicide may be considered.
* Even touching the site may start an attack of pain.

■ TRIGEMINAL NEURALGIA
Pain in the face in an area supplied by the trigeminal nerve [diagram] can be very severe.
* Stabbing, intermittent facial pain.
* Can be triggered by touch, or for no reason.
* Attacks come and go.

Trigeminal neuralgia

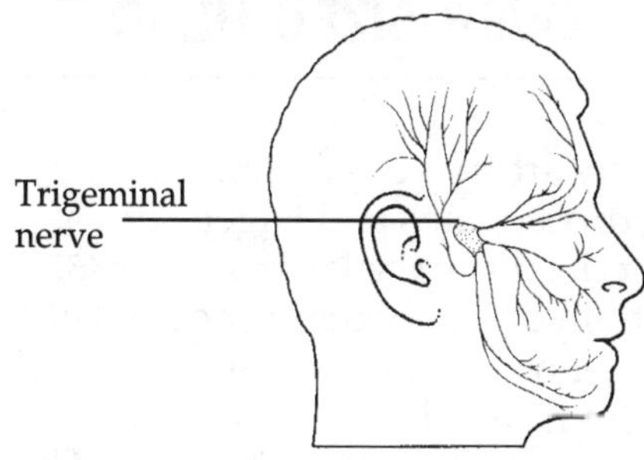

Many different treatments have been tried, some with more success than others.

RARE

■ MALIGNANT DISEASE
A doctor will consider the possibility of a cancerous tumor of the nose, mouth, sinuses or pharynx, particularly if the individual is an elderly smoker.

■ PAGET'S DISEASE
This disease *(see also page 437)* can cause local pain in the bones affected, including those of the face.

■ PSYCHOLOGICAL OR ATYPICAL
In a few individuals no cause of pain is ever found, despite full investigation and assessment. This pain is described as "atypical". Recent research by dental experts and pain specialists has found that tricyclics, a group of medications generally used to treat depression, can be helpful to patients with "atypical facial pain".

It is certainly worth trying these drugs before accepting that "only psychotherapy will help".

The Head

OVER-SIZED HEAD

There are two possibilities: hydrocephalus and Paget's disease. For details of the latter, *see page 437*.

In hydrocephalus, a problem of new-born and very young babies, there is inability to drain fluid from cavities within the brain. The result is increased pressure in the skull, with:
* Progressive enlargement of the head.
* Bulging fontanelles. (The "soft spot").

The increased pressure damages the brain and can cause:
* Intellectual impairment.
* Seizures.
* Physical impairment.
* Vulnerability to infection.

Hydrocephalus needs specialist treatment: the fluid can be drained away to another part of the body by a tube set permanently below the skin on the scalp.

BULGING OR SUNKEN PLACES ON HEAD

Babies have soft spots on their heads where the skull bones have not yet joined into a consistent bony covering. The smaller, posterior fontanelle closes soon after birth, while the larger one, the anterior fontanelle, usually closes by one and a half years of age.

The size of the fontanelles varies greatly from child to child. Your physician examines the fontanelle if your child is unwell. A bulging fontanelle can indicate raised pressure in the head — as in meningitis. However, the fontanelle will also bulge when the baby cries vigorously. Check on any changes or concerns regarding the fontanelle with your doctor.

PROBABLE
CRYING BABY
DEHYDRATION

POSSIBLE
PAGET'S DISEASE

RARE
HYDROCEPHALUS
RAISED INTRACRANIAL PRESSURE

PROBABLE

■ CRYING BABY
Vigorous crying will raise intra-cranial pressure and cause the soft spot to bulge. Harmless. Calm the baby.

■ DEHYDRATION
A baby who is short of fluid, typically after a bout of diarrhea, will show:
* Sunken eyes.
* Sunken fontanelle.
* Loss of skin elasticity.
* Listless, apathetic behavior.
* Dry lips and mouth.

Dehydration is a serious condition in any baby or child; if you suspect it, see a doctor urgently. It can be effectively treated.

POSSIBLE

■ PAGET'S DISEASE
See page 437.

RARE

■ HYDROCEPHALUS
See under OVER-SIZED HEAD, page 110.

■ RAISED INTRACRANIAL PRESSURE
A tumor or infection raises the pressure inside the skull. It is normal for the fontanelles to bulge outwards when a baby cries or strains, say when coughing. But if the fontanelle bulges permanently, there may be other symptoms such as vomiting and headache. See a physician.

When the fontanelle has closed, around 18 months, it cannot bulge. After this time the main signs of raised intracranial pressure will be vomiting and headache.

BLOOD VESSELS STAND OUT IN HEAD

If thickened or painful to the touch, they can be a sign of temporal arteritis; *see page 113.*

HEAD TWISTING TO ONE SIDE

Stiff neck? *See STIFFNESS OR PAIN IN NECK, page 135.* A common cause is torticollis, also considered in detail on *page 136 under WRY NECK.*

HEADACHE AND FITS OR CONVULSIONS

See CONVULSIONS, page 383.

HEADACHE

It is rare for headache to be the symptom of serious disease, such as a brain tumor. Even the most vicious, throbbing headache is in all likelihood benign: the headache that signifies a brain tumor will almost always be accompanied by other symptoms. Most headaches that doctors evaluate are caused by tension or sinus problems.

However, any headache that continues or gets worse over several days needs medical assessment.

PROBABLE
TENSION HEADACHE
SINUSITIS
MENSTRUATION- OR MENOPAUSE-RELATED
INFECTION
UNCORRECTED VISION

THE HEAD

POSSIBLE

MIGRAINE
CLUSTER HEADACHE
TEMPORAL ARTERITIS
EYE, EAR, NOSE, THROAT, OR DENTAL DISEASE
DRUGS/MEDICATIONS
TOXIC FUMES
HYPOGLYCEMIA

RARE

MENINGITIS
SUBARACHNOID HEMORRHAGE
BRAIN TUMOR
SUBDURAL HEMORRHAGE
BRAIN ABSCESS
HIGH BLOOD PRESSURE

PROBABLE

■ TENSION HEADACHE
A common cause of headache resulting from stress. The source of stress or tension is not always obvious. Environmental stressors such as noise, lights, stale air undoubtedly play a larger role than they used to.
* May be intermittent for weeks and months in a previously well person.
* Normal periods between headaches.
* Band-like, crushing pain around head.
* May have tender neck or forehead muscles.
* No other physical abnormalities present.
* Disappears after a variable length of time.
* May be linked with depression.

■ SINUSITIS
See page 56. Any inflammation of the sinuses (air-spaces in the facial bones) can cause headache.
* Constant low-grade, throbbing pain.
* Increased by turning the head or bending.

■ MENSTRUATION- OR MENOPAUSE-RELATED
Monthly changes in hormone levels or during the years of "the change" can cause headaches. Your physician may be able to advise you on treatment.

■ INFECTION
Viral infections of any kind produce multiple symptoms of which headache, often dull and persistent, is one. Other symptoms are:
* Fever.
* Muscle and joint pain.
* Feeling sick.

These are in addition to other, more specific, symptoms, typically sore throat.

■ UNCORRECTED VISION
If poor vision is uncorrected, the strain on the eye muscles can cause headache, especially after reading or driving If a child complains of headache at school or after, have the eyes checked.

POSSIBLE

■ MIGRAINE
Recurrent, severe headaches, often but not always accompanied by visual disturbance. Often starts in adolescence. Many different symptoms are described, including:
* Vision affected before the headache starts.
* Occasional numbness or weakness of one limb before the headache starts.
* Pain starts on one side of the head, but may spread.
* The pain throbs.
* A wish to avoid light.
* Vomiting may occur.
* May last for a couple of days, but normally four to 12 hours.

The cause is not not fully understood but probably related to abnormal blood flow in the head. Good relief is available from modern medications — see your physician.

■ CLUSTER HEADACHE
* Commonest in men.
* Tends to be one-sided.
* Often severe.
* May occur at night.
* Occurs several times within a period of a few weeks, then disappears, returning some months later.
* Unpleasant but not serious.

■ TEMPORAL ARTERITIS
Inflammation of the temporal artery which runs along the side of the forehead. Common in the elderly.

Temporal arteritis

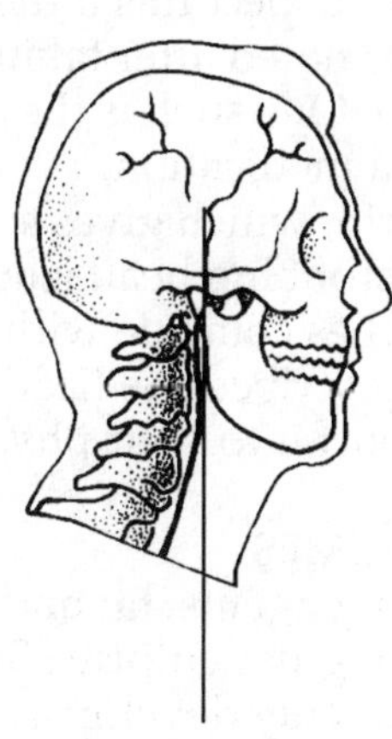

* Severe pain on side of the face.
* Skin over the artery may be inflamed.
* Artery is thickened and can be painful to touch.
* There may be fever and feeling unwell.

If suspected, urgent medical treatment is needed, as the eye may become involved.

■ EYE, EAR, NOSE, THROAT, OR DENTAL DISEASE
See those sections for full detail. All these organs can produce pain that is referred to the head. The pain may be dull and persistent. These possibilities should therefore be excluded if a headache persists for longer than expected.

■ DRUGS/MEDICATIONS
Including cigarettes and alcohol. The system is poisoned by the body's inability to eliminate the broken-down by-products.

THE HEAD

Some prescription medications can cause headache, too. You can reasonably suspect this if the headache is noted after taking the medication. One such is the anti-angina medication, nitroglycerin, which gives some people a throbbing headache.

If headaches coincide with taking a prescribed medication, always report it to your physician.

■ TOXIC FUMES

Dry-cleaning agents, tar and diesel fumes are regular culprits. Some people suddenly develop a sensitivity to fumes, even having worked with them for years.

Low-grade poisoning with carbon monoxide from a faulty furnace or automobile tail pipe can cause headaches.

RARE

■ MENINGITIS

An infection of the membranes that enclose the brain and spinal cord. If you suspect it, see a doctor immediately.

* Severe headache.
* Stiff neck; bending the neck worsens the pain.
* Reduced level of consciousness.
* Photophobia — extreme sensitivity to light.
* Vomiting.
* Fever.
* Very sick.
* A rash may appear.

■ SUBARACHNOID HEMORRHAGE

A leakage of blood from a diseased blood vessel in the brain. The following may occur:

* Sudden onset of severe headache — often described as being like a blow on the back of the head or the worst headache ever experienced. However:
* The headache may have a slower, more subtle, onset.
* Vomiting.
* Stiff neck.
* Mental confusion.
* Speech difficulties.
* Limb weakness.
* Visual disturbances.
* Convulsions.

If suspected, see a physician urgently.

■ BRAIN TUMOR

Because the adult skull is rigid, a growth within it can increase the internal pressure, giving rise to headache. However, not every brain tumor has this effect.

Brain tumors can be primary — a pituitary tumor is an example — or secondary, that is, having spread from elsewhere in the body, for example from a primary breast cancer. There will almost always be a range of symptoms:

* Headache often present when you wake in the morning.
* Gradually increasing, dull headache.
* Vision may be affected.
* Seizures may occur.
* Change in personality.
* Vomiting.
* Impaired consciousness.
* Pulse becomes slower.
* Weakness in the face or in a limb.
* Respiration rate becomes slower.

Urgent medical assessment is needed. The symptoms can often be relieved, even if the tumor itself cannot be removed.

■ SUBDURAL HEMORRHAGE
Blood collects between the layers of tissue covering the brain, causing raised pressure. May happen in the elderly after an (apparently) insignificant fall or injury. Symptoms may develop some weeks later and include:
* Headache, often minor.
* Periods of sleepiness and unconsciousness.
* Increased confusion.
* Possibly speech difficulties.
* Possibly seizures.

Any of these symptoms, except for the first, should be urgently evaluated by a physician.

■ BRAIN ABSCESS
Infection enters the brain in one of several ways: a broken skull-bone with overlying skin damage; from ear, throat, sinus and lung infection; or occasionally from facial infection.
* Symptoms of the initial infection, for example, earache.
* Progressive headache.
* Progressive drowsiness.
* Fever.
* Vomiting.
* Feeling unwell.
* Loss of appetite.
* Seizures.

Needs urgent medical attention.

■ HIGH BLOOD PRESSURE
Does not usually cause headache. Unusually high level, called "malignant hypertension" will cause:
* Headache.
* Visual disturbance.

HEADACHE WITH HIGH FEVER

The commonest illnesses which produce fever combined with headache are common viral infections such as influenza and glandular fever. There are, however, several unusual but dangerous infections such as Rocky Mountain Spotted Fever which may also be responsible for similar symptoms. Don't read this summary without also reading the sections on fever, *pages 440-51.*

PROBABLE

COMMON INFECTIONS, *see FEVER, pages 440-51*

POSSIBLE

TEMPORAL ARTERITIS, *page 113*
SINUSITIS, *page 56*
DISEASES OF EYE, EAR, NOSE, THROAT, TEETH, *see pages 13-29, 116-31 and 93-5*
MALARIA, *page 453*
ROCKY MOUNTAIN SPOTTED FEVER, *page 247*

RARE

MENINGITIS, *page 385*
BRAIN ABSCESS, *this page*
BRUCELLOSIS, *page 448*
TYPHUS FEVER, *page 453*
WEIL'S DISEASE, *page 453*
LYME DISEASE, *page 247*

THE HEAD/ THE THROAT

HEADACHE PLUS CHILLS AND FEVER

See FEVER, pages 440-51

HEADACHE: BABIES AND CHILDREN

Babies and children can get headaches for the same reasons as adults. But in seeking the cause, you should consider two other factors:

First, babies and young children find it difficult to be exact about where pain is coming from. "Head pain" is often earache or sore throat. So, explore every possibility before settling for headache.

Second, complaining of headaches can be characteristic of a child who is unhappy or under stress: typically he or she is having time a bad time at school. If you can detect no other symptoms, consider stress and try to find the cause. You may need help from a teacher or school counselor.

RECURRING HEADACHE

See HEADACHE WITH HIGH FEVER, page 115.

SLURRED OR UNCLEAR SPEECH

Hoarseness is covered separately on *page 118*. Listed here are the main causes of impaired speech; but bear in mind that impaired speech is not always a feature of these conditions, and that their other symptoms are usually more obvious. Look up specific entries elsewhere in the book for further details.

PROBABLE

ALCOHOL AND DRUGS
SEPTAL DEVIATION
INJURY
COMMON COLD
ADENOIDS
STUTTERING
LISPING AND ROLLING Rs
EXHAUSTION

POSSIBLE

CLEFT PALATE
NEUROLOGICAL DISEASE
CHRONIC SINUSITIS
BENIGN TUMORS

RARE

MALIGNANT TUMORS OF THE NOSE

THE THROAT

PROBABLE

■ ALCOHOL AND DRUGS
Temporary slowness and slurring.

■ SEPTAL DEVIATION
Muffled or nasal quality to speech.
See page 61.

■ INJURY
Muffled or nasal quality to speech.
See page 54.

■ COMMON COLD
Muffled or nasal quality to speech.
See page 454.

■ ADENOIDS
Muffled or nasal quality to speech.
See page 60.

■ STUTTERING
Tends to begin as a child begins to learn to talk, from two years onwards.

■ LISPING AND ROLLING Rs
Not necessarily a speech impairment, but a variation of normal. Common when children first learn to speak, and tends to disappear by the age of six. If marked or persistent, speech therapy may be appropriate. Indeed, early attention from a speech therapist can prevent speech disorders from becoming permanent.

■ EXHAUSTION
Prolonged lack of sleep or working without rest for long periods can cause slurred speech.

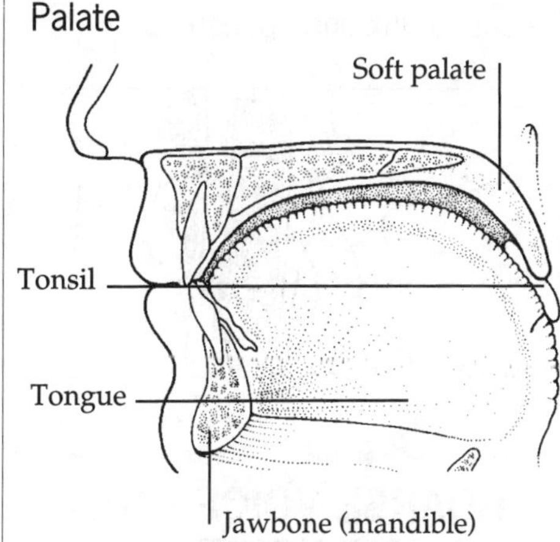

POSSIBLE

■ CLEFT PALATE
See page 88.

■ NEUROLOGICAL DISEASE
Any disease that can affect control of the tongue, soft palate and related structures will give slurred and unclear speech. Motor neurone disease, multiple sclerosis and Parkinson's disease are examples.

■ CHRONIC SINUSITIS
May give a muffled or nasal quality to speech. *See page 130.*

■ BENIGN TUMORS
Including nasal polyps, may give a muffled or nasal quality to speech. *See page 58.*

RARE

■ MALIGNANT TUMORS OF THE NOSE
See CANCER OF THE NOSE, page 59.

THE THROAT

Throat, larynx and speech

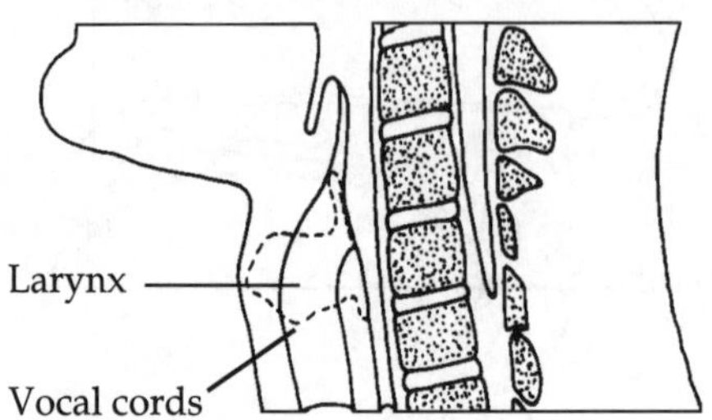

HOARSE VOICE - OR NO VOICE

The causes of hoarseness or loss of voice can be divided into three main categories: those affecting the vocal cords themselves; those affecting the nerves supplying them; and those caused by other disease of the larynx. All cases of hoarseness lasting more than 10 days must be reported to a physician.
See also PROBLEMS WITH SWALLOWING PLUS HOARSE VOICE, page 122.

PROBABLE
SMOKING, DRINKING, EXCESSIVE TALKING/SHOUTING/SINGING
LARYNGITIS
COMMON COLD

POSSIBLE
VOCAL NODULES
SURGERY
MYXEDEMA
EPIGLOTTITIS
CANCER OF THE LARYNX
INHALATION

RARE
FOREIGN BODIES
THORACIC AORTIC ANEURYSM
CANCER
AFTER RADIOTHERAPY
SARCOIDOSIS
MYASTHENIA GRAVIS

PROBABLE

■ SMOKING, DRINKING, EXCESSIVE TALKING/SHOUTING OR SINGING
All are capable of inflaming the vocal cords.
* Hoarseness.
* Sore throat.
* Settles in three to four days.

Resting the voice (not talking) is the only treatment. Smoking and drinking should cease.

■ LARYNGITIS
See page 126.

■ COMMON COLD
May occasionally involve the larynx, resulting in hoarseness.
See also page 454.

POSSIBLE

■ VOCAL NODULES
Typically in singers pitching their voice higher than their natural range.
* Progressive hoarseness.

The nodules often need to be removed by surgery.

■ SURGERY
Surgery to the neck, particularly to the thyroid gland, may damage the recurrent laryngeal nerve. Recovery takes a few weeks but the hoarseness can be permanent. If so, there are methods of improving the speech.

After any operation where a breathing tube as been passed down the throat, slight hoarseness and a sore throat is usual.

■ MYXEDEMA
The result of an underactive thyroid gland. Many other symptoms such as dry skin and hair, weight gain, cold intolerance plus deep, gruff voice.

■ EPIGLOTTITIS
See page 139.

■ CANCER OF THE LARYNX
See page 125.

■ INHALATION
Of smoke or chemicals can cause temporary hoarseness.

RARE

■ FOREIGN BODIES
See page 122.

■ THORACIC AORTIC ANEURYSM
The aorta is the main artery in the chest. An aneurysm is a swelling out of the artery wall due to weakness. This can cause hoarseness by local pressure on the recurrent laryngeal nerve.

■ CANCER
Any malignant tumor in the chest, but especially on the esophagus or lung, may press on or invade the recurrent laryngeal nerve causing hoarseness.

However, this symptom is usually one of the last to occur.
See NOTICEABLE BLOOD VESSELS IN THE NECK, SWOLLEN LYMPH NODES IN NECK, PROBLEMS IN SWALLOWING, pages 131, 137 and this page.

■ AFTER RADIOTHERAPY
Radiotherapy is sometimes used to treat cancer of the larynx, leaving the patient hoarse.

■ SARCOIDOSIS
A disease (cause unknown) giving enlarged lymph nodes and deposits in various tissues, including larynx, hence hoarseness.

■ MYASTHENIA GRAVIS
See page 122.

CLEARING THE THROAT

See MUCUS IN THE THROAT, page 129.

PROBLEMS WITH SWALLOWING

PROBABLE
TONSILITIS
PHARYNGITIS

THE THROAT

POSSIBLE
GLOBUS
ESOPHAGITIS
ACHALASIA

RARE
CONGENITAL ATRESIA OF THE ESOPHAGUS
CANCER OF THE ESOPHAGUS
CANCER OF THE STOMACH

PROBABLE

■ TONSILITIS AND PHARYNGITIS,
See pages 138 and 124.

POSSIBLE

■ GLOBUS
Sometimes occurs in people with a history of anxiety-related illness: a certain belief that there is a lump or something stuck in the throat; sensation of choking, excess mucus, can usually eat and drink normally. Requires full medical examination and, if all is normal, strong reassurance.

■ ESOPHAGITIS
See page 121.

■ ACHALASIA
A narrowing of the esophagus at the lower end. Appears in young adults.
* Difficulty in swallowing.
* Regurgitation of undigested food into the mouth .
* Vomiting.
* Loss of weight.
* Occasionally, chest infections with fever.

RARE

■ CONGENITAL ATRESIA OF THE ESOPHAGUS
At birth:
* All feeds regurgitated.
* Frothy saliva from mouth.
* Difficulty breathing while being fed.
*Episodes of cyanosis (blueskin).
* Pneumonia.

■ CANCER OF THE ESOPHAGUS AND CANCER OF THE STOMACH
See page 121.

PROBLEMS WITH SWALLOWING PLUS REGURGITATION OR VOMITING

PROBABLE
ESOPHAGITIS
HIATAL HERNIA

POSSIBLE
PEPTIC STRICTURE
ACHALASIA

RARE
CANCER OF THE ESOPHAGUS
STOMACH CANCER
OTHER CANCERS
THORACIC AORTIC ANEURYSM
PHARYNGEAL POUCH

PROBABLE

■ ESOPHAGITIS
Caused by stomach acid regurgitating.
* Burning pain on swallowing.
* Food and fluid regurgitated.
* Bitter taste in mouth.
* Heartburn.
* Pain in middle of chest, at front or at back, or down arms.
* Food "sticks" behind breast bone.
* Aggravated by hot or spicy foods and alcohol.
Relieved by antacids.

■ HIATAL HERNIA
See page 143.
Caused by a weakness of the muscles at the lower end of the esophagus.
* Same symptoms as esophagitis.
* Worse on bending or lying down.

POSSIBLE

■ PEPTIC STRICTURE
A narrowing of the esophagus caused by long-standing reflux esophagitis.
* Food regurgitated with fluid.
* Heartburn.
* Associated with weight loss after prolonged period.
* Chest infections associated with regurgitation.
* May be associated with hiatal hernia; *see page 143*.
* May be a long-standing history of reflux esophagitis.

RARE

■ PHARYNGEAL POUCH
See page 135.

■ CANCER OF THE ESOPHAGUS
Commonest in 50-plus age group.
* Difficulty in swallowing.
* Liquids swallowed more easily than solids.
* Some regurgitation of food.
* Rarely pain.
* Weight loss.
* Poor appetite.
* Fatigue.
* Anemia (particularly in women).
* Hoarse voice.
* Occasional chest infection with fever — due to regurgitation into the lungs.

■ STOMACH CANCER
Similar symptoms to esophageal cancer, but there may also be:
* Abdominal pain.
* Poor appetite, developing earlier.
* A feeling of fullness soon after eating very little.
* Symptoms of indigestion which persist, do not respond to usual treatment, or become more severe.
* Feeling bloated.
* A previous ulcer.
* Anemia.
* In later stages, occasional difficulty in swallowing.

■ OTHER CANCERS
Secondary tumors or large primary tumors in the chest, can compress the esophagus, causing:
* Difficulty in swallowing.
* Weight loss.
* Poor appetite.

* Weakness.
All in addition to the symptoms of the primary tumor.

■ THORACIC AORTIC ANEURYSM
See page 119.

PROBLEMS WITH SWALLOWING PLUS HOARSE VOICE

Hoarseness which continues in the absence of other symptoms can be a sign either of laryngeal polyps or of cancer. Early treatment will significantly improve the outcome. Seek your physician's advice as early as possible.

PROBABLE
LARYNGITIS

POSSIBLE
FOREIGN BODY IN ESOPHAGUS

RARE
MYASTHENIA GRAVIS
CANCER OF THE ESOPHAGUS

PROBABLE

■ LARYNGITIS
See page 126.

POSSIBLE

■ FOREIGN BODY (FOR EXAMPLE A FISH BONE) IN ESOPHAGUS
* Pain and discomfort on swallowing.
* Hoarseness.
* Feeling of "something in the throat".

RARE

■ MYASTHENIA GRAVIS
A disease causing weakness and tiring of the muscles.
* Muscular weakness.
* Drooping eyelids.
* Double vision.
* Hoarse, weak voice.
* Difficulty in swallowing.
* Possibly weight loss.

■ CANCER OF THE ESOPHAGUS
See page 121.

PROBLEMS WITH SWALLOWING PLUS WEIGHT LOSS

This combination of symptoms is likely to be an indication of serious illness. Seek help soon, since early intervention will significantly improve your chances of recovery. Smoking and drinking to excess will increase the risk of esophageal problems and cancer of the stomach.

PROBABLE
ESOPHAGEAL STRICTURE
CANCER OF THE ESOPHAGUS

POSSIBLE
ESOPHAGEAL BENIGN TUMOR
MULTIPLE SCLEROSIS
MOTOR NEURONE DISEASE
PARKINSON'S DISEASE
PSEUDOBULBAR AND BULBAR PALSY

RARE
CHAGAS' DISEASE
MYASTHENIA GRAVIS
SCLERODERMA
SYSTEMIC LUPUS ERYTHEMATOSUS (SLE)
CANCER OF THE STOMACH

PROBABLE

■ ESOPHAGEAL STRICTURE
See PEPTIC STRICTURE, page 121.
The symptoms are the same, but can be caused by, for instance, accidental or deliberate swallowing of toxic chemicals.

■ CANCER OF THE ESOPHAGUS
See page 121.

POSSIBLE

■ BENIGN TUMOR OF THE ESOPHAGUS
Such as a fibroma, leiomyoma or hemangioma.
* Intermittent difficulty in swallowing.
* Sensation of "something" in the esophagus.
* Health otherwise good.
* Minimal weight loss, unless tumor is large.

■ MULTIPLE SCLEROSIS
In addition to motor and sensory changes *(see page 405):*
* Difficulty in swallowing.
* Some risk of regurgitation of food into lungs.
* Gradual weight loss.

■ MOTOR NEURONE DISEASE
Progressive muscular weakness with:
* Difficulty in starting to swallow because of poor tongue muscle control.
* Risk of inhaling food or fluids.
* Gradual weight loss.
See also page 406.

■ PARKINSONS'S DISEASE
In addition to the tremor, mask face and slowness of movement:
* Difficulty in starting to swallow.
* Occasional choking.
* Weight loss.

■ PSEUDOBULBAR AND BULBAR PALSY
These conditions are usually set off by a stroke (pseudobulbar palsy) or motor neurone disease (bulbar palsy). They cause:
* Difficulty in speech.
* Difficulty in swallowing.
* Regurgitation of food into nose.
* If prolonged, weight loss.

THE THROAT

RARE

■ CHAGAS' DISEASE
Common in South America. Caused by infection with *trypanosoma cruzi*. Symptoms are similar to those of ACHALASIA; *see page 120.*

■ MYASTHENIA GRAVIS
See page 122.

■ SCLERODERMA
A disease which can affect many organs and which will usually have been diagnosed already. Commonest in women in their 30s and 40s.
* Associated with pain because of esophagitis; *see page 121.*
* Slow weight loss.

■ SYSTEMIC LUPUS ERYTHEMATOSUS (SLE)
See page 448.

■ CANCER OF THE STOMACH
See page 121.

PROBLEMS WITH SWALLOWING PLUS PAIN

PROBLABLE

TONSILITIS
PHARYNGITIS
LARYNGITIS

POSSIBLE

CANDIDIASIS
ESOPHAGITIS
ESOPHAGEAL SPASM
ULCERS OF TONGUE AND MOUTH
GLOSSITIS
HERPES SIMPLEX

RARE

CANCER OF THE ESOPHAGUS
CANCER OF THE LARYNX

PROBABLE

■ TONSILITIS
See page 138.

■ PHARYNGITIS
The pharynx lies behind the tonsils at the back of the mouth, above the voice box and throat.
* Pain on swallowing.
* Back of throat is noticeably red.
* Possibly enlarged lymph nodes — similar to tonsilitis, but tonsils not inflamed.

■ LARYNGITIS
See page 126.

POSSIBLE

■ CANDIDIASIS
* Discomfort making swallowing difficult.
* White patches seen at the back of the throat and sides of mouth.
* Commonest in children, the immuno-suppressed and the elderly.

■ ESOPHAGITIS
Similar to reflux esophagitis, but the main symptom is:
* Burning pain behind the breast bone within a few seconds of swallowing plus:
* Spread of pain to the arms.
* Heartburn.
* Aggravated by spicy foods or alcohol.

■ ESOPHAGEAL SPASM
Spasm of the muscles of the esophagus.
* Chest pain caused by eating or emotional stress.
* The condition can be mild or severe.
* Pain varies in intensity during an attack.
* Can be painless.
* Difficulty in swallowing may come and go with the pain.

■ ULCERS OF TONGUE AND MOUTH *See pages 96 and 97.*

■ GLOSSITIS
Swollen, painful tongue, occasional fever, sometimes associated with Vitamin B2 deficiency, *page 84*.

■ HERPES SIMPLEX
A viral infection causing pain and formation of fluid-filled spots or ulcers. May be present in mouth, throat or esophagus.
* Severe pain associated with the herpes sore.
* Vesicles and intensely painful ulcers seen in mouth.
* Feeling very unwell.
* Fever.

RARE

■ CANCER OF THE ESOPHAGUS
See page 121.

■ CANCER OF THE LARYNX
* Persistent hoarseness.
* Occasionally pain on swallowing because of spread or ulceration.

PROBLEMS WITH SWALLOWING PLUS FEVER

PROBABLE
TONSILITIS
LARYNGITIS

RARE
LUDWIG'S ANGINA
CANCER OF THE ESOPHAGUS

PROBABLE

■ TONSILITIS
Tonsils at the back of the mouth, either side of the throat, become inflamed.
* Enlarged tonsils.
* Occasional white spots on tonsils.
* Reddening in the throat.
* Pain on swallowing.
* Occasionally, associated cough.
* Fever.
* Enlarged lymph glands in neck may be tender.

THE THROAT

■ LARYNGITIS
Infection involving the larynx — the "voice box" in the neck.
* Hoarse voice, or difficulty in speaking at all.
* Fever.
* Pain on swallowing, but less severe than with tonsilitis.

RARE

■ LUDWIG'S ANGINA
Severe infection of the floor of the mouth.
* Severe pain.
* Can cause breathing difficulty — because of swollen upper airways.
* Pain on swallowing.
The condition is usually associated with poor oral hygiene, and problems with infected teeth or gums.

■ CANCER OF THE ESOPHAGUS
See page 121.

SWOLLEN THROAT

See SWOLLEN LYMPH NODES IN NECK, page 137.

LUMP IN THROAT

See PROBLEMS WITH SWALLOWING, pages 119-25.

SORE THROAT

Common reasons for a sore throat are covered under *PROBLEMS WITH SWALLOWING PLUS PAIN, page 124.*

If you think you have this symptom in isolation, *see SWOLLEN LYMPH NODES IN THE NECK, page 137; ISOLATED LUMPS AND SWELLINGS IN OR ON THE NECK, page 133; STIFFNESS OR PAIN IN THE NECK, page 135; PROBLEMS WITH SWALLOWING PLUS PAIN, page 124 and ULCERS IN MOUTH, page 127.*

It is however most likely to occur along with fever. *See below.*

SORE THROAT WITH FEVER

PROBABLE
COMMON COLD — UPPER RESPIRATORY TRACT INFECTION
TONSILITIS
LARYNGITIS
PHARYNGITIS

POSSIBLE
INFECTIOUS MONONUCLEOSIS
DENTAL INFECTION

RARE
GLOSSITIS
LUDWIG'S ANGINA
ADVERSE DRUG REACTION

Smoking
Smokers are likely to suffer from worse symptoms if they have any of the conditions listed below. They are also likely to take longer to recover than non-smokers; and are at greater risk of developing complications, such as secondary infections of the ears or lungs.

PROBABLE

■ COMMON COLD
See page 454.

■ TONSILITIS
See page 138.

■ LARYNGITIS
See page 126.

■ PHARYNGITIS
See page 124.

POSSIBLE

■ INFECTIOUS MONONUCLEOSIS (MONO)
See page 139.

■ DENTAL INFECTIONS
See page 138.

RARE

■ GLOSSITIS
See page 125.

■ LUDWIG'S ANGINA
See page 126.

■ ADVERSE MEDICATION REACTION
Sore throat, inflammation of the mucus membranes of the mouth and fever are the commonest symptoms of adverse medication reactions.

ULCERS IN MOUTH

PROBABLE
APHTHOUS ULCER
HERPES SIMPLEX
INJURY

POSSIBLE
ERYTHEMA MULTIFORME

RARE
CANCER OF THE MOUTH OR THROAT
SYPHILIS
PEMPHIGUS
CROHN'S DISEASE
BEHCET'S SYNDROME
LEUKEMIAS/MYELOMAS
TUBERCULOSIS

PROBABLE

■ APHTHOUS ULCER/CANKER SORE
* Small and multiple (or larger and solitary).
* Anywhere in mouth or on tongue, typically behind lower lip at the front.
* Extremely painful; aggravated by acid fruits.
* May be aggravated by sharp dentures or other dental problems.
* Often appears at times of stress.

Most heal after a few days, though larger ones take longer.

THE THROAT

Treatments for canker sores are often unsatisfactory. Pain relieving gel or tablets may be bought from the pharmacy.

■ INJURY
An ulcer will develop after an injury or burn of the lining of the mouth or throat. Pizza ulcer on the roof of the mouth is common.

■ HERPES SIMPLEX
See page 125.

POSSIBLE

■ ERYTHEMA MULTIFORME
Irregular red marks. May be associated with a reaction to drugs or an infection. Commonest in children and young women.
* Itchy rash anywhere on body; not unlike measles rash.
* Pale-centered wheals, sometimes called "target lesions".
* Sore throat.
* Headache.
* Fever.
* Ulceration in the mouth and throat.

There is a severe form of the condition, called Stevens-Johnson syndrome.

RARE

■ CANCER OF THE MOUTH OR THROAT
May occur anywhere in mouth or throat. Tobacco users at risk, especially pipe-smokers, tobacco-chewers. Suspicion is aroused by:
* Large ulcers lasting more than two weeks.
* Ulcer with irregular shape.
* Ulcers on surfaces of polyps.
* Ulcers with raised edges.
* Feeling unwell.
* Bad breath.
* Enlarged lymph nodes in neck .

■ SYPHILIS
Ulcers in the throat can mean primary, secondary or tertiary syphilis. Ulcers are likely to be:
* Single.
* Shallow.
* Hard at the base.
* Painless.
* Non-bleeding.

And they have:
* A raised, reddened margin.
* Enlarged lymph nodes in the neck may be present.

■ PEMPHIGUS
A skin disease in which fluid-filled sacs appear on the skin at sites of pressure and trauma.
* Fluid-filled sacs in the mouth.

These burst, forming:
* Ulcers which may remain for weeks.

■ CROHN'S DISEASE
The following symptoms always accompany other signs of gut disease.
* Aphthous-type ulcers. *See page 127.*

Recurrent diarrhea, with or without abdominal pain and weight loss, in an otherwise healthy person who has canker sores suggests the possibility of Crohn's disease.

■ BEHCET'S SYNDROME
Most common, though still rare, in some Middle Eastern countries.
* Recurrent major ulceration in

mouth and throat.
Followed by:
* Ulcers on the genitals.
* Eye inflammation.

■ LEUKEMIAS/MYELOMAS
* Ulceration in the mouth.
* Persistent sore throat.
* Infections.
* Feeling unwell.
* Bruise easily.

See also page 424.

■ TUBERCULOSIS
* Small ulcers.
* Sore throat.
* Difficulty in swallowing.
* Excessive salivation.

See also page 447.

MUCUS IN THE THROAT

PROBABLE
VASOMOTOR RHINITIS
ALLERGIC RHINITIS
CHEST INFECTION

POSSIBLE
SINUSITIS
NASAL POLYPS

RARE
CANCER OF THE NASAL FOSSA OR NASOPHARYNX

PROBABLE

■ VASOMOTOR RHINITIS
More or less constant production of mucus in the nasal passages.
* Clear discharge from front of nose. The mucus also dribbles into the throat from the back of the nose.
* Brought on by by change of environment or atmosphere.
* Difficulty in breathing through nostrils.
* Not associated with other symptoms of *ALLERGIC RHINITIS* ; *see below.*

■ ALLERGIC RHINITIS
You are likely to have a known allergy, typically to pollen, dust or animals.
* Clear discharge from front of nose and into throat.
* Difficulty in breathing through the nostrils.
* Watery eyes.
* Sneezing.
* Wheezing.

A family history of asthma, eczema or hay fever is likely in people with this condition.

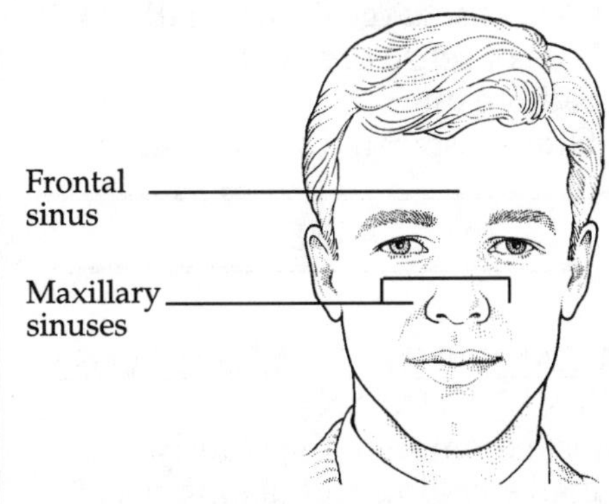

THE THROAT

■ CHEST INFECTION
Particularly in patients with chronic lung problems, for example, bronchitis, cystic fibrosis, bronchiectasis. Smokers are also a high-risk group.
* Persistent coughing up of green or yellow mucus.
* Fever
* Feeling unwell.
* Sometimes, difficulty breathing.
Normally requires antibiotics.

POSSIBLE

■ SINUSITIS
Any of the nasal sinuses may become infected causing local pain/discomfort.
* Persistent nasal discharge (green or yellow).
* Headache.
* Pain over affected sinus.
* Fever.
* Bad breath.
Usually requires antibiotics.

■ NASAL POLYPS
Polyps are fleshy growths almost never malignant. Often multiple.
* Can sometimes be seen by looking into the back of the nose.
* Obstruction in nose.
* Clear discharge occasionally.
* Loss of sense of smell.
* Bad breath.
Often associated with allergies.

RARE

■ CANCER OF THE NASAL FOSSA OR NASOPHARYNX
Most common in the elderly.
* Foul smelling and tasting nasal discharge.
* Persistent pain.
* Bad breath.
* A lump may be seen in the mouth or nose; or a facial swelling may develop.
* Toothache may develop.
* Bloodstained nasal discharge or sputum.

WHITE SPOTS VISIBLE IN MOUTH AND THROAT

PROBABLE
CANDIDIASIS
TONSILITIS

POSSIBLE
KOPLIK'S SPOTS
LICHEN PLANUS
LEUKOPLAKIA

RARE
KERATOSIS PHARYNGIS

PROBABLE

■ CANDIDIASIS
Otherwise known as thrush or monilia. Most commonly seen in new-born babies or infants. (It has been known for parents to mistake thrush for milk on the inside of a baby's cheek; but the white patches are hard to remove and doing so will cause the baby some discomfort.)
* White patches in mouth.

* Associated reddening.
* Lips, tongue and cheek may be painful.
* Patches may be dislodged, but not always easily.

Often associated with antibiotic therapy, general ill-health and immuno-suppression.

■ TONSILITIS
See page 138

POSSIBLE

■ KOPLIK'S SPOTS
A sure sign of measles *(see page 444)*.
* White spots inside the mouth opposite the molar teeth.
* Spots are about the size of a grain of salt with surrounding reddening.

Other symptoms of measles are:
* A red rash starting by the ears spreading over seven days to the body and limbs.
* Runny nose.
* Reddened eyes.
* Cough.

■ LICHEN PLANUS
Irregular, small, shiny patchy changes in the skin, occurring all over the body, including the genital area. Commonest in the middle-aged.
* Multiple fine white lines on lips, tongue and cheek.
* White spots in the same region.
* Sometimes ulcers between the spots and lines.

■ LEUKOPLAKIA
* White patches on the tongue or lining of the mouth.
* Cannot be scraped off.
* Occasionally disappear leaving a red base.
* Possibly localized hardening under the patch.

Associated with smoking (particularly pipe-smoking), and rubbing dentures. Also, it is increasingly found in people with AIDS.

RARE

■ KERATOSIS PHARYNGIS
* Small white or creamy lumps seen on tonsil surface.
* Frequently no other symptoms.

Persistent, white patches in the mouth can be a sign of serious illness, and should not be ignored.

Consult your physician if:
* Patches persist.
* They cannot be removed easily.

NOTICEABLE BLOOD VESSELS ON THE NECK

Newly developed, visible blood vessels are a sign of underlying disease that need careful investigation, and probably tests, before treatment can be started.

PROBABLE
HEART FAILURE

THE NECK

POSSIBLE
MALIGNANT TUMOR WITHIN THE CHEST
PERICARDIAL EFFUSION

RARE
BENIGN TUMOR WITHIN THE CHEST
CONSTRICTIVE PERICARDITIS

PROBABLE

■ HEART FAILURE
The heart fails to pump blood adequately, typically after a heart attack. May be associated with one or more of the following:
* Prominent symmetrical veins on each side of the neck, that are more obvious when the patient lies flat.
* The prominence varies with respiration and heart beat.
* Shortness of breath worse on lying flat.
* Shortness of breath on walking.
* Bluish discoloration of face.
* Swelling of ankles and legs.
Requires medical treatment.

POSSIBLE

■ MALIGNANT TUMOR WITHIN THE CHEST
Malignant tumors (primary or secondary) within the chest can compress the great veins inside the chest, causing:
* Symmetrical prominent veins on head neck and upper chest unaffected by body position.
* Face may appear congested and reddened.
* The face, neck and upper chest may be swollen.
* Breathing may be normal.
In addition, there may well be the following general symptoms of:
* Weight loss.
* Poor appetite.
* Weakness.
* Feeling unwell.

■ PERICARDIAL EFFUSION
Fluid distends the sac around the heart. May be caused by infection, auto-immune disease, tumor or after a heart attack and can cause:
* Shortness of breath whenlying flat.
* Prominent neck veins (symmetrical).
* Tightness in the chest, varying with movement.
* Fever (with infection).
* Feeling unwell.

RARE

■ BENIGN TUMOR WITHIN THE CHEST
Large benign tumors within the chest can compress the great veins inside the chest giving rise to the same symptoms as malignant tumor(s) — *see this page.*

■ CONSTRICTIVE PERICARDITIS
Increasing rigidity of the sac round the heart. Caused by tuberculosis, or other infection or injury, often many years earlier.
* Rapid pulse (sometimes irregular).
* Low blood pressure.
* Tiredness.

* Prominent neck veins — more prominent on breathing in.
* Fluid in the belly.
* Liver enlargement.
* Shortness of breath.

ISOLATED LUMPS OR SWELLINGS IN OR ON NECK

Isolated lumps may be associated with a number of structures in the neck in addition to the lymph nodes (*see page 137: read with this*). These include the skin, and the salivary or thyroid glands. A few are present from birth.

PROBABLE
BOIL
SEBACEOUS CYST
LIPOMA

POSSIBLE
GENERAL THYROID ENLARGEMENT
ISOLATED THYROID NODULE (BENIGN)
SUBMANDIBULAR DUCT STONE

RARE
CERVICAL RIB
GENERAL THYROID ENLARGEMENT (MALIGNANT TUMOR)
ISOLATED THYROID NODULE (MALIGNANT)
THYROGLOSSAL CYST
PHARYNGEAL POUCH
STERNOMASTOID TUMOR
SUBMANDIBULAR TUMOR

THE NECK

PROBABLE

■ BOIL
A skin infection commonly originating in a hair follicle or follicles.
* Painful.
* Localized reddening.
* Skin warm to the touch.
* Localized swelling.
* A yellow center that may discharge pus.

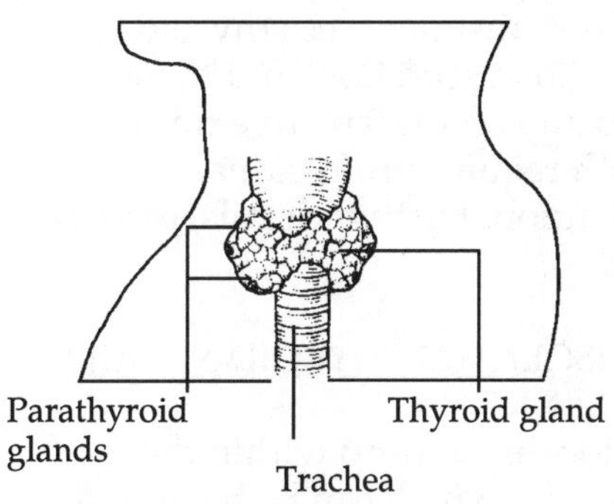

■ SEBACEOUS CYST
* Feels firm.
* Superficial.
* Painless (unless infected).
* Present for many years.
* Slowly increases in size.
* Has a central point — the opening to the blocked sweat gland that causes the cyst.

■ LIPOMA
A benign fatty tumor which can be superficial or extend under the skin. Same characteristics as a sebaceous cyst except:
* No central point.
* Usually feels soft.

The Neck

POSSIBLE

■ DIFFUSE THYROID GLAND ENLARGEMENT
The thyroid gland lies on both sides of the neck below the Adam's apple.
* Swelling moves up and down on swallowing.
* General swelling — no separate lumps.
* No other symptoms.

Other causes of diffuse thyroid swelling can be divided into those causing excess thyroid hormone secretion, and those causing an underactive thyroid. Both require professional attention. Further details, *pages 479 and 461.*

■ ISOLATED THYROID NODULE — BENIGN
A localized lump within the thyroid, which can be benign or malignant - *see this page.*
* Can be felt either side of the neck below the Adam's apple.
* Moves up and down on swallowing.

May be associated with signs of overactive or underactive thyroid; *see above.*

■ SUBMANDIBULAR DUCT STONE
Beneath the jaw, each side of the tongue, are two salivary glands, the submandibular glands. Stones may form in the ducts of the glands, or the body of the gland, causing:
* Painless swelling (normally on one side).
* The swelling increases when eating and
* Reduces between meals.
* Swelling can sometimes be felt in the mouth, under the tongue.
* Can become infected.

Needs medical attention.

RARE

■ CERVICAL RIB
See page 136.

■ GENERAL THYROID GLAND ENLARGEMENT (MALIGNANT TUMOR)
Features of thyroid enlargement plus:
* Irregular symmetric enlargement.
* May no longer move up and down on swallowing.
* Trachea (wind pipe) may be compressed, causing difficulty in breathing.

■ ISOLATED THYROID NODULE — MALIGNANT
A localized lump within the thyroid gland.
* Moves up and down on swallowing.

May have no other symptoms, but can cause:
* Hoarseness.
* Pain.
* Drooping of one eyelid (Horner's syndrome).

■ THYROGLOSSAL CYST
* Lies in the middle of the neck at the front.
* Near the surface.
* Moves up if the tongue is stuck out.
* Painless.

■ PHARYNGEAL POUCH
A swelling on one side of the neck caused by a defect in the upper esophagus.
* Varies in size.
* Causes variable difficulty in swallowing.
* Enlarges while eating or drinking.
* May "gurgle" as fluid empties from it.
* Old food may regurgitated.
* Can be emptied by direct pressure on it.
* Not painful, but can be uncomfortable as it increases in size.

■ STERNOMASTOID TUMOR
Present from birth — not a true tumor:
* Lump sited in the middle of the muscle at the side of the neck.

■ SUBMANDIBULAR TUMOR
May be benign or malignant.
* One-sided enlargement of gland.
* Progressive.
* May become painful.
* Lymph nodes may be involved.

STIFFNESS OR PAIN IN NECK

PROBABLE
ACUTE STIFF NECK
ACUTE NECK SPRAIN
WHIPLASH INJURY
WRY NECK (TORTICOLLIS)

POSSIBLE
CERVICAL SPONDYLOSIS
CERVICAL RIB
RHEUMATOID ARTHRITIS

RARE
CERVICAL SPINE INFECTION
MENINGITIS
ENCEPHALITIS
PROLAPSED CERVICAL DISC
SPINAL CORD TUMORS

PROBABLE

■ ACUTE STIFF NECK
* Associated with sleeping in awkward position; also with exposure to cold.
* Pain on movement localized to neck.
* Neck movements limited by pain and muscle spasm.

■ ACUTE NECK SPRAIN
* Associated with sudden twisting/turning or bending.
* Extreme pain on any movement.
* Pain in upper back and head.
* Marked muscle spasm limiting neck movement.

■ WHIPLASH INJURY
Typically present after an automobile accident.
* Pain in neck and upper back.
* Neck held stiffly.
* Pain may have taken a few hours to develop after injury.
* Pain and stiffness may persist for weeks.
* May have pain, weakness and

THE NECK

tingling in arms.
* Reduced range of neck movement.
* May have dizziness.

■ WRY NECK (TORTICOLLIS)
* Head pulled down on affected side.
* Chin points towards the opposite shoulder.
* The affected muscle is a solid band.
* Neck movements are considerably restricted.

Typically, the condition occurs on waking: suddenly, you cannot move your neck freely. Wears off in a day or two. Often occurs in children.

POSSIBLE

■ CERVICAL SPONDYLOSIS
Caused by wear and tear of the lower cervical intervertebral discs. Sufferer is typically middle-aged.
* Pain in neck and back.
* Painful over neck.
* Worse on waking.
* Slight limitation of movement.

Occasionally:
* Pain in arms.
* Numbness in arms.
* Weakness in arms.

■ CERVICAL RIB
Some people are born with an extra rib, or with fibrous material which constricts nerves and arteries in the neck. Symptoms may appear in the late twenties.
* May feel a lump in the neck.
* Neck is rarely painful.
* Pain behind collar bone.
* Pain on the inner side of the arm

Prolapsed lower cervical intervertebral disc

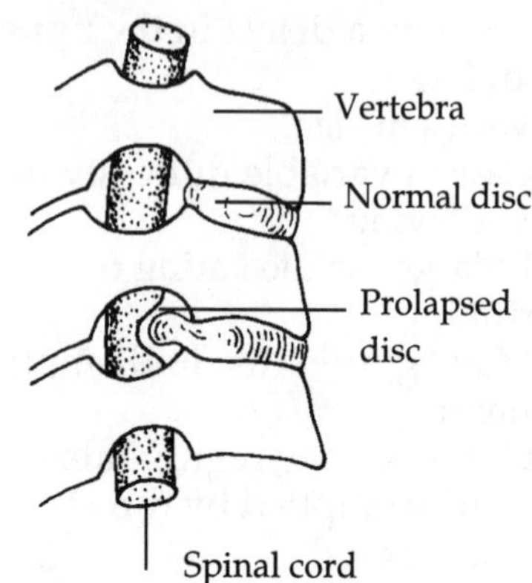

after or when carrying groceries.
* Intermittent coldness and blueness of fingers.

■ RHEUMATOID ARTHRITIS
Patients with rheumatoid arthritis may have joint problems in the neck.
* Pain is common.
* Range of movement is reduced.
* Weakness, numbness and tingling may be present in upper and
occasionally lower limbs.

RARE

■ CERVICAL SPINE INFECTION
Tuberculous infection still occasionally occurs.
* Mild neck pain.
* Pain on any movement.
* Head may be held in hands.
* Stiffness, with reduced movement.

Occasionally there may be sudden paralysis as the spinal cord gets involved.

■ ENCEPHALITIS
Inflammation of the brain which can be caused by viruses and bacteria often carried by ticks.
* Headache.
* Stiff neck.
* Often a rash.
* High fever.
* Muscle pain.
* Nausea.
Requires urgent medical care.

■ MENINGITIS
Infection of the lining of the brain and spinal cord. Usually other marked symptoms, such as fever, will be present.
* Neck stiffness — inability to bend the neck forward because of pain and muscle spasm.
* Headache.
* Feeling unwell.
* Fever
* Fine purple rash.
If meningitis is suspected, call a physician immediately.

■ PROLAPSED CERVICAL DISC
May be caused by sudden movements, and damage or rupture of the intervertebral discs. There is a sudden onset of symptoms which may include:
* Neck pain and stiffness.
* Pain and altered sensation in the arms.
* Weakness in the arms.
* Muscular spasm of the neck and upper back.
* Symptoms may resolve and then return.
Needs medical attention.

■ SPINAL CORD TUMORS
Progressive onset of symptoms may include:
* Altered sensation in arms and legs.
* Areas of numbness.
* Weakness in arms and legs.
* Wasting of muscles.
* Ability to pass urine may be affected.

Lymph nodes of the neck

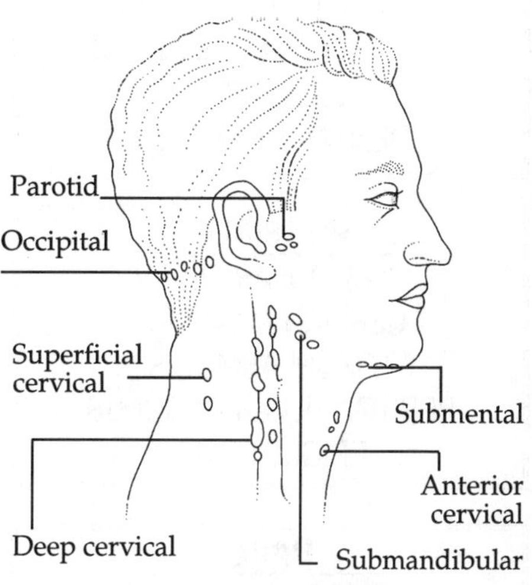

SWOLLEN LYMPH NODES IN NECK

Most people have temporarily enlarged lymph nodes (also known simply as glands) in the neck at some time. This is generally associated with infection or inflammation, either locally, or of the whole body. Sometimes just one is enlarged, giving a single swelling. Occasionally, recurring or persistent enlargement may indicate more serious underlying disorders such as chronic infection or cancer.

Enlarged lymph nodes need to

The Neck

be distinguished from other lumps in the neck, such as enlarged salivary glands — *see ISOLATED NECK LUMPS OR SWELLINGS IN OR ON NECK, page 133.*

PROBABLE
COMMON COLD
LOCAL INFECTION OR INFLAMMATION
TONSILITIS
DENTAL INFECTION

POSSIBLE
GLANDULAR FEVER
GERMAN MEASLES
TOXOPLASMOSIS
PERITONSILLAR ABSCESS
EPIGLOTTITIS

RARE
TUBERCULOSIS
CANCER
LEUKEMIAS/LYMPHOMAS
HIV/AIDS

PROBABLE

■ COMMON COLD

Or upper respiratory tract infection (URTI). These can occur alone or in combination:
* Tender lymph nodes enlarged symmetrically below ears and under jaw.
* Fever.
* Feeling sick.
* Sore throat
* Cough.
* Runny nose.
* Earache.

Usually cures itself.

■ TONSILITIS
* Tonsils enlarged
* Throat looks red.
* Tender lymph nodes enlarged below and behind jaw.
* Often enlarged more on one side than the other.
* White spots often apparent on tonsil surface (pus draining from tonsil).
* Fever.
* Feeling unwell.

Could require antibiotics. Your physician may take a culture from the tonsils, if it is likely to be a strep. infection. Frequent attacks may need referral to an ENT specialist.

■ LOCAL INFECTION OR INFLAMMATION (EG ACNE, IMPETIGO, SEBACEOUS CYST)
* Nearest lymph nodes will be enlarged and may be painful.
* Pain and tenderness in scalp.
* If a lump is present it may be an infected sebaceous cyst.
* If an area is scaly/reddened/weeping/itchy, consider impetigo, dermatitis, eczema/psoriasis — see your physician to distinguish which.

■ DENTAL INFECTION

Diseases of the gums or teeth may be associated with lymph node enlargement.
* Enlarged tender nodes which tend to be those nearest the affected tooth.
* Toothache.
* Bleeding gums (gingivitis).
* Teeth with loose fillings.
* Dental abscess (painful tooth/gums and local swelling).

POSSIBLE

■ GLANDULAR FEVER — INFECTIOUS MONONUCLEOSIS
Caused by infection with the Epstein-Barr virus and known as "mono". A disease of children and young adults.
* Generalized lymph node enlargement and tenderness, but neck nodes, including those at the back of the head, may be worst affected.
* Fever.
* Sore throat.
* Can have abdominal discomfort.
* Feeling unwell.
* Symptoms may last for a few days to a few weeks.
* Characteristic changes in the blood: your physician may confirm
the diagnosis with a blood test.
* Spleen may become enlarged.

■ GERMAN MEASLES
Rubella. Commonest in children.
* Runny nose.
* Red rash, mainly on body.
* Enlarged, tender neck lymph nodes, particularly over the back of the scalp, just above the neck.
* In teenage and adult females there may be pains in the joints of the hands.

■ TOXOPLASMOSIS
A parasite which infects many of us without obvious signs or symptoms. Mostly cures itself in one to three weeks. Acquired by eating infected, raw or lightly cooked meat (or through contact with cat faces). Only about 20 percent of people affected actually have symptoms.
* Fever.
* Enlarged lymph nodes — neck nodes predominant — which may also be tender.
* Feeling unwell.

Diagnosis is confirmed by blood test or by removing a lymph node and examining it under a microscope. Often a problem for AIDS patients.

If a pregnant mother develops toxoplasmosis there is a risk of the baby being damaged. Brain and eyes are primarily affected. In many countries there is routine screening for toxoplasmosis, but not in the USA.

Avoiding toxoplasmosis in pregnancy:
– Never eat raw or uncooked meat.
– Wash all fruit, vegetables and salads well.
– Do not empty cat litter trays. (If you must do so, wear protective gloves.)
– Wear gloves for gardening.

■ PERITONSILLAR ABSCESS
Similar signs to tonsilitis, but:
* Pain on opening mouth also present because abscess or "quinsy" has developed. Requires surgical drainage.

■ EPIGLOTTITIS
* Very painful throat.
* Voice often hoarse or faint.
* Pain on swallowing.
* Lymph nodes may be enlarged.
* Fever.

A physician should see any

THE NECK

child suspected of having epiglottitis immediately.

RARE

■ TUBERCULOSIS
* Isolated non-tender lymph node enlargement.
* Redness.
* Skin overlying node(s) breaks down.
* Intermittent fever.

Skin tests and blood tests, or biopsy of the node, confirms the diagnosis. Drug treatment required.

■ CANCER OF THE MOUTH OR UPPER RESPIRATORY PASSAGES (INCLUDING LARYNX)
All these cancers can cause enlarged lymph nodes, often as a result of the cancer spreading. These are diseases especially of smokers in the 50-plus age range.
* Persistently enlarged but painless lymph nodes.
* Other lump developing in mouth/tongue or palate.
* Change in voice.
* Weight loss.
* Feeling unwell.
* Persistent pain in mouth or neck.
* Dentures not fitting.
* Anemia.

■ CANCER ELSEWHERE IN THE BODY
* Enlarged painless lymph nodes above the collar bone may suggest spread of a tumor from within the chest or abdomen, but would normally be accompanied by other symptoms from those areas.

■ LEUKEMIAS
Some or all of the following in combination:
* Enlarged painless lymph nodes in the neck or elsewhere.
* Persistently feeling unwell.
* Pale skin, due to anemia.
* Shortness of breath.
* Fatigue.
* Bruising.

■ LYMPHOMAS
May have no symptoms apart from:
* Painless, generalized enlargement of lymph nodes.

Later stages include:
* Fever.
* Weight loss.
* Anemia.

■ HIV/AIDS
HIV stands for the human immunodeficiency virus, which may infect people for years without making them ill. Eventually, however, it leads to AIDS.
* Enlarged lymph nodes.
* Fever.
* Feeling unwell.

Anyone in a high-risk group for HIV infection should report persistently enlarged lymph nodes to their physician or public health clinic. Effectiveness of treatment depends on early diagnosis.

Persistent symptoms
If enlarged lymph nodes persist in the neck for more than two weeks, and particularly if other symptoms are present, you must see your physician.

The Abdomen – Digestive and Urinary Systems

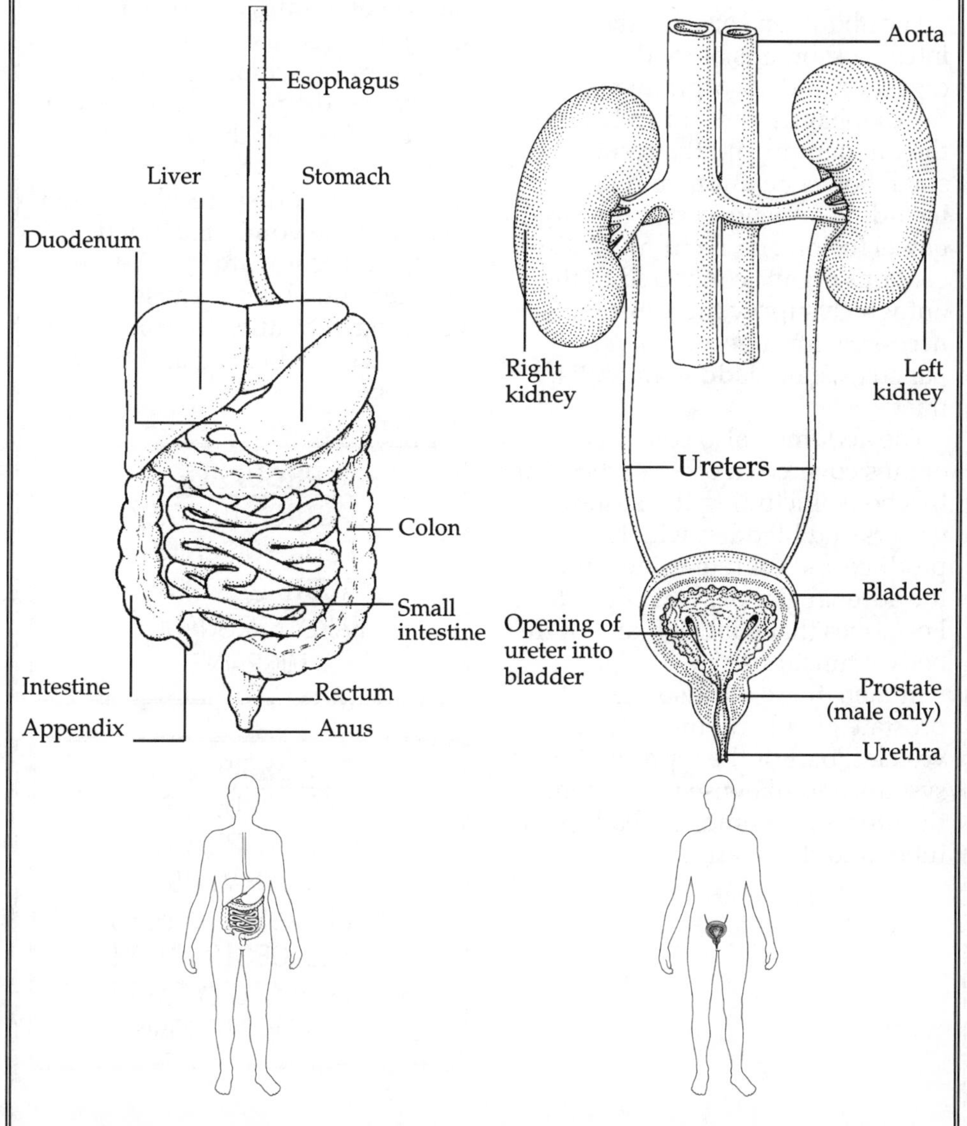

ABDOMEN: DIGESTIVE SYSTEM

THE ABDOMINAL CAVITY INTRODUCTION

It lies below the rib cage and above the pelvic bones. The terms belly, stomach and gut are often used. The latter two are really organs that lie within the abdominal cavity.

The abdomen contains the intestines: organs of food digestion and absorption; part of the esophagus, the stomach, then the duodenum and the rest of the small bowel (jejunum and ileum, including appendix) and the large bowel (colon and rectum). It also contains organs connected to the gut which supply the substances necessary for digestion: liver, pancreas, gall bladder and biliary tract.

The abdomen also contains organs covered in other sections of this book, including the kidneys, ureters and bladder, which produce and excrete urine; and the adrenal glands, which produce hormones that control many of the body's functions.

In men, there are also the prostate gland and the seminal vesicles, part of the reproductive system; and likewise in women, the uterus or womb, the Fallopian tubes and the ovaries.

VOMITING

Vomiting can be forceful or it can be passive, as when one regurgitates food into the mouth.

Sometimes bitter gastric or duodenal juices are vomited, sometimes undigested food, and sometimes blood (either fresh or old — sometimes called "coffee grounds" because of its appearance). Vomiting blood always needs medical attention. In order to discover the underlying cause, you have to take precise note, however disagreeable, of the nature of the vomit. Excluded from this section are the all-too-familiar and obvious causes of vomiting: too much to drink, too much rich food to eat; and travel sickness.

PROBABLE

GASTROENTERITIS/
FOOD POISONING
ACUTE GASTRITIS
EARLY PREGNANCY
MIGRAINE

POSSIBLE

PEPTIC ULCER
HIATUS HERNIA AND
ESOPHAGITIS
ESOPHAGEAL VARICES
BOWEL OBSTRUCTION
POST-GASTRECTOMY SYNDROME
PYLORIC STENOSIS

POSSIBLE continued
PANCREATITIS
BULIMIA
HEPATITIS
DRUG/ALCOHOL WITHDRAWAL
APPENDICITIS
MEDICATIONS
HEART ATTACK
POISONS

RARE
STOMACH CANCER
BRAIN TUMORS
RENAL FAILURE
BOTULISM
CHOLERA
GLAUCOMA

Terminology
"Gastric contents" means typical vomit: partially digested and undigested food, pinkish-yellow, frothy, foul-smelling.

"Duodenal contents" means bile-stained (green), thin fluid, mixed with slime and clear secretions.

PROBABLE

■ GASTROENTERITIS/ FOOD POISONING
Gastric or duodenal contents. Likely to be viral or can occur as part of food poisoning. Abdominal pain may be a feature.

Vomit is likely to contain partially-digested and undigested food, and will look like "typical vomit" at first. After several vomits, clear, greeny-yellow liquid and slime.
See page 167.

■ ACUTE GASTRITIS
Gastric and duodenal contents. May contain fresh or old blood, which appears as streaks of red or brown staining or looking like coffee grounds. This is likely after a very heavy drinking bout.

Abdominal pain might be a feature. *See page 171.*

■ EARLY PREGNANCY
Gastric and duodenal contents. Other symptoms of pregnancy will be pronounced:
* Nausea on waking.
* Tendency to acid stomach and heartburn.

See also page 148.

■ MIGRAINE
Gastric and duodenal contents. *See page 113.* Other migraine symptoms will be present.

POSSIBLE

■ PEPTIC ULCER
Gastric and duodenal contents.
See page 170.

■ HIATUS HERNIA and ESOPHAGITIS
* A feeling like regurgitation.
* A feeling of acid in the lower throat; bitter taste.
* Symptoms of heartburn.
* If severe, vomiting undigested food; also,
* Vomiting old blood, sometimes fresh.

Abdomen: Digestive System

■ ESOPHAGEAL VARICES
Fresh or old blood. *See page 158.*

■ BOWEL OBSTRUCTION
* Pain in belly that comes and goes.
* No wind or feces passed rectally.
* Abdomen becomes swollen.
* You feel bloated.

Gastric and bowel contents, occasionally like diarrhea.

See also page 150.

■ POST-GASTRECTOMY SYNDROME
See page 168.

Duodenal contents.

■ PYLORIC STENOSIS
This is a narrowing of the outlet from the stomach. Usually only affects babies of about one month old or older individuals with long-standing ulcers. Vomiting is very forceful. Most common in boys.

Gastric contents.

■ PANCREATITIS
See PAIN IN THE ABDOMEN AND DIARRHEA, page 167.

Gastric contents.

■ BULIMIA
See ANOREXIA NERVOSA, page 423.

■ HEPATITIS
See page 154.

■ DRUG/ALCOHOL WITHDRAWAL
Vomiting associated with trembling, sleeplessness, confusion, rapid pulse, wide eye pupils. *See page 378.*

■ APPENDICITIS
Loss of appetite, belly pain usually on right side, vomiting and may have diarrhea. *See page 164.*

■ MEDICATIONS
A variety of medications can cause vomiting: digoxin, anti-cancer drugs, antibiotics, aminophyline or theophyline (used for asthma). See your physician if you suspect a new medication.

■ HEART ATTACK
The symptoms of a heart attack can often include sweating, nausea and vomiting with or without chest pain.

■ POISONS
Young children may eat or drink plants or household cleaners, causing repeated vomiting. If you suspect these as a cause, take the child to the nearest emergency room immediately.

RARE

■ STOMACH CANCER
Vomiting can be a late feature of stomach cancer and may be present with other signs of cancer, such as feeling sick, marked weight loss and anemia.

Gastric and bowel contents.
* Likely to follow a progressive feeling of fullness after eating small quantities.

Also STOMACH DISEASE, page 164.

■ BRAIN TUMORS
See BRAIN SECTION, page 114.

Gastric contents.

■ RENAL FAILURE
Acute or chronic.
* Mental confusion.
* Headache.
* Breath smelling of urine.
* Vomiting gastric contents.
* Coma.

■ BOTULISM
A dangerous but extremely rare form of food poisoning.
* Feeling sick.
* Nausea.
* Dizziness.
* Vomiting gastric and duodenal contents.
* Abdominal cramp and diarrhea.
* Breathing problems.
* Pupils wide open.
* Collapse leading to coma.

■ CHOLERA
See page 168.

■ GLAUCOMA
Sometimes vomiting is a symptom of glaucoma in the elderly.
See page 16.

VOMITING BLOOD

See ABDOMINAL PAIN PLUS VOMITING BLOOD, page 171.

VOMITING AND HEADACHE

See especially MIGRAINE, page 113; also other causes of headache and headache with fever, pages 111-16.

REGURGITATION

See VOMITING, page 142.

PROMINENT BLOOD VESSELS ON THE ABDOMEN

Unusually large surface veins sometimes develop on the skin of the abdomen. They may be caused by blockage of vessels; pressure from inside the belly; or local pressure from tumors.

Other symptoms that may be present if any of these causes apply are:
* Leg swelling, sometimes one-sided.
* Lower belly veins most prominent.
* Distended veins radiating out from the umbilicus.

Some conditions that can cause these symptoms are:

Acute pancreatitis – page 149.
Cirrhosis of the liver – see page 150.
Malignant ascites – see page 150.
Ovarian cyst – see page 170.
Cancer of the kidney – see BLOOD IN URINE, page 181. A kidney tumor blocks the main vein in the abdomen.

Abdomen: Digestive System

GENERALIZED SWELLING OF THE ABDOMEN IN BABIES AND CHILDREN

PROBABLE
NORMAL VARIANT
CONSTIPATION

POSSIBLE
CYSTIC FIBROSIS
CELIAC DISEASE
PREMATURITY

RARE
HIRSCHSPRUNG'S DISEASE

PROBABLE

■ NORMAL VARIANT
The pot-bellied child is simply made that way and because the belly bulges in childhood, it will not necessarily do so in adult life.

■ CONSTIPATION
In some toddlers and children there is a strong psychological element to constipation. It may develop at potty-training, when the child resists parental pressure to pass stools; and it can develop into a life-long habit.

Clothes may get soiled with feces — "apparent diarrhea" — as a result of hardened stools building up in the rectum: watery material leaks past the solid mass.

See also CONSTIPATION, page 161.

POSSIBLE

■ CYSTIC FIBROSIS
Most symptoms of this hereditary disease are caused by abnormal body secretions.
* Failure to grow, but healthy appetite.
* Thin, with distended belly.
* Recurrent chest infections.
* Large amounts of smelly feces.
* Finger end swelling.
* Occasionally the rectum may slip out through the anus (rectal prolapse).

■ CELIAC DISEASE
Caused by an allergy to gluten, a component of cereals. Normally, the child will be underweight and will not grow as expected.
* Often, the child has a fair complexion.
* Child is unhappy.
* Appetite is poor.
* Muscles are wasted.
* Belly is distended.
* Occasional diarrhea and vomiting.

Treatment is a gluten-free diet for life, and a complete recovery can be expected.

■ PREMATURITY
Premature babies may become constipated with bowel distension due to the presence of meconium, the greenish bowel contents present at birth. This stage usually passes quickly.

RARE

■ HIRSCHSPRUNG'S DISEASE
Part of the bowel fails to develop proper nerve tissue and fails to work correctly, resulting in the progressive distension of the large bowel by feces. Large quantities may be retained. Symptoms of constipation appear soon after birth. Can be corrected surgically.

GENERALIZED SWELLING OF THE ABDOMEN

Described by doctors as distension. The common causes are fat, wind, feces, fluid or, in a woman, a baby.

There are *many* causes of abdominal swelling: some are harmless, and some suggest serious disease.

It is important to consider whether symptoms associated with abdominal swelling are new and uncomfortable (such as pain and indigestion) or have built up slowly, possibly during a period when your life-style altered (for example, reduced exercise, "comfort eating", family crisis or bereavement). Usually it will be clear to you whether your symptoms are part of a long, even lifelong, history of abdominal discomfort, or are new and therefore more likely to suggest an illness.

PROBABLE
OBESITY
GAS
POOR MUSCLE TONE
CONSTIPATION
HORMONAL BLOATING

POSSIBLE
PREGNANCY
IRRITABLE BOWEL SYNDROME
DIVERTICULAR DISEASE
HEART FAILURE
PERFORATED BOWEL
BOWEL CANCER
SWOLLEN BLADDER
PANCREATITIS

RARE
CIRRHOSIS OF THE LIVER
MALIGNANT ASCITES
OVARIAN CYST
BOWEL OBSTRUCTION
ULCERATIVE COLITIS

PROBABLE

■ OBESITY
An obvious, and extremely common problem, but worth considering in its own right. Fat does not just accumulate below the skin, it accumulates in the body cavities. The abdomen is the largest body cavity and it can hold large amounts of fat.

Abdomen: Digestive System

■ GAS
Doctors call it flatus. Produced by the fermentation of food in the gut. Most of us are aware of those foods that cause most gas.

■ POOR MUSCLE TONE
Many women develop protruding abdomens after childbirth. Often, intensive exercise is needed to get the abdominal wall muscles to return to their original tone.

Men can also find that they acquire a "beer belly", either when they stop exercising or when they indulge in the steady consumption of beer, sodas and junk food.

■ CONSTIPATION
Most people have regular bowel movements for most of their lives. Constipation is a term people use if they believe they are not passing stools either easily or frequently enough. In fact, constipation should be divided into three types.

First, that in which hard, pellet-like or rock-like stools are passed, a common condition caused by change in diet and/or lifestyle, often in younger people and in children.

Second, there are people who have bowel movements at long intervals — say every week or two. This has been their pattern for a long time, but they describe themselves as constipated. In fact, there is nothing essentially wrong: they are a variant of normal.

The third is constipation of sudden onset, often in the elderly. Sometimes it is impossible even to pass gas. This suggests an underlying problem; report it to a physician; it must be investigated.

■ HORMONAL BLOATING
Some women have a swollen belly related to the menstrual cycle or hormone replacement therapy. Fluid retention is thought to be the cause.

POSSIBLE

■ PREGNANCY
Again, an apparently obvious diagnosis, but some women are taken unawares by pregnancy. An enlarging abdomen, increased weight, missed periods, heartburn, fullness and discomfort of the breasts, with or without morning sickness in a sexually active woman in the reproductive years are sound reasons for getting a pregnancy test.

■ IRRITABLE BOWEL SYNDROME
Many people have bowel symptoms which, after investigation, are nothing to do with any specific abnormalities of the bowel. Irritable bowel syndrome (IBS) could then be suspected: it is a well-defined syndrome or set of symptoms, probably caused by abnormal motility of the gut. It tends to come and go, and to be related to anything that affects the gut's activity, for example, stress, change of diet, unusual food. The typical picture is:

* Intermittent abdominal pain.
* Bowel upsets (diarrhea and constipation).
* Passage of mucus.
* Abdominal distension.
* Gas.

Medication can help.

ABDOMEN: DIGESTIVE SYSTEM

■ DIVERTICULAR DISEASE
A diverticulum is a small pouch on the wall of the bowel. Most people develop them as they get older, but only a few will get symptoms. These usually arise if one of the diverticula becomes inflamed.
* Change of bowel habit.
* Steady or crampy abdominal pain, often on the left side.
* Abdominal distension.
* Pellet-like stools.
* Occasional passage of dark to bright red blood from the rectum.

If the inflammation becomes severe, with:
* Fever.
* Intense pain.
* A tender lump in the abdomen.

This condition is then called diverticulitis. It usually settles down with antibiotic treatment.

Decreasing the amount of food you eat allows the gut to rest and will also help.

■ HEART FAILURE
Severe untreated heart failure can result in the accumulation of fluid in the abdominal cavity in addition to several other symptoms. *See page 208.*

■ PERFORATED BOWEL
The major symptom of this condition is pain, which will dominate any discomfort or swelling of the abdomen.

Most commonly the appendix bursts. Gut contents leak into the abdominal cavity. This material contains organisms that can cause peritonitis — inflammation of the abdominal cavity. If treatment is delayed, it can be fatal.

The symptoms are similar whichever part of the gut perforates.
* Sudden onset of severe pain.
* Fever.
* Very tender abdomen (muscles of the abdominal wall appear rigid).
* Vomiting.
* Pale, sweating face, sunken eyes.
* Eventually, distension of the abdomen caused by leakage of gas and contents from the gut.
* Shock may develop. *See page 408.*

■ BOWEL CANCER
Includes cancer of colon and rectum. This can block the intestine, either gradually or suddenly. Though a common symptom is a change in bowel habit (type or frequency of stool), swelling (distension) of the abdomen may be caused by a build-up of food, fluid, feces or gas. Other possible symptoms may include:
* Crampy, abdominal pain.
* Symptoms can come and go.
* Slime or mucus in stool.
* Diarrhea.
* Blood in stools.

■ SWOLLEN BLADDER
See page 163.

■ PANCREATITIS
Abdominal pain will be a major symptom of this condition. It is inflammation of the pancreas, which lies at the back of the abdominal cavity and produces chemicals, known as enzymes, which help with digestion of food. There are mild or very severe, and sometimes fatal forms. People who drink excessive amounts of

Abdomen: Digestive System

alcohol, or who have a history of gall bladder disease are at increased risk. Features include:
* Continuous, central abdominal pain.
* Pain may radiate to the back.
* Vomiting.
* Feeling sick.
* Slight jaundice may appear a couple of days after the first attack.
* Bruising/discoloration around the umbilicus or flanks after two to three days.

Can become chronic and lead to the formation of cysts in the belly.

RARE

■ CIRRHOSIS OF THE LIVER

An irreversible degeneration of the liver that has many causes. Perhaps the most well known is alcohol abuse. Features of advanced cirrhosis are:
* Feeling sick, weakness.
* Weight loss.
* Loss of appetite.
* Swelling of the ankles.
* Abdominal distension due to fluid in the abdominal cavity — ascites.
* Vomiting, sickness.
* Vomiting blood, blood in stools.
* Jaundice.
* Mental deterioration.
* Easy bruising.
* Red vascular marks on skin (spider nevi).
* Clubbing of the nails. *See page 296.*

In men:
* Enlargement of the breasts.
* Shrinkage of the testes.

Other causes of cirrhosis, of which there are several different types, include:

Active chronic hepatitis.
Hemochromatosis.
Wilson's disease.
Primary biliary cirrhosis.
Budd-Chiari syndrome.
Chronic cardiac failure.

In most cases the individual is aware of the primary diagnosis before cirrhosis develops.

■ MALIGNANT ASCITES

Cancer of any organ within the abdominal cavity may lead to the formation of fluid in the abdominal cavity, or ascites. In addition to the symptoms of the original cancer individuals may develop:
* Tense, distended abdomen.
* Swelling of the ankles.
* Shortness of breath (due to pressure on the diaphragm).

■ OVARIAN CYST

Very occasionally, a large cyst may develop on an ovary, causing abdominal distension. It requires surgery.

■ BOWEL OBSTRUCTION

Blockage can occur for many reasons. The features are similar:
* Crampy, often central abdominal pain (site dependent on cause).
* Abdominal distension: if low, ileum or colon/rectum obstruction is likely.
* Vomiting may be an early feature of stomach or jejunal obstruction, later involving the ileum. It tends to be a late feature of colon obstruction.
* Constipation — no bowel movement and often no gas.
* Loops of bowel may be seen

undulating under the skin surface as they try to overcome the obstruction.
* Perforation may eventually occur *(see PERFORATED BOWEL, page 149)*.
Urgent medical attention is needed. Causes include:
Strangulated hernia
* Hernia (rupture) in groin may become painful and not be able to be pushed back.
Cancer
* Other features of cancer may have been present before, for example, altered bowel habit (constipation/diarrhea), weight loss,
loss of appetite, anemia.
Inflammation
For example, Crohn's disease, diverticular disease.
* A fibrous internal band, sometimes referred to as adhesions, common after abdominal surgery.
* Bowel gets twisted internally around fibrous tissue present from, or after, birth.
Volvulus
* Bowel twists on itself, causing a blockage.
Gall-stone
* Occasionally a gall-stone passes into the bowel and gets jammed in the narrowest part (the end of the ileum).

■ ULCERATIVE COLITIS
Chronic inflammation of the colon. Main features:
* Diarrhea.
* In acute attacks, blood, mucus and pus is passed.
* Abdominal pain and fever in acute cases.
* As a complication of some cases, abdominal swelling.

OVERALL SWELLING OF THE ABDOMEN PLUS DIARRHEA

PROBABLE
OBESITY
GAS

POSSIBLE
CONSTIPATION
IRRITABLE BOWEL SYNDROME
DIVERTICULAR DISEASE
FACTITIOUS DIARRHEA
CROHN'S DISEASE

RARE
BOWEL CANCER
ULCERATIVE COLITIS

PROBABLE

■ OBESITY
■ GAS
See pages 147 and 148.

POSSIBLE

■ CONSTIPATION
Occasionally someone, especially an elderly person, can become so constipated that other gut contents leak out of the rectum past the impacted mass of feces. This gives the impression of diarrhea.

■ IRRITABLE BOWEL SYNDROME

Abdomen: Digestive System

■ DIVERTICULAR DISEASE
See pages 148 and 149.

■ FACTITIOUS DIARRHEA
Some people take laxative medicine as a matter of habit and yet complain of diarrhea. They may be doing so in order to lose weight, but sometimes they cannot explain why they take laxatives so often, or they may deny it altogether. So, this is worth considering for any individual who complains of diarrhea, yet is otherwise well. Some laxatives cause associated abdominal distension and discomfort.

■ CROHN'S DISEASE
Tends to occur in young adults.
* Intermittent, crampy pain with or without diarrhea.
* With or without weight loss.
* Spontaneously resolves and relapses.
* Sometimes taken for a "grumbling appendix".
* Occasionally intestinal obstruction due to narrowing of bowel.

Medication treatment and/or surgery may be needed. *See also page 128.*

RARE

■ BOWEL CANCER
See page 149.

■ ULCERATIVE COLITIS
See page 151.

OVERALL SWELLING OF THE ABDOMEN PLUS CONSTIPATION

PROBABLE
GAS
CONSTIPATION

POSSIBLE
IRRITABLE BOWEL SYNDROME
DIVERTICULAR DISEASE

RARE
BOWEL CANCER

PROBABLE

■ GAS
■ CONSTIPATION
See pages 148 and 161.

POSSIBLE

■ IRRITABLE BOWEL SYNDROME
■ DIVERTICULAR DISEASE
See pages 148 and 149.

RARE

■ BOWEL CANCER
Most bowel cancer originates in the rectum, colon or cecum. It is

possible to divide symptoms into right colon + cecum and left colon + rectum. *See also BOWEL OBSTRUCTION, page 150.*

Right colon plus cecum:
* Vague lower abdominal pain.
* Pain may localize to right side.
* Mass in right side of abdomen.
* Change in bowel habit; often diarrhea, occasionally constipation.
* Anemia and associated symptoms (*see page 420*) due to slow blood loss.

Left colon plus rectum:
* Increasing constipation.
* Intermittent diarrhea.
* Crampy abdominal pain and distension.
* Blood present when passing stools.
* Mass in left side of abdomen.

Any persistent change in bowel habit in someone over 40 must be assessed by a physician.

QUICKLY FEELING FULL ON EATING

■ POST-GASTRIC SURGERY
If surgery to remove a diseased stomach leaves only a small part behind, relatively small meals make you feel full.

■ STOMACH CANCER
See STOMACH DISEASE, page 164.

WORMS

There are four types of worm that most commonly affect humans. In developed countries, the only type of worm normally seen is the pinworm.

Pinworms are a common infestation among schoolchildren. Many children will have them at some time. Typically, a child wakes with an itchy anus at night and may be very distressed. Small, white, thread-like worms can be seen on the skin of the anus, and, less easily, in the stools.

Treatment is simple, with medicine which should normally be taken by all family members. The commonest source of pinworm infestation is garden soil. Washing hands and scrubbing nails helps prevent infection or re-infection. Wash sheets, pajamas and underwear in hot water every day until infestation is cleared.

PROBABLE

■ PINWORM
* Anal irritation.
* May prevent sleep.
* Worms observed in stools.

POSSIBLE

■ ROUNDWORMS — ASCARIS LUMBRICOIDES
* May be no symptoms.
* Worm observed in stools.

ABDOMEN: DIGESTIVE SYSTEM

* Occasionally abdominal pain.
* Occasionally the lungs become inflamed.
* Occasionally an allergic skin reaction develops; *see page 257*.

■ HOOKWORMS
* May cause chronic bleeding from small intestine.
* Anemia.
* Malaise.
* Diarrhea.

■ TAPEWORMS
* Abdominal discomfort.
* Increased appetite.
* Segments of worms seen in stools.

All types of worm infestation should be assessed and treated by a physician.

TAR-LIKE STOOLS

See BLOOD FROM THE RECTUM , page 157.

PALE-COLORED FECES

Feces are normally colored brown by a mixture of the body's bile pigments and bacteria. Certain conditions hinder this pigmentation; and sometimes bile is excreted instead in the urine, which then appears dark brown or yellow. There may also be jaundice and sometimes itching.

Jaundice occurs when pigments which are normally excreted in bowel or urine waste products build up in the body to such an extent that they color the eyes and skin with a yellow tinge.

PROBABLE
GALL STONES
HEPATITIS

POSSIBLE
CANCER OF THE PANCREAS
PANCREATITIS
CIRRHOSIS OF THE LIVER
LIVER TUMORS

RARE
JAUNDICE OF PREGNANCY
BILIARY ATRESIA
SCLEROSING CHOLANGITIS
CANCER OF THE BILE DUCTS

PROBABLE

■ GALL STONES
See CHOLECYSTITIS, page 173.

■ HEPATITIS
Several different types of virus cause hepatitis. Some are more dangerous than others and so suspected hepatitis needs professional attention. In some cases, the disease is so mild it is assumed to be a cold or flu.
* Lethargy.
* Loss of appetite.
* Loss of desire for cigarettes and alcohol.

* Nausea.
* Joint pains.
* Itching.
* Variable rash.
* Right-sided upper abdominal pain.
* Fever.
* Diarrhea.

The pale stools, dark urine and jaundice may appear after a few days. In mild cases, jaundice may not occur.

POSSIBLE

■ CANCER OF THE PANCREAS
See DISEASED PANCREAS, page 165.

■ PANCREATITIS
See page 167.

■ CIRRHOSIS OF THE LIVER
See page 150.

■ LIVER TUMORS
See LIVER DISEASE, page 164.

RARE

■ JAUNDICE OF LATE PREGNANCY
Occurs in a small proportion of women. Usually complete recovery.

■ BILIARY ATRESIA
Failure of the biliary tract to develop properly in a fetus.
* Jaundice a few days after birth.
* Retarded growth.
* Cirrhosis develops.
* Malabsorption.

Liver transplants offer hope.

■ SCLEROSING CHOLANGITIS (ADULT)
For some unknown reason the bile ducts grow fibrous and shrink.
* Progressive jaundice.
* Itching.
* Liver failure after a few years.

■ CANCER OF THE BILE DUCTS
Very rare. Causes jaundice with pale feces and dark urine associated with other signs of cancer, such as weight loss.

DIARRHEA

Can be difficult to define: perhaps the most useful criterion is whether the passage of stools is loose enough or frequent enough to be inconvenient.

Diarrhea may be watery; green-yellow; bloody (bright red, dark or tarry); a normal color; or mixed with mucus and pus. Strictly speaking, blood passed via the anus is not diarrhea, but as it is often difficult to tell it from liquid stool, it is also included under this heading.

PROBABLE
GASTROENTERITIS
IRRITABLE BOWEL SYNDROME
DIVERTICULAR DISEASE

ABDOMEN: DIGESTIVE SYSTEM

POSSIBLE
FACTITIOUS DIARRHEA
CROHN'S DISEASE
ULCERATIVE COLITIS
BOWEL CANCER
CELIAC DISEASE
PANCREATITIS
BACILLARY DYSENTERY
SPRUE
AIDS-RELATED DIARRHEA
HYPERTHYROIDISM
POST-GASTRECTOMY SYNDROME

RARE
CARCINOID SYNDROME
CHOLERA
TYPHOID

PROBABLE

■ GASTROENTERITIS
* Loose, runny, watery. *See page 167.*

■ IRRITABLE BOWEL SYNDROME
Slightly loose normal stool. *See page 148.*

■ DIVERTICULAR DISEASE
Normal stool, but may be blood-streaked, or with dark blood mixed in. *See page 149.*

POSSIBLE

■ FACTITIOUS DIARRHEA
Loose, but normal. *See page 152.*

■ CROHN'S DISEASE
Loose, but normal. *See page 152.*

■ ULCERATIVE COLITIS
Loose stools with blood, mucus and pus. *See page 151.*

■ BOWEL CANCER
Loose, but normal, and may be blood-streaked. *See page 149.*

■ CELIAC DISEASE
Loose, pale and bulky. *See page 146.*

■ PANCREATITIS
Loose pale, bulky, smelly. *See page 167.*

■ BACILLARY DYSENTERY
Loose, bloody, pus and mucus. *See page 168.*

■ SPRUE
A condition of poor food absorption by the bowel that starts with an initial attack of diarrhea.
* Persistent diarrhea.
* Stools are bulky, pale and fatty.
* Progressive weight loss.
* Loss of appetite.
* Anemia.
* Fluid retention.
* Inflamed tongue.

Requires medical treatment.

■ AIDS-RELATED DIARRHEA
AIDS patients commonly have diarrhea and abdominal pain as symptoms. Tests are needed to decide whether these symptoms are related to AIDS alone or to bacterial infection.

■ HYPERTHYROIDISM
Loose, but normal. *See page 479.*

■ POST-GASTRECTOMY SYNDROME
After the removal of part of the stomach (a gastrectomy), diarrhea is a common complaint. Fortunately, since the introduction of modern ulcer-curing medications, gastrectomy is no longer as common an operation as it once was.

RARE

■ CARCINOID SYNDROME
See page 168.

■ CHOLERA
Profuse, watery. *See page 168.*

■ TYPHOID
Loose, watery. *See page 168.*

BLOOD FROM THE RECTUM

This can appear in several forms: fresh, bright red; darkish, coming from the colon; or "tarry" coming from even higher up the gut. In general, any disease that can cause bleeding in the gut can produce either vomited blood, and/or blood passed in stools.

PROBABLE
HEMORRHOIDS
ANAL FISSURE

ABDOMEN: DIGESTIVE SYSTEM

POSSIBLE
POLYPS
DIVERTICULAR DISEASE
BOWEL CANCER
BLEEDING PEPTIC ULCER
MEDICATION-INDUCED

RARE
ESOPHAGEAL VARICES
INTUSSUSCEPTION
JEJUNAL DIVERTICULUM
MECKEL'S DIVERTICULUM

PROBABLE

■ HEMORRHOIDS
These are lumps of tissue that may push out from the anal canal: a very common problem.
* Bright red bleeding after a bowel movement, seen in the toilet and on the tissue.
* Pain is not a symptom of uncomplicated hemorrhoids.
* Fleshy lumps felt protruding from the anus after a bowel movement, which go back inside on their own or can be pushed back inside.
* However, some hemorrhoids remain permanently protruding.

Hemorrhoids are normally caused by a diet which is abnormally low in fiber or by pregnancy, which puts pressure on the veins around the rectum. You can usually cure 90 percent of hemorrhoids by increasing the amount of fiber in your diet, ideally by adding bran.

ABDOMEN: DIGESTIVE SYSTEM

Severe cases may need injection or, rarely, surgical removal.

■ ANAL FISSURE
See page 159.

POSSIBLE

■ POLYPS
Intestinal polyps (growths of the tissue lining the gut), which are initially benign growths, may cause anemia, or episodes of rectal bleeding. As they grow, the risk of cancerous change increases. *See also BOWEL CANCER, page 149.*

■ DIVERTICULAR DISEASE
See page 149.

■ BOWEL CANCER
See page 149.

■ BLEEDING PEPTIC ULCER
This can cause a black, tarry motion, in association with other symptoms. Sometimes a black stool is the first and only sign of a significant episode of bleeding from an ulcer. The stool is black because the blood is altered by its passage through the gut. *See page 170.*

■ MEDICATION-INDUCED
Certain medications (particularly steroids and non-steroidal anti-inflammatory medications, including aspirin) may cause gastric bleeding. Initial symptoms may include vomiting blood or tarry stools.

RARE

■ ESOPHAGEAL VARICES
Delicate, distended veins in the lower end of the esophagus. They may be associated with cirrhosis of the liver *(see page 150)*. They may cause massive vomiting of blood and also bleeding from the rectum or the appearance of black stools. This condition can be fatal because of sudden blood loss.

■ INTUSSUSCEPTION
This condition is extremely painful and a medical emergency. It produces a form of bowel blockage. It is an abnormality which occurs when the gut tries to expel unwanted tissue such as polyps.

In children it is the commonest form of bowel obstruction, but no one knows why it occurs.

Inflamed lymph nodes may cause the gut to push back into itself.

* Severe, crampy, abdominal pain.
* Thighs and knees drawn up because of pain.

Intussusception

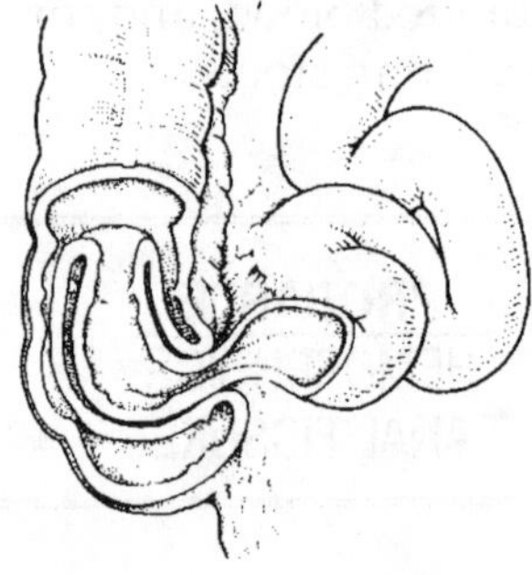

* Blood-stained stools and mucus are passed.
* Vomiting.
* Swollen belly.

■ JEJUNAL DIVERTICULA
Like the colon, the jejunum may develop multiple diverticula. *See DIVERTICULAR DISEASE, page 149.*
* Tarry stools.
* Often pain-free.
* Sometimes diarrhea due to altered digestion and absorption.

■ MECKEL'S DIVERTICULUM
This is like an extra appendix but originates in the ileum. Very rarely, it can cause bleeding. *See page 170.*

PAIN AROUND ANUS OR IN RECTUM

PROBABLE
ANAL FISSURE

POSSIBLE
ANAL ABSCESS

RARE
FISTULA-IN-ANO

PROBABLE

■ ANAL FISSURE
A small tear in the surface tissue of the anal canal, mainly caused by the passage of hard feces. Can cause bleeding in infants and children. May have been caused by injury (perhaps during anal intercourse).
* Local pain, worse after passing a stool.
* Pain stops the individual wanting to move their bowels, and they can become constipated.
* Occasional bleeding (bright red) may be noted (in toilet or on tissue).

Pain-relieving creams may help healing, which will often occur spontaneously.

POSSIBLE

■ ANAL ABSCESS
The anus or anal canal and rectum are common sites for infection, because of the moist environment and the many bacteria present in feces.

However, if you do develop symptoms of an abscess in or around this area, there may be underlying disease. If abscesses or infection recur, medical assessment and treatment are needed.
* Localized throbbing pain (either around the anus or in the rectum).
* Local tender swelling.
* Reddening of the skin if near the surface.

ABDOMEN: DIGESTIVE SYSTEM

* Often fever.
* Often feeling sick.
* Often a fast pulse rate.

Possible underlying diseases that should be considered are diabetes mellitus *(see page 484)* and Crohn's disease *(see page 152)*.

RARE

■ FISTULA-IN-ANO
May be the final result of an abscess which has burst from bowel to skin creating a false track.
* Persistent fecal discharge on skin near anus.

ITCHING ANUS

Itching is usually a sign of inflammation, infection or infestation of the skin's surface. It can occur as a result of an underlying illness in the rest of the body, which makes the skin more vulnerable to this sensation in one particular area.

PROBABLE
OCCUPATIONAL HAZARD
PINWORM
HEMORRHOIDS
YEAST INFECTION

POSSIBLE
PRURITUS ANI
ANAL FISSURE
FISTULA-IN-ANO
PILONIDAL SINUS

RARE
DIABETES MELLITUS

PROBABLE

■ OCCUPATIONAL HAZARD
The anal area is moist and is prone to infection and irritation. People who sit all day (particularly driving trucks and automobiles) and who have stressful jobs, may get this problem.

Regular washing and proper drying will reduce itching. (*See below.*) On the other hand, excess washing and wiping can damage the skin surface, also causing minor irritation and itching. A mild cortisone cream can be helpful; get a physician's advice.

■ PINWORM
See page 153.

■ HEMORRHOIDS
See page 157.

■ YEAST INFECTION
Because this area is continuously moist and damp, it is vulnerable to yeast and fungal infections such as thrush, which is caused by the yeast *candida.* Simple anti-fungal creams can cure the condition. However, it may recur.

POSSIBLE

■ PRURITUS ANI
Some people scratch the anal region as a matter of habit, or when tense. Constant scratching

causes inflammation, cracking, itching and discomfort.

■ ANAL FISSURE
See page 159. Individuals with anal fissures sometimes complain of local itching or irritation.

■ FISTULA-IN-ANO
See page 160. Those with anal fistulas occasionally complain of local irritation and itching.

■ PILONIDAL SINUS
A small hole underneath the skin between the buttocks, thought to be created by a hair growing into and under the skin. It can cause recurrent infection and itching.

RARE

■ DIABETES MELLITUS
See page 484. Some diabetics complain of an itching perianal region, for which no local cause is found.

CHANGE IN BOWEL HABIT

See CONSTIPATION, this page and DIARRHEA, page 155 . Any change in bowel habit which does not have a simple explanation, such as a sudden change in diet, should be reported to your physician.

CONSTIPATION

A diagnosis as well as a symptom. For details on constipation as a diagnosis, *see page 148*.

PROBABLE
INADEQUATE DIET
PREGNANCY
ANAL FISSURE
MEDICATION SIDE-EFFECT

POSSIBLE
DIVERTICULAR DISEASE
BOWEL OBSTRUCTION
BOWEL CANCER
PREMATURITY
IMMOBILITY

RARE
CROHN'S DISEASE
HIRSCHSPRUNG'S DISEASE

PROBABLE

■ INADEQUATE DIET
A diet too low in fluids and/or too low in fiber will cause constipation.

■ PREGNANCY
There are two main causes for constipation in pregnancy.
* Decreased movement of the gut.
* The pressure of the growing womb on the colon.

See page 148.

ABDOMEN: DIGESTIVE SYSTEM

■ ANAL FISSURE
See page 159.

■ MEDICATION SIDE-EFFECT
Many painkillers, in particular codeine and morphine, contain substances which may cause constipation. Many other medications also cause constipation as a side-effect.

POSSIBLE

■ DIVERTICULAR DISEASE
■ BOWEL OBSTRUCTION
See pages 149 and 150.

■ BOWEL CANCER
See page 149.

■ PREMATURITY
See page 146.

■ IMMOBILITY
Anyone relatively immobile or bedridden (for example, the elderly, or anyone who has had a head injury, stroke or progressive neurological disease) is prone to constipation.

RARE

■ CROHN'S DISEASE
See page 152.

■ HIRSCHSPRUNG'S DISEASE
See page 147.

A SWELLING FELT WITHIN THE ABDOMEN

Any organ inside the abdomen can, if diseased, appear as a swelling, a lump or a mass. You might notice this yourself, or your physician may do so at a routine examination .

This is such a general symptom that it makes sense to list only the principal possible causes.

You must a see a physician if you suspect any of these problems. Pregnancy is excluded from the possibilities.

PROBABLE
INGUINAL AND FEMORAL HERNIAS
UMBILICAL HERNIA

POSSIBLE
ENLARGED BLADDER
AORTIC ANEURYSM
CANCER OF THE COLON OR RECTUM
GALL BLADDER
PROBLEMS OF THE OVARIES
STOMACH DISEASE

RARE
APPENDICITIS
KIDNEY DISEASE
LIVER DISEASE
DISEASED PANCREAS
DISEASED SPLEEN
DISEASED UTERUS

ABDOMEN: DIGESTIVE SYSTEM

PROBABLE

■ INGUINAL AND FEMORAL HERNIAS
Hernias are protrusions of bowel through weak spots in the muscular wall of the abdomen. They may be noticed as lumps in the groin. Inguinal hernias are very much more common than femoral hernias.
* May make a gurgling sound.
* Can be pushed back into the abdomen.
* May disappear at night, reappearing once you are up and about.
* In men, hernias may extend into the scrotum.

Hernias gradually enlarge.

Sometimes the bowel gets trapped in the hernia, causing bowel obstruction *(see page 150)*. If this happens, the following may be noticed:
* The hernia becomes painful.
* It cannot be pushed back.
* Intermittent abdominal pain.
* Possibly vomiting.

Surgery may be needed.

■ UMBILICAL HERNIA
Symptoms are the same as for inguinal and femoral hernias, *above*, but are less likely to obstruct the gut. They are commonest in babies and infants. They usually disappear as the abdominal muscles develop.

POSSIBLE

■ ENLARGED BLADDER
Caused by *ENLARGED PROSTATE, page 190*.
* Mid-line swelling in the lower abdomen above the pubic bone.
* Constant pain.
* Inability to pass urine.
* Possibly dribbling of urine.

Needs urgent medical attention.

■ AORTIC ANEURYSM
Swelling of the body's main artery. It may burst without warning.
* Abdominal pain.
* A swelling in middle of abdomen which pulsates in time with the heart beat.
* Back pain.
* Sometimes, sudden collapse.

Often the individual is unaware of the aneurysm until the sudden onset of severe pain. Can be helped by surgery.

■ CANCER OF THE COLON OR RECTUM
See BOWEL CANCER, page 149.

■ GALL BLADDER
The gall bladder may become enlarged for two main reasons. If it is caused by infection:
* Upper right abdominal pain.
* May be a tender mass just below the right rib margin.
* Pain may be made worse by breathing in.
* Fever.
* Feeling sick.

If it is a tumor (of the pancreas, bile ducts or gall bladder):
* Jaundice.
* Non-painful mass in right upper abdomen.
* Pale stools.
* Dark urine.
* Other signs of malignant disease may be present, such as weight loss.

Abdomen: Digestive System

■ PROBLEMS OF THE OVARIES
Ovarian cysts (*page 170*) and cancer of the ovaries can produce abdominal swelling; in the case of ovarian cancer the swelling may be large with weight loss despite the swelling.

■ STOMACH DISEASE
Generally the only reason, in an adult, for the stomach to be so enlarged that you can feel it would be a tumor. Stomach cancer is rare under age 45. Symptoms include:
* Loss of appetite.
* Indigestion and abdominal pain.
* Weight loss.
* Anemia.
* Upper abdominal midline mass.
* Occasionally vomiting, if the pylorus is blocked.
* Even more occasionally, vomiting blood.

Sometimes the individual goes to a physician complaining of jaundice and a swollen bladder *(see page 163)* both the result of the tumor having already spread.
* Hypertrophic pyloric stenosis. Mostly in baby boys. The stomach outlet is blocked by thickened intestinal muscle which can sometimes be felt. *See page 144.*

RARE

■ APPENDICITIS
Inflammation of the appendix. A lump is rarely a noticeable feature of appendicitis; however, if appendicitis is not diagnosed at an early stage, a lump may subsequently appear a few days later which can be felt in the right side of the abdomen.
* Right-sided lower abdominal pain — often starts over the navel or umbilicus, and then moves down and to the right.
* Pain worse on pressing over appendix.
* There may be fever.
* Loss of appetite.
* Nausea and sometimes vomiting.
* Feeling sick.
* If an abcess forms, a lump can be felt in the right lower abdomen; this is called an appendix mass.

■ KIDNEY DISEASE
Kidney enlargement may be noticed on the right or left sides of the abdomen and in the loin, and may be felt as a mass.

Enlargement is occasionally caused by tumor, polycystic disease or urine flow blockage *(see relevant entries in ABDOMEN: URINARY SYSTEM)*.

■ LIVER DISEASE
The liver lies under the right rib cage but extends across the midline. The individual may feel or see the enlargement as a mass moving in and out with breathing. The main reasons for enlargement are:

Cirrhosis
See page 150.

Cancer
Several types of cancer can spread to the liver, including breast and lung. Rarely, the liver is the original site of the tumor, known as a hepatoma.

Infection
The liver may become infected by a number of organisms and liver abscesses may develop.
* Up and down fever.
* Sweating.
* Right upper abdominal pain.
* Enlarged, sore liver.
* Sometimes jaundice.
* Feeling sick.

Hydatid disease
Infection from a tapeworm: causes cysts to form in the liver.
* Often, no symptoms.
* Occasionally the liver is enlarged because of a big cyst.

■ DISEASED PANCREAS
The pancreas lies at the back of the abdomen and may enlarge through inflammation or cancer.

Cancer of the pancreas:
* Abdominal pain.
* Loss of weight.
* Nausea.
* Jaundice.
* Pale stools.
* Dark urine.
* Occasional vomiting.

Pancreatitis
See page 149. Acute pancreatitis sometimes develops a complication called a pseudocyst: a large cyst which may be felt as a mass in the middle of the abdomen.

■ DISEASED SPLEEN
The spleen may be felt as a mass in the abdomen when enlarged two to three times its normal size. Its tip can be felt under the left rib margins. It may be enlarged by any viral infection, but if it is noticed as a mass; the main causes would be:

Malaria *See page 453.*

Chronic myeloid leukemia
* Anemia.
* Discomfort in abdomen due to large spleen.
* Night sweats.
* Fever.
* Loss of weight.
* Occasional generalized itchiness.

Myelofibrosis
Often in association with other illnesses such as cancer.
* Anemia.
* Weakness.
* Enlarged spleen.
* Gout.

Cirrhosis *See page 150.*

Blood diseases
In certain blood diseases the red cells are fragile and get easily destroyed in the spleen: Sickle Cell disease, Spherocytosis.

Cancer
Certain types of cancer: lymphoma, Hodgkin's disease.

■ DISEASED UTERUS
See CANCER OF THE WOMB, page 353.

Abdomen: Digestive System

RIGID ABDOMEN

See PERFORATED BOWEL, page 149.

PAINFUL ABDOMEN

See all symptoms involving abdominal pain, this page and pages 167-74.

CONSTANT VERY SEVERE PAIN IN THE ABDOMEN

Constant severe belly pain requires urgent medical evaluation. The causes listed are not common but require immediate attention.

POSSIBLE
PERFORATED BOWEL
MESENTERIC VASCULAR THROMBOSIS
PANCREATITIS

RARE
RUPTURED AORTIC ANEURYSM

POSSIBLE

■ PERFORATED BOWEL
See page 149.

■ MESENTERIC VASCULAR THROMBOSIS
The main blood vessels to the intestines (gut) are blocked.
* Severe pain, starting suddenly.
* Bloody stools.
* Vomiting.
* Shock.
* Occasionally, abdominal distension.

■ PANCREATITIS
Sometimes, pancreatitis starts suddenly with very severe upper abdominal pain; *see page 149.*

RARE

■ RUPTURED AORTIC ANEURYSM
See AORTIC ANEURYSM, page 163.

SEVERE BUT INTERMITTENT ABDOMINAL PAIN

This suggests a different set of causes to those of constant severe pain; *this page.*

PROBABLE
KIDNEY STONES

POSSIBLE
BOWEL OBSTRUCTION
BILIARY COLIC

ABDOMEN: DIGESTIVE SYSTEM

PROBABLE

■ KIDNEY STONES
See page 184.

POSSIBLE

■ BOWEL OBSTRUCTION
See page 150.

■ BILIARY COLIC
Caused by gall stones temporarily blocking a bile duct.
* Intense pain lasting from minutes to hours.
* Pain is in upper abdomen, and may pass to shoulder tip.
* Vomiting.
* Individual is pale and sweaty.
* Possibly jaundice.
* Possibly fever or chills.

DIARRHEA PLUS ABDOMINAL PAIN

PROBABLE
GASTROENTERITIS
IRRITABLE BOWEL SYNDROME

POSSIBLE
BOWEL CANCER
CROHN'S DISEASE
ULCERATIVE COLITIS
PANCREATITIS
BACILLARY DYSENTERY

RARE
PERNICIOUS ANEMIA
CHOLERA
TYPHOID
POST-GASTRECTOMY SYNDROME
CARCINOID SYNDROME

PROBABLE

■ GASTROENTERITIS
Otherwise known as food poisoning. Can also be caused by viral infections. Very common. Episodes rarely last more than 24 to 36 hours and cure themselves.
* Abdominal pain.
* Vomiting.
* Watery diarrhea.
* Muscle/joint pains.
* Headache.
* Occasional fever.

■ IRRITABLE BOWEL SYNDROME
See page 148.

POSSIBLE

■ BOWEL CANCER
■ CROHN'S DISEASE
■ ULCERATIVE COLITIS
See pages 151 and 153.

■ PANCREATITIS
Inflammation of the pancreas, often resulting in permanent and irreversible damage. Alcohol abuse is the commonest cause. You must stop drinking.
* Pain worsened by food and alcohol. Often very persistent.
* Poor food absorption, due to lack of digestive enzymes, causes fatty diarrhea.

ABDOMEN: DIGESTIVE SYSTEM

* Weight loss.
* Diabetes develops; *see page 485.*
* Sometimes associated with jaundice, pale stools and dark urine.

■ BACILLARY DYSENTERY
Caused by person-to-person spread of a bacterial infection.
* Fever.
* Abdominal pain.
* Watery diarrhea.
* After one to three days, bloody diarrhea with mucus.

Most cases cure themselves, although antibiotics may help.

RARE

■ PERNICIOUS ANEMIA
The lining of the stomach stops producing acid and other essential substances. Occurs in people over 30 years of age. Often familial.
* Anemia, slow onset.
* Sore tongue.
* Tingling and/or numbness of extremities (peripheral neuropathy)
* Fever.
* Abdominal pain.
* Diarrhea.
* Mild jaundice.

■ CHOLERA
Common in some countries with inadequate water and sewer systems. Caused by an organism present in water when water supplies are contaminated.
* Initially, mild diarrhea.
* Then large volumes of diarrhea.
* Vomiting.
* Abdominal pain.
* Thirst.
* Muscle cramps.
* Slight fever.

Treatment aimed at minimizing dehydration.

■ CHOLERA
Only 5 percent of those infected with the chólera organism will develop symptoms. Today's infections are much less severe than those seen earlier in this century.

■ TYPHOID FEVER
Caused by one of the salmonella organisms. In the first week:
* Increasing fever.
* Abdominal pain.
* Headache.
* Cough.

In the second week:
* General sickness.
* Apathy.
* Fever.
* Abdominal swelling.
* Diarrhea.
* "Rose" spots on abdomen.

Fatal in some cases, but antibiotics can change the course of the disease.

■ POST-GASTRECTOMY SYNDROME
Gastrectomy is surgical removal of the stomach. After a meal, within two or three hours, there may be:
* Upper abdominal distension.
* Faintness.
* Weakness.
* Palpitations.
* Sweating.
* Diarrhea.

■ CARCINOID SYNDROME
Carcinoid tumors may appear in any part of the gut. They cause many symptoms, due to the

chemicals they secrete, including:
* Facial flushing.
* Explosive, watery diarrhea.
* Abdominal pain.
* Asthmatic wheeze.
* Pain in the abdomen and weight loss.
* Sweating.

ABDOMINAL PAIN AND PROGRESSIVE LOSS OF WEIGHT

This combination needs to be taken seriously. Your physician will consider the following possibilities. They are not listed in order of probability: diagnosis depends upon accompanying symptoms.

CROHN'S DISEASE, *page 128.*
ULCERATIVE COLITIS, *page 151.*
PANCREATITIS, *page 167.*
CANCER OF THE PANCREAS, *page 165.*
CANCER OF THE STOMACH, *page 164.*
CANCER OF THE BOWEL, *page 152.*
SPREAD OF CANCER TO THE LIVER, *page 164.*

ABDOMINAL PAIN PLUS VOMITING

PROBABLE
GASTROENTERITIS
MESENTERIC ADENITIS

POSSIBLE
PEPTIC ULCER
APPENDICITIS
KIDNEY STONES
OVARIAN CYST
SALPINGITIS (PID)
BILIARY COLIC
STOMACH CANCER
PANCREATITIS

RARE
MECKEL'S DIVERTICULUM
BOWEL OBSTRUCTION
PORPHYRIA

PROBABLE

■ GASTROENTERITIS
See page 167.

■ MESENTERIC ADENITIS
Often mistaken for appendicitis in children; *see page 164.* This condition is caused by enlargement of lymph glands in the stomach, usually caused by a viral infection. Typically, there are common cold symptoms, plus:
* Pain and soreness in the right lower abdomen; pain may also be present throughout the abdomen.
* Fever.
* Nausea and vomiting.

If operated on, enlarged glands are found with a normal appendix. The adenitis settles on its own.

Abdomen: Digestive System

POSSIBLE

■ PEPTIC ULCER

The term covers ulcers of the stomach and duodenum. There is a wide range of symptoms which vary considerably from person to person:
* Pain in the epigastrium (upper middle part of the abdomen).
* Pain comes and goes.
* Heartburn may be present.
* Pain may radiate to the back.
* Pain may be present for a few weeks at a time.
* Night waking because of pain is common.
* Possibly nausea and vomiting.
* Food can either improve or worsen the pain.

Ulcers can bleed, causing anemia and tarry stools or vomiting blood. *See BLOOD FROM THE RECTUM, page 157 and ABDOMINAL PAIN PLUS VOMITING BLOOD, page 171.*

They can also perforate — *see PERFORATED BOWEL, page 149.*

■ APPENDICITIS

See page 164.

■ KIDNEY STONES

See page 184.

■ OVARIAN CYST

Ovarian cysts may be attached to the ovary on a stalk. If the cyst rotates, it will tighten the stalk, causing severe pain.
* Sudden lower abdominal pain.
* Vomiting.
* Cyst may bleed into the abdominal cavity.

May mimic appendicitis if on the right ovary.

Ovaries and Fallopian tubes

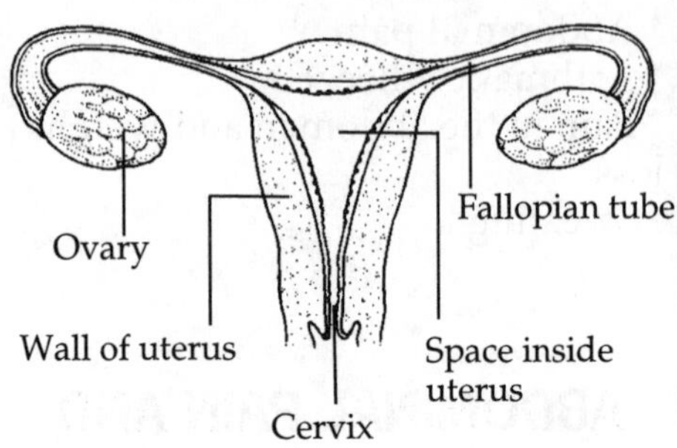

■ SALPINGITIS (PID)

Infection or abscess on a Fallopian tube — one possibility in the wider picture of *PELVIC INFECTION,* known as PID, *page 349.*

■ BILIARY COLIC

See page 167.

■ STOMACH CANCER

See STOMACH DISEASE, page 164.

■ PANCREATITIS

see pages 149 and 150.

RARE

■ MECKEL'S DIVERTICULUM

A diverticulum is an out-pouching — a little sac; this type occurs in the ileum.

Symptoms mimic appendicitis if it becomes inflamed *(see page 164)* and may also cause:
* Anemia.
* Intestinal obstruction.
* Rectal bleeding.

■ BOWEL OBSTRUCTION

See pages 150 and 151.

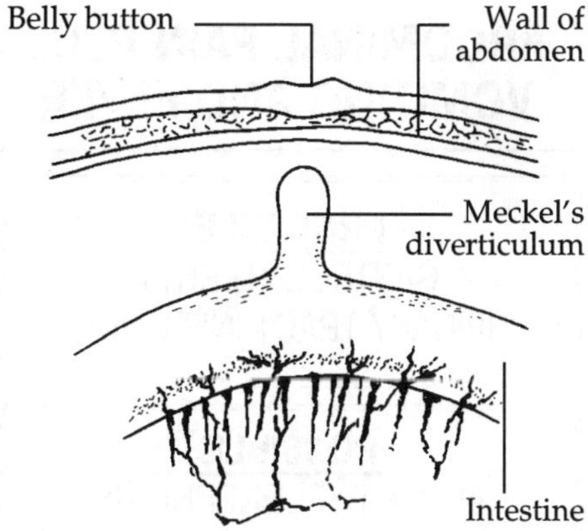

Belly button
Wall of abdomen
Meckel's diverticulum
Intestine

■ PORPHYRIA
A group of metabolic diseases. The following are the commonest features:
* Intermittent abdominal pain.
* Vomiting.
* Constipation.
* Fever.
* Fast pulse.
* Neurological abnormalities.

ABDOMINAL PAIN PLUS VOMITING BLOOD

A rare combination, but if you have both these symptoms, you must see your physician. Bleeding may continue even without vomiting, putting you in danger until the source is detected and the bleeding stopped.

PROBABLE
MALLORY-WEISS TEAR
ACUTE GASTRITIS

POSSIBLE
PEPTIC ULCER
MEDICATION-INDUCED

RARE
CANCER OF THE STOMACH
HIATUS HERNIA AND ESOPHAGITIS

PROBABLE

■ MALLORY-WEISS TEAR
A small tear in the lining of the upper stomach caused by vomiting. First noticed in studies of alcoholics.
* Vomiting frequent
* Fresh blood may be vomited.
* Tarry stools.

Normally self-healing without further treatment.

■ ACUTE GASTRITIS
Inflammation of the lining of the stomach caused by food, medications, alcohol or infection.
* Indigestion.
* Occasionally blood is vomited.

This usually looks like coffee grounds; the blood is altered by the gastric juices.

POSSIBLE

■ PEPTIC ULCER
See page 170.

■ MEDICATION-INDUCED
Some medications, particularly steroids and non-steroidal anti-inflammatory medications,

including aspirin, can cause gastric bleeding. This may be experienced as vomiting up blood or passing tarry stools (melena).

Non-steroidal anti-inflammatory medications. These were originally introduced to treat arthritis, and they are now widely used as general pain-killers. Their side-effects on the intestine are significant: indigestion and bleeding. Elderly people who take them continuously are at greatest risk.

RARE

■ CANCER OF THE STOMACH
See STOMACH DISEASE, page 164.

■ HIATUS HERNIA AND
■ ESOPHAGITIS
Inflammation of the esophagus caused by reflux of stomach contents.
* Heartburn.
* Difficulty in swallowing.
* Bitter fluid comes into mouth.
* Vomiting.
* Nausea.
* Occasional anemia.
* If very severe, may cause tarry stools or vomiting blood.

ABDOMINAL PAIN PLUS VOMITING AND FEVER

PROBABLE
GASTROENTERITIS
URINARY TRACT INFECTION

POSSIBLE
ACUTE PYELONEPHRITIS
PELVIC INFLAMMATORY DISEASE
APPENDICITIS
CHOLECYSTITIS

RARE
INTESTINAL OBSTRUCTION
PANCREATITIS
MECKEL'S DIVERTICULITIS
PORPHYRIA

PROBABLE

■ GASTROENTERITIS
See page 167.

■ URINARY TRACT INFECTION
See page 183.

POSSIBLE

■ ACUTE PYELONEPHRITIS
See KIDNEY INFECTION, page 183.

■ PELVIC INFLAMMATORY DISEASE *See page 352.*

■ APPENDICITIS
See page 164.

ABDOMEN: DIGESTIVE SYSTEM

Gall stones

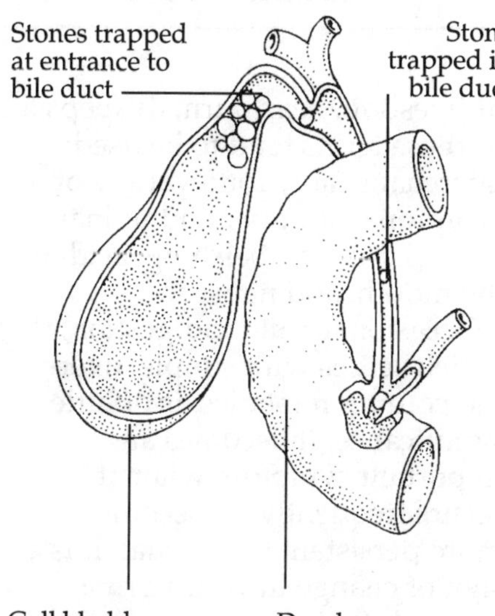

■ CHOLECYSTITIS
The gall bladder may become inflamed and infected because of gall stones, which form from fats, calcium and pigment. Many people have them, but they often remain unnoticed unless the individual develops cholecystitis.
* Upper right abdominal pain.
* Tenderness just below the right rib margin.
* Pain may be made worse by breathing in.
* Fever.
* Feeling unwell.
* Vomiting.
* Jaundice may develop if stones block biliary tract.

See a physician without delay.

RARE

■ BOWEL OBSTRUCTION
■ PANCREATITIS
See pages 150 a nd 149.

■ MECKEL'S DIVERTICULITIS
See page 170.

■ PORPHYRIA
See page 171.

ABDOMINAL PAIN, VOMITING AND JAUNDICE

PROBABLE
CHOLECYSTITIS
BILIARY COLIC

POSSIBLE
PANCREATITIS
HEPATITIS

RARE
CANCER OF THE PANCREAS
CANCER OF THE STOMACH

PROBABLE

■ CHOLECYSTITIS
See this page.

■ BILIARY COLIC
See page 167.

ABDOMEN: DIGESTIVE SYSTEM

POSSIBLE

■ PANCREATITIS
See page 149.

■ HEPATITIS
See page 180.

RARE

■ CANCER OF THE PANCREAS
See page 165.

■ CANCER OF THE STOMACH
See STOMACH DISEASE, page 164.

APPARENT CONSTIPATION ALTERNATING WITH DIARRHEA

This is a possible combination, but it is best to explore the possibilities in detail by separately reading *CONSTIPATION, page 161 and DIARRHEA, page 155 and CHANGE IN BOWEL HABIT, page 161.*

CONSTIPATION AND ABDOMINAL PAIN

Explore the full possibilities by reading
CONSTIPATION, page 161
and *ABDOMINAL PAIN, pages 166-174.*

INDIGESTION

Indigestion, heartburn, dyspepsia — these terms tend to be used interchangeably for a variety of symptoms of upper abdominal pain, flatulence, belching, acid in the mouth, and nausea.

Occasional, mild indigestion, which settles with simple, over-the-counter remedies, is of little significance. It becomes an important symptom when it recurs frequently, or becomes more persistent than usual. It is a sign of change in your normal pattern of tolerance to food and carries a clear message: seek medical advice.

PROBABLE
NON-ULCER DYSPEPSIA
ESOPHAGITIS AND HIATUS HERNIA
PEPTIC ULCER
PREGNANCY

POSSIBLE
GALL STONES

RARE
CANCER OF THE STOMACH
CANCER OF THE ESOPHAGUS
ACHALASIA
PANCREATITIS

Abdomen: Digestive System

Digestive system

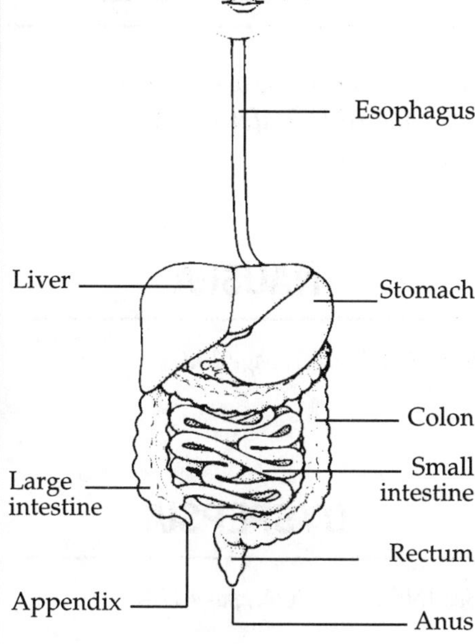

PROBABLE

■ NON-ULCER DYSPEPSIA
A term used to describe groups of symptoms such as:
* Upper abdominal pain.
* Nausea.
* Flatulence and belching when there is no evidence of an ulcer after special tests. Can be associated with poor eating habits and stress.

■ ESOPHAGITIS AND HIATUS HERNIA
See page 172.

■ PEPTIC ULCER
See page 170.

■ PREGNANCY
See page 148.

POSSIBLE

■ GALL STONES
See page 173.

RARE

■ CANCER OF THE STOMACH
See STOMACH DISEASE, page 164.

■ CANCER OF THE ESOPHAGUS
See page 121.

■ ACHALASIA
See page 120.

■ PANCREATITIS
See page 167.

CRAMPING PAINS IN THE ABDOMEN

See all combinations of symptoms involving ABDOMINAL PAIN, pages 166-74.

LOSS OF APPETITE

See page 473.

FLATULENCE OR BELCHING

See INDIGESTION, page 174.

ABDOMEN: DIGESTIVE SYSTEM

DIARRHEA, BLOODY

See DIARRHEA, page 155 and BLOOD FROM THE RECTUM, page 157.

DIARRHEA PLUS VOMITING

See DIARRHEA, page 155 and *VOMITING, page 142;* also *GASTROENTERITIS, page 167*, one of the common causes.

"STOMACH ACHE"

See all combinations of symptoms involving ABDOMINAL PAIN, pages 166-74.

NAUSEA

See VOMITING, page 142.

DYSPEPSIA

See INDIGESTION, page 174.

HEARTBURN

See INDIGESTION, page 174.

INCONTINENCE

Lack of control over the act of urination so that accidental or unplanned leakage occurs. This is a common problem. Any irritation or inflammation may predispose to some degree of leakage. Age often worsens these problems. Can be associated with leakage of feces.

PROBABLE
ENLARGED PROSTATE
BLADDER NECK OBSTRUCTION
URINARY TRACT INFECTION
IRRITABLE BLADDER
STRESS INCONTINENCE

POSSIBLE
CYSTOCELE
RECTOCELE
UTERINE PROLAPSE
STROKE
EPILEPSY
MULTIPLE SCLEROSIS

RARE
SPINAL CORD INJURY
CAUDA EQUINA SYNDROME

PROBABLE

■ ENLARGED PROSTATE
See page 187.

■ BLADDER NECK OBSTRUCTION
See page 187.

■ URINARY TRACT INFECTION
See page 183. Especially in the elderly.

■ IRRITABLE BLADDER
See page 188.

■ STRESS INCONTINENCE
Often in women who have had children.
* Leakage of urine when coughing, laughing or sneezing.
* Leakage when straining.

POSSIBLE

■ CYSTOCELE AND RECTOCELE
These two conditions are common in women who also suffer from stress incontinence — above. They are caused by weakness of the vaginal wall, which allows the bladder (cystocele) or rectum (rectocele) to bulge into the vagina. This distortion of anatomy (often felt as a bulge) can cause leakage of urine.

■ UTERINE PROLAPSE
The structures that keep the womb (uterus) in place stretch after multiple childbirths and with age. In some this allows the womb to drop down into the vagina where it may often be seen or felt.
* Red lump at vagina.
* Sometimes bleeds.
* Discharge may be present.
* Associated with urinary leakage.
* May be pushed back internally.
* Comes back out on straining/coughing/sneezing.

Abdomen: Urinary System

■ STROKE
Anyone who has suffered a stroke may develop incontinence or difficulty in urination.
Sometimes the bladder over-fills with urine, but because of lack of sensation no pain is felt, although the individual may appear restless and sweaty. Some overflow incontinence may develop.

■ EPILEPSY
In major epileptic seizures *(see page 384)*, symptoms include:
* Jerking movements.
* Tongue biting.
* Urinary incontinence (the entire bladder empties spontaneously during the fit).

■ MULTIPLE SCLEROSIS
See page 405. Early symptoms reported to a doctor can include:
* Weakness or numbness in a limb.
* Heaviness in a limb.
* "Jumping" legs.
* Muscular spasms.
* Impaired vision.
* Hesitancy, frequency, incontinence and retention of urine may all be present.
* Altered sensation in limbs and trunk.

RARE

These diseases can be associated with very sudden loss of bladder control — together with other symptoms.

■ SPINAL CORD INJURY
* Weakness of the limbs below the level of damage.
* Sensory loss below the level of damage.
* Loss of bladder control — usually resulting in retention of urine.
Urgent medical attention is required.

■ CAUDA EQUINA SYNDROME
Meaning damage to the lowest part of the spinal cord. Can be caused by bone damage, tumor or a "slipped disc".
* Back pain.
* Loss of sensation at the lower back and around the buttocks and anus.
* Leg weakness.
* Loss of bladder control.
Urgent medical attention is required.

NEED TO URINATE URGENTLY OR OFTEN

This symptom usually suggests that the bladder itself is irritated. The commonest cause is urine infection — cystitis. *See page 182; also PROBLEMS WITH URINATING, page 186.*

URINATING TOO MUCH, OR TOO OFTEN

The obvious cause is drinking too much tea, coffee or alcohol. These all stimulate the production of urine and can make you want to urinate during the night.

PROBABLE
URINARY TRACT INFECTION

Abdomen: Urinary System

POSSIBLE
ENLARGED PROSTATE
DIURETICS
DIABETES MELLITUS

RARE
DIABETES INSIPIDUS
CHRONIC RENAL FAILURE
ALDOSTERONISM
HYPERCALCEMIA

PROBABLE

■ URINARY TRACT INFECTION
See page 183. Causes frequent urination, rather than excessive volume.

POSSIBLE

■ ENLARGED PROSTATE
See page 187. Again, causes frequent urination, rather than excessive volume.

■ DIURETICS
A range of medications given to reduce high blood pressure or to treat heart failure. Their intended effect is to increase the amount of urine passed, in order to reduce the amount of fluid in the system and so lower the blood pressure. May increase frequency of urination.

■ DIABETES MELLITUS
See page 486. Young people who are just developing the disease may suddenly experience:
* Increased volume of urine (polyuria).
* Increased thirst (polydipsia).
* Rapid weight loss.
* Feeling sick.
* Other symptoms such as vomiting, muscle cramps, abdominal pain, blurred vision.

If untreated, coma and death may follow. In the elderly, onset is slower and eye, nerve or kidney symptoms may be the first signs.

RARE

■ DIABETES INSIPIDUS
See page 486. Don't confuse it with diabetes mellitus, above. It may arise spontaneously or after injury to the head (typically after surgery or an accident); because of brain tumors; or because of significant infection. The main symptom is:
* Enormous volumes of urine — about 9 pints passed daily.

■ CHRONIC KIDNEY FAILURE
Any disease resulting in kidney failure *(see INABILITY TO URINATE, page 189)* can cause excess urine at some stage.

■ ALDOSTERONISM
Caused by a tumor of the adrenal gland. The blood chemistry becomes abnormal, leading to:
* Muscle weakness.
* Excessive urination.
* Excessive thirst.
* High blood pressure.

ABDOMEN: URINARY SYSTEM

■ HYPERCALCEMIA
High levels of calcium in the blood may be caused by a number of conditions and diseases including:
* Abnormalities of the parathyroid glands (*see diagram page 133*).
* Excess Vitamin D.
* Sarcoidosis: an illness of body tissues leading to the deposit of material, described as sarcoid, in various sites in the body.
* Malignant bone tumors (primary or secondary).
* Thyrotoxicosis: an illness caused by having too much thyroid hormone.
The symptoms of excess calcium in the blood are:
* Poor appetite.
* Nausea.
* Vomiting.
* Thirst.
* Polyuria (passing urine more often than normal).
* Constipation.
* Muscle fatigue.

URINE LOOKS DARK

PROBABLE
CONCENTRATED URINE

POSSIBLE
HEPATITIS
FOOD OR MEDICATION

RARE
CANCER OF THE PANCREAS
HEMAGLOBINURIA
"CRUSH" SYNDROME
MELANOMA
ALKAPTONURIA

PROBABLE

■ CONCENTRATED URINE
If you have been physically very active or out in the sun, without also increasing your fluid intake, you may notice that your urine is a dark yellow color, and that it is passed in small amounts. In the absence of other symptoms, this is normal. By increasing your fluid intake, or by avoiding the heat or exercise, urine will soon return to normal.

POSSIBLE

■ HEPATITIS
Inflammation of the liver. There are several different types, some, particularly hepatitis B, are more serious than the others. If you suspect hepatitis, you must see a doctor. General symptoms may include:
* Fever.
* Feeling sick.
* Poor appetite.
* Nausea.
* Muscle and joint pains.
* Jaundice.
* Dark urine: it can be dark yellow, orange or brown.
* Stools become pale.

■ FOOD OR MEDICATION
Several foods and medications can cause discoloration of different hues.
Examples are:
* Orange — rhubarb, senna.
* Red — beets, blackberries.
* Green/blue — methylene blue dye.

After stopping the food or medication, urine should be back to normal within about 24 hours.

RARE

■ CANCER OF THE PANCREAS
A malignant tumor of the pancreas which blocks the bile ducts. This means that yellow bile is passed out in the urine.
* Jaundice.
* Dark yellow/orange/brown urine.
* Pale stools.
* Abdominal and back pain.
* Weight loss, no appetite.

■ HEMAGLOBINURIA
In contrast to hematuria (which is the medical term for blood in urine *(see this page)*, hemoglobinuria means broken down red blood cells in the urine, coloring the urine brown. It is caused by several different diseases or conditions such as: hemolytic anemias, thrombocytopenic purpuras, cardiac disease (for example, after valve replacement), malaria, septicemias.

Discolored urine is unlikely to be the first or only symptom of these conditions, and in most cases the individual will already be under medical care.

■ "CRUSH" SYNDROME
See page 191.

■ MELANOMA
A melanoma is a skin cancer *(see page 244)*. In some advanced cases, the pigment melanin gets into the urine and colors it dark brown or black.

■ ALKAPTONURIA
This is a metabolic disease, where the body fails to deal correctly with certain chemicals in the blood, which are then excreted in urine. It becomes progressively darker if left standing.

BLOOD IN URINE

The significance of blood in the urine varies greatly from the simple and easily treated to the severe and life-threatening. It should never be ignored as a symptom and is more serious if it recurs. Red blood cells in the urine (the medical term is hematuria) may come from any part of the urinary tract — the kidneys, the ureters (which connect the kidneys to the bladder), the bladder and the urethra *(see illustration, page 183)*. Blood may also appear in urine because of generalized disease.

It may become apparent in several ways. The urine may appear the color of blood (frank hematuria), or in smaller quantities it may only color it pinkish, or give it a smoky or cloudy appearance. Occasionally clots of blood are passed with minimal coloring of the rest of the urine. Also, blood may appear only at the beginning or end of urination.

The male and female urinary tracts differ in that the male has a prostate gland and two seminal vesicles (*see illustration, page 183*). In females of child-bearing age, menstrual loss of blood may sometimes be mistaken for blood in the urine. In this case, the bloody discoloration disappears as menstruation ends.

Some foods, particularly beets, can discolor the urine.

PROBABLE
CYSTITIS
URINARY TRACT INFECTION
KIDNEY INFECTION
(PYELONEPHRITIS)

POSSIBLE
KIDNEY STONES
PROSTATITIS
BENIGN TUMORS
OF BLADDER/KIDNEY
ENLARGED PROSTATE
CANCER OF THE PROSTATE
CHRONIC NEPHRITIS
INJURY
EXERCISE

RARE
CANCER OF THE BLADDER/KIDNEY
WILM'S TUMOR (CHILDREN)
ENDOCARDITIS
ANTICOAGULANT THERAPY
BILHARZIA

PROBABLE

■ CYSTITIS
Inflammation of the bladder lining, giving symptoms of urine infection.
* Frequent passing of urine.
* Burning or scalding as you urinate.
* Strong desire to urinate with little result.
* Having to rush to pass urine with urgency.
* Dull ache in lower belly; may persist or worsen after urination.
* Fever; backache.
* Dark, cloudy or blood-stained urine.

Medical attention is recommended.

Children
Blood in the urine should always be taken seriously. Medical evaluation will be required. While an adult may commonly suffer an infection causing blood to appear in the urine, this is not acceptable in children. Any urine infection in a child is an unusual event. It may be the first sign of an abnormality in the structure of the urinary tract.

■ URINARY TRACT INFECTION

Symptoms as for cystitis; in addition, there may be more severe symptoms such as:
* High fever.
* Pain in the back, loin, groin, front of abdomen.
* Vomiting, nausea.
* Sweating.

Will require antibiotics.

Bacterial resistance

Increasingly, the bacteria causing urinary infections (and cystitis) do not respond to commonly prescribed antibiotics. To treat your problem effectively your physician may recommend sending a urine sample to the laboratory before treatment starts. If symptoms do not clear during or after antibiotic treatment, inform your physician.

■ KIDNEY INFECTION

Medical term: pyelonephritis.

Symptoms as for cystitis, plus:
* Severe fever.
* Loin pain.
* Tenderness and pain in the loin and side of abdomen.
* General feeling of being unwell.

Cystitis symptoms may not be marked, particularly in the early stages, when the symptoms may be confined largely to the upper abdomen; for example:
* Pain, vomiting, nausea.

Severe and advanced cases (also termed acute nephritis) will show diminished urine output, swelling of face and ankles, headache and other symptoms as above.

Requires urgent treatment.

Bladder

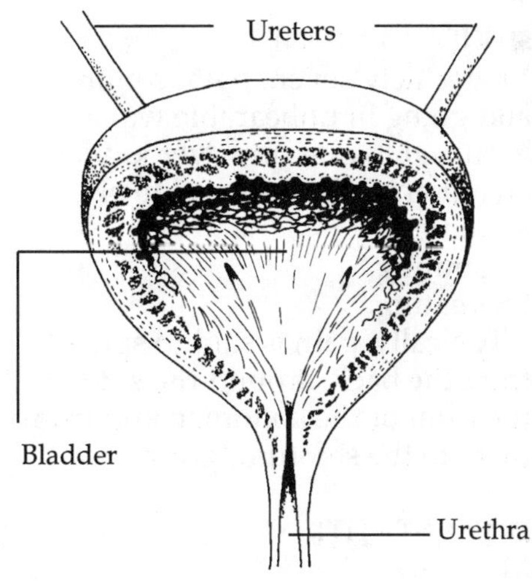

Male urinary and reproductive system

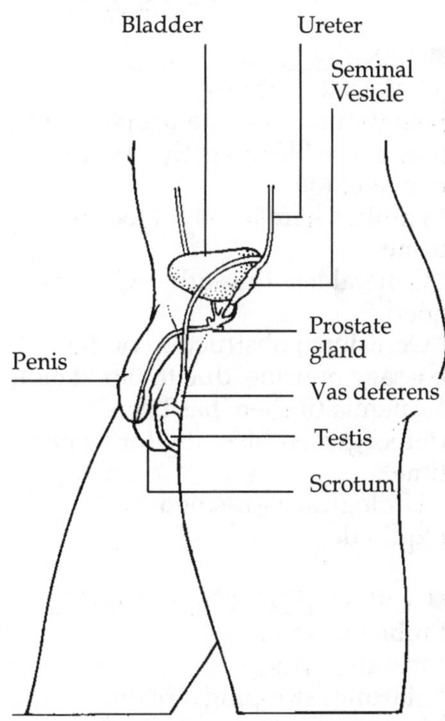

Abdomen: Urinary System

POSSIBLE

■ KIDNEY STONES
* Extremely severe pain, coming and going in unbearable waves, localized to one side over kidney area (loin and extreme side of abdomen).
* Vomiting.
* Sweating.

Typically, pain is said to spread from the back, around the side to the front of the abdomen and from there to the scrotum/groin area.

■ PROSTATITIS
Men only.
* Fever.
* Pain in the rectal area behind scrotum.
* Difficulty in passing urine.
* Sensation of passing hot urine.

■ BENIGN TUMORS OF BLADDER/KIDNEY
Benign tumors of the urinary tract may cause bleeding. Symptoms may include:
* Painless hematuria (blood in urine).
* General health is otherwise good.
* Occasional obstruction of the passage of urine, due to blood clot.
* Anemia (if there has been unrecognized bleeding for some time).

Urological assessment is required.

■ ENLARGED PROSTATE (MEN)
Problems with:
* Passing urine.
* Starting/stopping stream.
* Holding on to pass urine later.
* Dribbling.

Inability to pass urine (retention of urine) requires medical intervention and catheterization (drainage through a tube).

■ CANCER OF PROSTATE
As for enlarged prostate. Diagnosis is frequently made only during operative intervention for enlarged prostate symptoms. After about 80 years of age, nearly every male has evidence of cancer of the prostate. It lies dormant in the gland, seldom causing severe problems at that age.

■ CHRONIC NEPHRITIS
Passing large amounts of urine at night.
* Anemia.
* Swelling.
* Shortness of breath.

■ INJURY
Injuries to the back, abdomen or pelvis (such as a blow or a fall) may damage underlying structures. If you have any blood in your urine after such an injury, whether in large or small quantities, you will need a full medical assessment in order to rule out serious damage.

■ EXERCISE
It is now widely recognized that certain types of prolonged, repeated exercise — in particular, contact sports and running — may cause transient appearances of blood in the urine.

RARE

■ CANCER OF THE BLADDER/KIDNEY
Commonest in adults over 50.
* Painless hematuria — blood in urine.
* Pain in the loin.
* Swelling in loin or abdomen.
* Occasionally bone pain, due to spread of the tumor.
* Fever.
* Loss of weight.
* Anemia.

Simple tests to examine the cell content of urine, can reveal the presence of malignant cells.

■ WILM'S TUMOR (CHILDREN)
The child has:
* One-sided, abdominal swelling.
* Painless blood in urine.
* Loss of appetite.
* Anemia.
* Pain in late stages only.

Modern medications and medical techniques have revolutionized the treatment of this disease. Early diagnosis is important.

■ ENDOCARDITIS
Infection of the heart valves; may affect the kidneys. Multiple symptoms appear. The person will be very ill. Symptoms include:
* Rash.
* Joint pains.
* Finger clubbing *(see page 296)*
* Fever.
* Chest pain.

■ ANTICOAGULANT THERAPY
People who are taking anticoagulants (blood-thinning medication) may notice blood in their urine. They should consult their physician immediately to check the dose of the medication.

■ BILHARZIA
Or schistosomiasis. Caused by an organism that inhabits water. Common in Africa, the West Indies, South America and Japan.
* Blood in urine.
* Pain on passing urine.
* Frequent passing of urine.

Cancer of the bladder can develop, as well as liver damage.

BLOOD IN URINE PLUS PAIN WHEN URINATING

The **probable** causes are: urinary tract infection; cystitis; kidney stone.

The **possible** causes are: acute pyelonephritis; prostatitis.

The **rare** cause is: bilharzia, above. All are covered under *BLOOD IN URINE, page 181.*

KIDNEY PAIN

The kidneys are situated at the sides of the abdomen, towards the back. This area is known as the kidney or loin area.

The most likely cause of pain in this area is infection. There are a number of other possible causes all of which are covered in *BLOOD*

ABDOMEN: URINARY SYSTEM

IN URINE, page 181, BLOOD IN URINE PLUS PAIN WHEN URINATING, page 185, and KIDNEY STONES, page 184.

PAIN WHEN URINATING

Pain when passing urine is almost always a sign of cystitis or urine infection. Rarely, it can be one of the symptoms caused by a kidney stone or sexually transmitted infection such as NSU; *see NON-SPECIFIC URETHRITIS, page 188 or GONORRHEA, this page.*

Also, the conditions listed under *BLOOD IN URINE, page 181* may all cause pain on passing urine as an early symptom, prior to the appearance of blood in the urine.

URINE LOOKS CLOUDY

Mainly blood, pus cells and micro-organisms have this effect. Other symptoms may well be noticed at the same time. Urine which is concentrated but normal often goes cloudy if left standing. Cloudy appearance does not always signify illness.

PROBABLE
URINARY TRACT INFECTION
CYSTITIS
KIDNEY STONE

POSSIBLE
ACUTE PYELONEPHRITIS
PROSTATITIS
GONORRHEA

PROBABLE

- URINARY TRACT INFECTION
- CYSTITIS
- KIDNEY STONES

See BLOOD IN URINE, page 181.

POSSIBLE

- ACUTE PYELONEPHRITIS
- PROSTATITIS

See BLOOD IN URINE, page 181.

- GONORRHEA

A sexually transmitted disease. Often has no symptoms in women, although vaginal discharge, pelvic inflammatory disease and pain on passing urine may be experienced.

If a man has genital symptoms (and he may not) there will be:
* Discharge from end of penis.
* Discomfort on passing urine.
* Cloudy urine.
* Reddening and pain around the glans of the penis and urethra.
* Enlarged lymph nodes in the groin.

PROBLEMS WITH URINATING

These include such symptoms as difficulty in starting to urinate; poor urine stream; and dribbling. The causes tend to be either obstruction to the passage of urine; or structural abnormalities of the urinary tract; pain on urinating due to other causes such as infection; neurological defects may also affect urination.

PROBABLE
ENLARGED PROSTATE
BLADDER NECK OBSTRUCTION
URINARY TRACT INFECTION
GONORRHEA
NON-SPECIFIC URETHRITIS

POSSIBLE
IRRITABLE BLADDER
URETHRAL STRICTURE
PROSTATITIS
KIDNEY STONES
MEDICATIONS

RARE
URETHRAL TUMORS
SPINAL CORD DAMAGE
NEUROLOGICAL DISEASE
STROKE

PROBABLE

■ ENLARGED PROSTATE (MEN)
The gland can be enlarged as a result of benign or malignant tumors. Symptoms may be similar in both cases:
* Difficulty starting to urinate.
* Poor stream.
* Terminal dribbling.
* Feeling as though the bladder has not emptied.
* Need to urinate in the night.
* Sudden desire to pass urine.
* Some blood in the urine.
* Sometimes, leakage of urine: overflow incontinence. *See below.*
* Later in the disease, acute obstruction occurs with inability to pass urine at all. Severe abdominal pain develops because of the distended bladder.

In some cases, the obstruction develops so slowly that the bladder compensates by enlarging over a period of weeks or months. There is minimal discomfort and the urine frequently leaks out, without the individual being able to control it. The bladder does not empty properly, which is often seen as abdominal swelling. This type of urine loss is called overflow incontinence. Medical and surgical treatment can help. Cancer of the prostate may also cause:
* Back pain.
* Bone pain.

■ BLADDER NECK OBSTRUCTION
Symptoms similar to an enlarged prostate, but occurring in a younger age group and, occasionally, in women. Caused by

Abdomen: Urinary System

overgrowth of the bladder muscle at its outlet to the urethra.

■ URINARY TRACT INFECTION
See page 183.

■ GONORRHEA
See page 186.

■ NON-SPECIFIC URETHRITIS
A common sexually transmitted disease caused by an organism called *Chlamydia.* Often there are no symptoms. If there are symptoms, men will have:
* Discomfort or itch on passing urine — making it difficult to urinate.
* Discharge (white, yellow) from penis.

Women will have:
* Pain/burning on passing urine.
* Occasional vaginal discharge.

The womb and Fallopian tubes can be infected.
See also PELVIC INFLAMMATORY DISEASE, page 352.

NSU or NON-SPECIFIC URETHRITIS
It is very important to have this disease treated. Both partners must receive treatment, since, even with a total absence of symptoms, *Chlamydia* may be present. Untreated chlamydial infections can cause infertility.

POSSIBLE

■ IRRITABLE BLADDER
A term encompassing different symptoms caused by irritation of sensory or motor nerves to the bladder. Other causes (such as infection) must be excluded first. Special tests are needed to confirm the diagnosis. Symptoms can be one or more of:
* Frequent desire to pass urine (for example every 30 minutes).
* Pain over the bladder.
* Difficulty in passing urine (small volumes) and the bladder still feels full.
* Sometimes retention of urine occurs.
* Occasionally leakage of urine.

■ URETHRAL STRICTURE
Urethral stricture is a narrowing of the outflow passage from the bladder. It is commoner in men than women and may be caused by previous infection (perhaps gonorrhea), surgery, damage by an instrument or a catheter.
* Poor stream.
* Needing to strain hard to empty the bladder.

■ PROSTATITIS
See page 184.

■ KIDNEY STONES
See page 184.

■ MEDICATIONS
See page 190.

RARE

■ URETHRAL TUMORS
Benign or malignant tumors may cause progressive obstruction of the urethra in men and women leading to:
* Poor stream.

* Need to strain harder than usual to pass urine.

- SPINAL CORD DAMAGE
- NEUROLOGICAL DISEASE
- STROKE

See INCONTINENCE, page 177.

URINE DRIBBLES

Meaning either a poor stream, or dripping when trying to stop the flow of urine. Can be a form of incontinence.

The following, all dealt with in detail under *PROBLEMS WITH URINATING, pages 187-9,* can all be occasional causes of dribbling.

PROBABLE

- ■ ENLARGED PROSTATE
- BLADDER NECK OBSTRUCTION
- URINARY TRACT INFECTION

POSSIBLE

- URETHRAL STRICTURE
- PROSTATITIS

RARE

- URETHRAL TUMORS

URINATING AT NIGHT

If you have a drink in the late evening, you know you will probably have to get up to urinate later on. It is only abnormal if it develops as a new symptom, or if the number of times you get up increases significantly.

The commonest causes are an enlarged prostate gland (in men) bladder irritability or infection (in women).

Medications are another important cause. Diuretics can often be taken, in the morning, to minimize this problem. *See also PROBLEMS WITH URINATING, page 187 and URINATING TOO MUCH, OR TOO OFTEN, page 178.*

INABILITY TO URINATE

The medical term is anuria, and it is a serious problem. Don't confuse it with passing small volumes of concentrated urine infrequently. Urination may stop for three main reasons: first obstruction in the urethra *(see illustration page 183)*; second, failure of the bladder muscle to contract; and third, both kidneys may stop producing urine, because they are diseased, or because of disease elsewhere.

The first two cases are described as retention of urine. In all three cases, but particularly in the last, there may be a period of hours or days when the volume of urine

Abdomen: Urinary System

gradually diminishes.

In the case of obstruction, there will be severe pain because of an increasingly distended bladder. Failure to excrete urine results in a build-up of toxic chemicals in the blood — and so it is, of course, a medical emergency.

PROBABLE
ENLARGED PROSTATE
KIDNEY STONES
URETHRAL STRICTURE

POSSIBLE
SURGERY OR INJURY
MEDICATIONS
PYELONEPHRITIS
MALIGNANT TUMORS
SHOCK
SEPTICEMIA

RARE
INJURY
SPINAL CORD DAMAGE
NEUROLOGICAL DISEASE
POISONING
BLOOD TRANSFUSION
"CRUSH SYNDROME"

PROBABLE

■ ENLARGED PROSTATE
Much the most common reason (in men) for a sudden inability to pass urine is an enlarged prostate gland causing an obstruction to the outlet from the bladder. You will feel pain as the bladder distends.

See page 187. All the other causes in this section are much less common.

■ KIDNEY STONES
See page 184. If a stone lodges in the urethra or at the neck of the bladder, it will block the passage of urine. In addition to urine failure:
* Pain because of distended bladder.
* Inability to pass urine.

In men, pain may radiate to the tip of the penis.

■ URETHRAL STRICTURE
See page 188.

POSSIBLE

■ SURGERY OR INJURY
Any event that causes uncontrolled blood loss, and thus low blood pressure, can damage the kidneys and prevent them from working. The elderly, and those with chronically raised blood pressure, are vulnerable to this type of kidney damage.

■ MEDICATIONS
A number of medications may unexpectedly cause retention of urine, particularly in patients with prostatic disease. Examples are: amitryptiline and imipramine.

■ PYELONEPHRITIS
See KIDNEY INFECTION, page 183.

In severe, untreated cases, the kidneys may be so badly damaged that they stop working. No urine is produced and the patient gets more and more sick, with:
* Weak pulse.
* Fever.
* Rigors.
* Vomiting.

■ MALIGNANT TUMORS
Any malignant tumor of organs in or near the pelvis can involve parts of the urinary tract, blocking the urethra, ureters, bladder or kidneys. Cancers of the colon, uterus, ovaries, bladder and prostate can all have this effect. But it is very rare for anuria to be the first symptom, and the diagnosis has usually been made long before.

■ SHOCK
See also page 408. If shock is untreated or untreatable, the kidneys fail to produce urine and gradually urine output ceases.

■ SEPTICEMIA
Infection of the bloodstream and whole body from any cause. It can lead to shock *(see page 408)*, which, if untreated or severe, results in acute kidney failure.
Possibly fatal.

RARE

■ INJURY
Direct injury to the urethra (particularly in men) occurs typically in automobile accidents where the pelvis has been fractured. This is a medical emergency which in most cases is promptly treated because the patient is already in hospital.
Very occasionally, a kick to the male scrotum, or crotch, may damage the urethra, or indeed the spinal cord.

■ SPINAL CORD DAMAGE
■ NEUROLOGICAL DISEASE
See page 178.

■ POISONING
A number of chemicals may directly damage the kidneys, causing kidney failure. These include mercury, arsenic and bismuth.

■ BLOOD TRANSFUSION
If a patient is given blood which is incompatible with his or her own, the result may damage the kidneys and cause kidney failure. This is one reason why such care is taken when giving blood, and why it is only given when needed.

■ "CRUSH SYNDROME"
Damaged leg muscles, sustained in a crushing injury to the lower limbs, causes toxins to enter the blood stream, resulting in direct damage to the kidneys.
Discolored urine may be a symptom. The longer the limb is crushed, the greater the risk.

The Heart, Chest, Lungs and Breathing

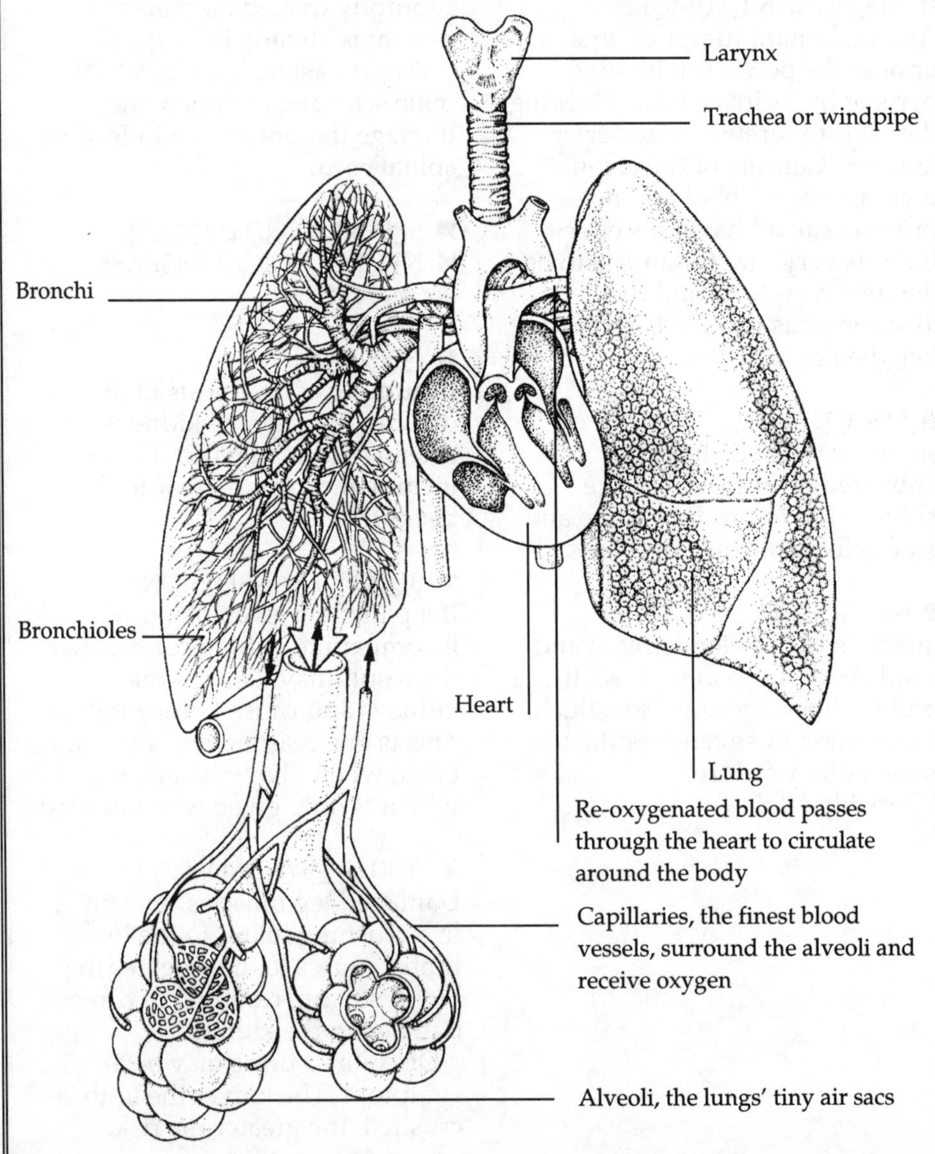

THE HEART INTRODUCTION

The heart is a superb pump: it gives decades of service, responding automatically to all the varied demands of growth, activity and stress, so that we are rarely aware of its action.

How does the heart work? Two major systems, both electrical, control the heart's activity; there is also a built-in mechanism that increases the heart's muscular effort in response to high demand.

Emotion and stress are communicated to the heart by a branch of the nervous system called the autonomic system. It is this system that, for example, sets the heart beating faster when you watch an exciting ball game, and continues to increase both its speed and power when you jump up and down and scream and yell.

Within the heart itself there are two electrical pacemakers that control the rate of heartbeat. The main one, the sino-atrial node, normally sets the rate, transmitting a regular firing signal down an electrical pathway to the second pacemaker, a relay station called the atrio-ventricular node. From there, the signal to contract is transmitted to the rest of the heart by other electrical tracts. The atrio-ventricular node may also act as a pacemaker should the sino-atrial node fail for some reason.

Clearly there are many opportunities for malfunction in this system. If there is a problem, heart-rhythms may be too fast, too slow or irregular. Occasional rhythm disorders are common and are not necessarily a sign of disease. These irregularities are felt in various ways: perhaps a thumping in the chest or a fluttering sensation; sometimes only skilled examination can detect a problem. This section looks at the possibilities.

Where irregularities decrease the pumping efficiency of the heart significantly, faintness, dizzy turns or, at worst, collapse may follow.

HEART MAKES EXTRA BEATS

This is a common symptom with an interesting explanation. What happens is that the heart beats twice in rapid succession. The extra beat goes unnoticed.

However, the next beat of the heart is delayed by a fraction of a second and it is this slight delay that you may be aware of. During the delay, blood continues to fill the heart, triggering an automatic mechanism that makes the heart beat more forcefully the fuller it gets. The next beat after the delay is, therefore, extra-powerful, and is felt as a thump in the chest. It is important to get medical advice about these symptoms, even though most will not be serious.

THE HEART

PROBABLE
UNEXPLAINED
TOO MUCH COFFEE OR TEA
ALCOHOL
CIGARETTE SMOKING
FEVER

POSSIBLE
ANXIETY
INDIGESTION

RARE
COMPLICATIONS OF HEART ATTACK
EXCESS DIGOXIN
RHEUMATIC CARDITIS
HYPERTHYROIDISM

PROBABLE

■ UNEXPLAINED
In the young or early middle-aged.
* Happens occasionally.
* Otherwise sound health.
* The extra beat causes no other symptoms: no faintness or chest pain.

■ TOO MUCH COFFEE OR TEA
The small amounts of caffeine in these drinks is responsible for the "lift" they provide. Taken in excess — an excess varies from person to person — the caffeine will cause:
* Rapid heart rate.
* Extra beats.
* Tremor.
* Anxiety.
* Increased output of urine.
Treatment is simply to reduce intake.

■ ALCOHOL
Alcohol has a direct effect on the heart. This increases with time and excessive use and can lead, in rare cases, to heart failure.

■ CIGARETTE SMOKING
Nicotine has a stimulant effect on the heart, increasing its rate and output. Extra beats are one reflection of this.

■ FEVER
Heart rate rises by about ten beats per 0.5 degree celsius rise in temperature and increases the chance of extra beats. Some infections, as well as causing fever, can irritate or damage the heart.

POSSIBLE

■ ANXIETY
Has its effect via the autonomic nervous system *(see THE HEART, INTRODUCTION, page 193)*, increasing the resting rate of the heart and the chances of extra beats. Other well-known symptoms include:
* Tension in neck, shoulders.
* Constant feeling of pressure in the head.
* Excess sweating, tremor.
* Constantly feeling that something dreadful is about to happen.

■ INDIGESTION
It is uncertain how this affects the heart. Probably it results from a reflex action in those nerves which serve both the digestive system and the heart, though there may be direct irritation of the heart by a

distended stomach. The features of indigestion are familiar.
* Bloating, belching.
* Acid, burning sensation after meals.
* Discomfort felt behind breast bone.

RARE

■ COMPLICATIONS OF HEART ATTACK
Extra beats are common in the days after a heart attack, often producing few symptoms. They have a different origin from benign extra beats, arising instead from spontaneous beating of the ventricles, the main pumping chambers of the heart. In hospital, it is usual to monitor the heart's electrical activity in the days after a heart attack looking for just such ventricular extra beats. They can be a warning of the sudden, uncontrolled activity of the ventricles which causes collapse and possibly sudden death.

■ EXCESS DIGOXIN
Digoxin is widely used to treat heart failure. In excess it causes:
* Nausea and vomiting.
* Very slow pulse, with extra beats.
* Fatigue.
* Red or green hallucinations.
* Abdominal pains.

Mild cases can be corrected by temporarily stopping digoxin. Severe cases need intensive treatment in hospital.

■ RHEUMATIC CARDITIS
Fortunately this once-common disease in children is now a rarity in the developed world, but is still prevalent elsewhere.
* Begins two to three weeks after a "strep" throat.
* Joint pains; stiffness flitting from limb to limb.
* Fever.
* Rashes rapidly coming and going.
* Rapid pulse, extra beats.
* Sudden, fidgety movements.

There is danger of permanent damage to the heart valves leading later to heart disease.

■ HYPERTHYROIDISM
Excessive amounts of thyroid hormone raise the resting heart rate and can cause extra beats.
See page 200.

HEART BEATS IRREGULARLY

Your physician can diagnose simple irregularities arrhythmias by listening to the heart with a stethoscope while feeling your pulse. Further tests would include an ECG (electrocardiogram) and wearing a Holter Monitor for 24 hours.

PROBABLE
SINUS ARRHYTHMIA
SICK SINUS SYNDROME

POSSIBLE
EXTRA BEATS

THE HEART

RARE
PULMONARY EMBOLUS

PROBABLE

■ SINUS ARRHYTHMIA
Careful observation of your own pulse will reveal a change in rhythm as you breathe. The autonomic pathways mentioned elsewhere slow the heart as you breathe out and let it run faster as you breathe in. In some people this is particularly noticeable and may cause alarm. It is not a disease but an exaggeration of a normal reflex. The reflex is especially noticeable in children.
* Otherwise well.
* Clear relationship to breathing.
* Rhythm changes by about ten beats per minute faster or slower.

■ SICK SINUS SYNDROME
The sino-atrial node is the trigger in the heart that fires the electrical signal which causes the heart to beat *(see THE HEART, INTRODUCTION, page 193)*. So vital is this area of the heart that it has its own blood supply, but with age that blood supply can become diseased, resulting in erratic functioning of the trigger.
* Pulse may vary between very fast or very slow.
* Symptoms vary from none at all to fainting to loss of consciousness.

Treatment is with medication or an electronic pacemaker.

POSSIBLE

■ EXTRA BEATS
Extra beats happening frequently will give the impression of an irregular heart beat. It is difficult to diagnose this situation without an ECG. Treatment aims to cure the underlying cause. *See HEART MAKES EXTRA BEATS, page 193.*

RARE

■ PULMONARY EMBOLUS
A blood clot blocking the circulation to part of the lung and usually arising from a clot in a vein in the calf.
* Sudden feeling of pressure in the chest.
* Breathlessness.
* Possibly sharp chest pain and coughing blood.
* Heart rhythms varying from fast but regular to irregular.

PALPITATIONS (INCLUDING RAPID REGULAR HEART RATE)

Strictly speaking, "palpitations" simply means an awareness of the beating of the heart but most people use it to mean not just awareness of the heart, but an awareness of some abnormality in the beat. So this symptom is subdivided into: **1** an awareness of a rapid but regular heartbeat; **2** irregular heartbeats; **3** rapid and irregular heartbeat. Extra heart beats (see the previous section) may also cause palpitations. There is much overlap between causes, so it is best to check in all relevant sections.

RAPID BUT REGULAR HEART RATE

PROBABLE
FEVER
EXERCISE
EMOTION
PAROXYSMAL TACHYCARDIA

POSSIBLE
PREGNANCY
ANEMIA
HEART FAILURE
HYPERTHYROIDISM
MEDICATIONS

RARE
ELECTRICAL CONDUCTION DISORDERS
BERI-BERI
BLEEDING
MYOCARDITIS
CARDIOMYOPATHY

PROBABLE

■ FEVER
Heart rate rises by ten beats per minute per 0.5 degree centigrade rise in temperature so that very high fevers will be accompanied by correspondingly high pulse rates. There is no specific treatment. Relief comes with the disappearance of fever.

■ EXERCISE
Any but the gentlest exercise will cause a modest rise in heart rate as the heart responds to the increased demand from the muscles and the lungs for larger quantities of oxygen-rich blood. Pulse rates above 120-130 per minute should be viewed with suspicion as a sign of over-exertion, under-fitness or some combination of the two. Chest pain appearing on exertion should always be checked with a physician *(see below)*.

■ EMOTION
Heart rate increases with excitement or acute emotional turmoil through the mechanism of the autonomic nervous system. Accompanying features include:
* Dry mouth.
* Rapid breathing.
* Tremor.

Such a response is normal in many circumstances such as fear, sexual arousal, sudden emotional shock. It is part of a co-ordinated system that prepares the body for exertion and to cope with stress. The response becomes abnormal if the individual begins to suffer from chronic anxiety, keeping his or her body in a constant state of increased arousal.

■ PAROXYSMAL TACHYCARDIA
A term used to cover all those otherwise unexplained episodes of rapid heart beat. There may be

underlying causes such as an excess of stimulants such as coffee, alcohol, cigarettes *(see HEART MAKES EXTRA BEATS, page 193)*; or from heart disease *(see this page)* or conduction disorders *(see this page)*. An ECG or Holter Monitor is used to diagnose this problem.
* Abrupt onset of rapid heart rate.
* Entirely regular rhythm.
* If rate is fast enough, faintness, lightheadedness.
* Stops as abruptly as it began.

Occasionally the rhythm is so fast or so prolonged that the heart becomes exhausted, causing breathlessness. This requires medical intervention to correct the rhythm.

POSSIBLE

■ PREGNANCY

There is a slight but sustained rise in heart rate during pregnancy, by about ten beats per minute. So if your usual rate is 70 per minute it can be expected to rise to 80 per minute. This is the way the heart copes with the demands of the growing womb, placenta and baby.

■ ANEMIA

In the anemic state there is less capacity to transport oxygen around the body. The heart compensates by increasing its speed of pumping. This will only be a noticeable feature in cases of severe anemia. Other symptoms are:
* Pale skin.
* Slight breathlessness.
* Fatigue.

Anemia alone is not a complete diagnosis. Further investigation is needed to find the cause.

■ HEART FAILURE

The early symptoms can be quite undramatic.
* Tiredness.
* Breathlessness on modest exertion.
* Increased heart rate.
* Swelling of ankles.
* Breathlessness lying flat.

Further tests are needed to determine the reason for the heart failure. *See also page 208.*

■ HYPERTHYROIDISM

The over-active gland can cause extra beats or a sustained rapid pulse. *See page 200.*

■ MEDICATIONS

There are several over-the-counter medications which can cause rapid heart rates in a few individuals, including cold remedies containing pseudoephedrine or phenylpropanolamine. Certain anti-asthmatic medications such as salbutamol may have a similar effect.

RARE

■ ELECTRICAL CONDUCTION DISORDERS

These can be thought of as short circuits in the heart which disrupt the usually smooth control of heartbeat *(see THE HEART, INTRODUCTION, page 193)*. They are relatively rare. There are surgical treatments available to cut

the abnormal electrical circuits responsible for the disorder; otherwise they are controlled by medication.
* Recurrent bursts of rapid heart rate.
* Characteristic changes on the electrocardiograph (ECG).

■ BERI-BERI
A deficiency of vitamin B1, common in Third World countries where polished rice is a staple diet. In the developed world it may occur in alcoholics with diets deficient in vitamins.
* Tender muscles.
* Rapid, bounding pulse.
* Often swollen ankles.
* Dementia, unsteady gait.

Rapid recovery is possible if it is recognized and treated early enough.

■ BLEEDING
Serious external bleeding is obvious, but internal bleeding can continue for several hours with few symptoms apart from:
* Increases in pulse rate.
* Thirst.
* Faintness on standing.
Eventually there will be:
* Pale skin.
* Cold extremities.
* Confusion, collapse.

■ MYOCARDITIS
Inflammation of the heart muscle, due to a variety of causes most of which are infections. Some possibilities are influenza, diptheria, some viruses and street drugs.
* Sudden onset of a feverish illness.
* Breathlessness, swelling of ankles.
* Breathlessness when lying flat.
* Rapid pulse.

The diagnosis requires blood tests, ECG recordings and, in difficult cases, biopsy of heart muscle.

■ CARDIOMYOPATHY
Another wide group of disorders where there is an non-inflammatory disturbance of the heart muscle. Many cases are congenital or else related to alcoholism, or due to coronary artery disease.
* Heart failure, tiredness, breathlessness.
* In young people, fainting episodes during exercise.
* Rapid heart rates which may be both regular and irregular.

Diagnosis is by ECG and heart biopsy. These disorders need medication treatment to reduce the risk of sudden serious heart rhythm disturbance.

RAPID, IRREGULAR HEARTBEATS

Most such rhythms are either atrial fibrillations or atrial flutters. Atrial fibrillation is common in old people. It may be the result of diseased coronary arteries, but frequently there are no other symptoms. The condition occasionally occurs in bursts in young people, when it is known as paroxysmal atrial fibrillation.

The basic defect is uncontrolled

The Heart

contraction of the atria, the small antechambers where blood first arrives in the heart. In fibrillation, the atria beat at rates upwards of 400 per minute, every one of those contractions sending off to the ventricles, the main pumping chambers, a signal to beat. Fortunately, only a fraction of these signals get through, but still enough to give a heart rate of between 100 to 150 beats per minute. The resulting heart rhythm is totally irregular and needs medical evaluation.

Not surprisingly, atrial fibrillation reduces the pumping efficiency of the heart and its symptoms can include breathlessness and swollen ankles. It also carries a small risk of sending off a blood clot which may cause a stroke or block arteries in the limbs. It is usual to treat fibrillation with medications which slow the rhythm and strengthen the heart.

Atrial flutter is a less common condition in which the atria beat at a regular rate of between 240-360 beats per minute. This is still too fast to trigger regular contractions of the ventricles, which beat at half or a quarter of the atrial rate (90-180 per minute). Though strictly speaking this is a *regular* rapid heart rhythm, frequently the rate keeps changing abruptly, going from 180 to 120 to 90 and back again, giving an impression of irregularity. Atrial flutter is a symptom of serious heart disease and needs hospital treatment.

Episodes lasting longer than a few minutes can exhaust the heart, sending the individual into rapid heart failure, of which increasing breathlessness is a symptom.

The causes below relate mainly to atrial fibrillation.

PROBABLE
ISCHEMIC HEART DISEASE
HYPERTHYROIDISM

POSSIBLE
MITRAL STENOSIS
ALCOHOL ABUSE
COMPLICATIONS OF HEART ATTACK

RARE
PNEUMONIA
ENDOCARDITIS
PERICARDITIS
ATRIAL SEPTAL DEFECT

PROBABLE

■ ISCHEMIC HEART DISEASE
Blockage or narrowing of the coronary arteries that supply the heart. This may produce no symptoms other than fibrillation but frequently there will also be angina; *see page 232.*

■ HYPERTHYROIDISM
Atrial fibrillation may be the only sign of an over-active thyroid gland, especially in the elderly. Thus it is routine to check for this condition, whose other symptoms include:

* Sweating.
* Tremor.
* Increased appetite.
* Protruding eyes.

POSSIBLE

■ MITRAL STENOSIS
The mitral valve separates the two left chambers of the heart. Stenosis means that the valve has become narrowed and stiff. The most common reason for this is the process of aging. Rheumatic fever can also be a cause. The condition gradually strains the heart, eventually causing heart failure.
* History of rheumatic fever years before.
* Mildest symptoms are just fibrillation.
* As the condition worsens, breathlessness, cough with bloodstained mucus.
* Eventually swelling of ankles.
* There may be a permanent purple flush over the cheek bones.

Medication is used to treat mild cases, with surgery to the valve being reserved for more severe cases.

■ ALCOHOL ABUSE
Long-term alcohol abuse weakens the muscle of the heart, allowing various rhythm disorders to result.

■ COMPLICATIONS OF HEART ATTACK
In the hours and days after a heart attack the injured heart can produce a variety of disordered rhythms. Monitoring and dealing with these ventricular rhythms is one major reason for observation in a coronary care unit after a heart attack.
* Rapid thumping in the chest.
* Faintness.
* As the condition worsens, loss of consciousness.

RARE

■ PNEUMONIA
This severe chest infection can occasionally set off atrial fibrillation, which disappears after recovery. *See page 214.*

■ ENDOCARDITIS
An infection of the valves of the heart which usually attacks valves that are already abnormal, for example, after rheumatic fever. Fibrillation is just one of a variety of symptoms.
* Night sweats.
* Feeling unwell.
* Clubbed fingernails.
* Breathlessness.
* Anemia.

Aggressive long-term antibiotic treatment is needed to eradicate the infection.

■ PERICARDITIS
Constriction of the heart by fluid or by fibrous material can give rise to fibrillation.
See PERICARDIAL EFFUSION, page 218.

■ ATRIAL SEPTAL DEFECT
There is a hole between the right and left sides of the baby's heart. This hole should close at birth, but occasionally remains open. Symptoms can take years to develop, or a murmur may be

detected on examination.
* Increased susceptibility to chest infections.
* Breathlessness.
* Palpitations including fibrillation are common.

HEART BEATS SLOWLY

By convention, this is taken as a rate of less than 60 beats per minute. Frequently it is an incidental finding in someone without symptoms, but very slow rates below 40 per minute are likely to cause dizziness, fainting and, in the elderly, confusion. There are two main causes of very slow rates. The pacemaker of the heart may be sending out a slow signal, or there is a block to the pacemaker rhythm so that the ventricles beat at a much slower rate than the signals sent from the pacemaker. An ECG or Holter Monitor is needed to diagnose these conditions effectively.

PROBABLE
FITNESS
MEDICATION-INDUCED
HEART BLOCK

POSSIBLE
HYPOTHYROIDISM
SICK SINUS SYNDROME
CONGENITAL

RARE
CARDIOMYOPATHY

Electrocardiogram (ECG) showing change in blood pressure as the heart contracts (systole) and relaxes (diastole)

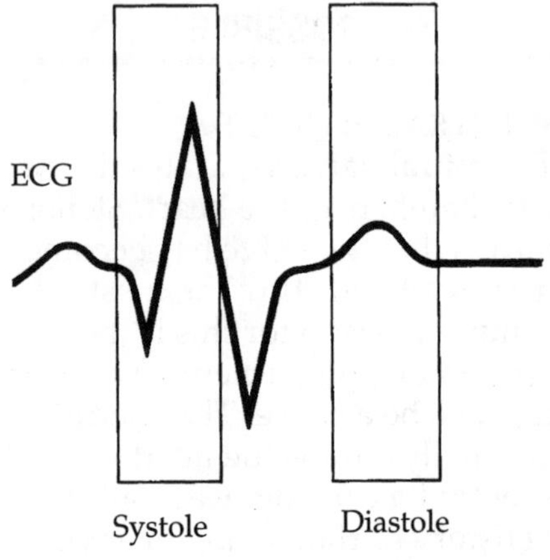

PROBABLE

■ FITNESS
A slow pulse is common in athletes and others who take regular physical exercise.

■ MEDICATION-INDUCED
Digoxin is one medication which causes a very slow pulse if given in high doses. Another widely-used class of medications called beta blockers slows the pulse to around 60 beats per minute but this is an intentional effect and is a sign of correct dosage. Beta blockers are used to treat high blood pressure and angina.

■ HEART BLOCK
Heart block comes from disease of the conducting pathways that transmit the pacemaker signal to the rest of the heart. The ventricles have their own pacemaker which

triggers them at 30 to 40 beats per minute, so there may be no dramatic symptoms, even with complete heart block. The usual reason for this problem is aging or poor blood supply to the heart. It can also happen after a heart attack. Symptoms, in increasing order of severity, include:
* None at all, but noticed on an ECG tracing.
* Awareness of a slow thudding heart beat.
* Tiredness.
* Dizzy spells.
* Recurrent abrupt loss of consciousness.

Treatment is with an artificial pacemaker to maintain regular contraction.

POSSIBLE

■ HYPOTHYROIDSM
An under-active thyroid gland, whose other symptoms include:
* Coarse dry skin.
* Sensitivity to the cold.
* Slow thought, tiredness.
* Gruff voice.

Treatment with thyroid hormone has to be life-long.

■ SICK SINUS SYNDROME
Caused by the effects of aging on the pacemaking area of the heart. This can cause rhythms from slow to fast and any combination in between.
* Palpitations.
* Dizzy spells.
* Tiredness.

See also page 196.

■ CONGENITAL
Some people are born with a slow pulse, but doctors would usually search for other signs of heart disease such as heart murmurs or abnormal ECG tracings.

RARE

■ CARDIOMYOPATHY
A general term for diseases of the heart muscle. The effect is to cause the rapid appearance of heart failure with either slow or rapid heart rates. *See also page 199.*

BREATHING INTRODUCTION

Why do we breathe? In order to provide the body's cells with the oxygen essential to their function. Also, to discharge carbon dioxide produced as a waste product of metabolism. Breathing is affected by all sorts of bodily disorders. Commonest of these are simple obstructions of the airways; heart disease is also significant.

Breathing also helps to regulate the body's acid-alkaline balance. The brain controls breathing, so diseases and medications that affect the brain may also affect breathing patterns.

This section begins with causes of sudden breathlessness, then continues with breathlessness appearing over relatively a long time period.

Causes tend to overlap, so you will see the same diagnoses coming up repeatedly. We make no apology for this: breathlessness is an alarming symptom, and some repetition is helpful.

HEIMLICH'S MANEUVER

There are references to this first-aid technique at several points in this section. It is named for the American physician who promoted this simple, life-saving procedure for someone who is choking as a result of inhaling food or other solid objects.

* Stand behind the person choking.
* Extend your arms in a hug around their upper abdomen.
* With clenched fists make a hard, fast squeeze just under the breast bone.

The maneuver forces a blast of air out of the lungs, sufficient to dislodge something stuck in the upper airway. For full details see any modern manual of first aid. All parents, teachers, and child-care personnel should learn this technique for use on babies and children.

See illustration on page 235.

RASPING, SNORING BREATHING

Also described as stertorous breathing. It is only occasionally a symptom of disease, usually just a nuisance.

Snoring is the result of vibration of the soft palate, which is at the back of the roof of the mouth. The cure is often a matter of trying out different sleeping postures, or changing the number or firmness of your pillows. *See page …*

PROBABLE
SNORING

POSSIBLE
ADENOIDS
STROKE
ALCOHOLIC STUPOR

RARE
SLEEP APNEA

PROBABLE

■ SNORING — *see page 204.*

POSSIBLE

■ ADENOIDS
These are pads of tissue at the back of the nose, similar to tonsils. In childhood, adenoids can grow so large that they obstruct nasal breathing. The child exhibits:
* Nasal speech.
* Snoring.
* Mouth breathing.
* Repeated ear infections.

Treatment is surgical removal of the adenoids, if there is no sign of a natural decrease in their size and symptoms persist.

■ STROKE
A blood clot or bleeding in the brain causing:
* One-sided paralysis.
* Coma.
* Stertorous breathing, typically if the individual goes into a deep coma.

■ ALCOHOLIC STUPOR
Drinking to the point of collapse frequently gives this symptom.

RARE

■ SLEEP APNEA
Partial obstruction of the trachea (a major airway), during sleep. This causes partial suffocation until the individual briefly awakes, snorts to relieve the obstruction, and goes back to sleep again. The typical picture is:
* Grossly overweight.
* Daytime drowsiness.

Occasionally people with this condition benefit from oxygen masks during sleep. Sometimes surgery is needed.

HOARSE, "WHEEZY" INTAKE OF BREATH

This is probably a stridor: *see FOREIGN BODY, PAGE 226.*

CHEST ABNORMALLY SHAPED

PROBABLE
CONGENITAL
ASTHMA

CHEST

POSSIBLE
CHRONIC OBSTRUCTIVE PULMONARY DISEASE (COPD)

RARE
RICKETS

PROBABLE

■ CONGENITAL
A spinal defect at birth. Twists of the spine (scoliosis) can gradually produce a mis-shapen chest. These can be treated if found early.
* Seen from behind, the spine is curved.
* Curve becomes more prominent on bending forward.

Another congenital abnormality gives a funnel-shaped chest with a depressed breastbone. This too can be corrected by surgery, which is recommended if there is a risk of the depression pressing on the heart.

■ ASTHMA
Chronic, severe asthma which is inadequately treated can result in a young adult who has:
* A broad, over-inflated chest.
* Prominent rib margins.
* Prominent breastbone, which gives a pointed appearance to the front of the chest.

The cause is thought to be years of extra effort by the muscles between the ribs, which have to work harder in asthma. They gradually pull the lower ribs into a prominent shape. This is seen less and less as asthma treatment improves. The condition rarely causes anything other than cosmetic problems and can be corrected surgically.

POSSIBLE

■ CHRONIC OBSTRUCTIVE PULMONARY DISEASE (COPD)
A general term covering chronic bronchitis and emphysema. The continual effort of breathing in these conditions can eventually, in adult life, cause a barrel-shaped chest. *See page 222.*

RARE

■ RICKETS
This disease, due to lack of vitamin D, can cause unsightly prominent joints where the ribs join the breast bone. Now a rarity in developed countries.

BREATHLESSNESS, RAPID ONSET

Considered here are attacks of breathlessness which happen rapidly, yet fall short of abrupt suffocation or asphyxia. There should be little difficulty in recognizing the seriousness of the situation, except perhaps with babies and children: you should be alert to drowsiness and breathlessness which interferes with feeding.

PROBABLE
ASTHMA
BRONCHIOLITIS
LUNG INFECTION

POSSIBLE
HEART FAILURE
ACUTE OR CHRONIC BRONCHITIS
PNEUMOTHORAX ANXIETY

RARE
ALLERGIC ALVEOLITIS

PROBABLE

■ ASTHMA

This common illness can occasionally turn suddenly and unpredictably into a life-threatening condition.

Muscle surrounds the airways right down into the lungs. Asthma results from excessive contraction of muscle, which narrows the airways and increases the effort required to move air into the lungs. As a cause of chronic breathlessness *ASTHMA* is covered in detail under *BREATHLESSNESS AND WHEEZE, page 211.* Severe, acute asthma is a potential killer. There is danger for the known asthmatic who underestimates the severity of an attack. There is also danger for someone whose first attack of asthma is severe, unrecognized and who has no medication available.

* Poor response to usual medication.
* Wheeze, especially breathing out.
* The chest feels "tight".
* Sweating, breathlessness, rapid pulse.
* Neck muscles strain in an attempt to increase breathing.
* As attack worsens, blue lips, tiredness, pallor, drowsiness.
* Confusion, coma.
* Deterioration can take several hours or just a few minutes.

Known asthmatics must seek, or be given, help if their regular treatment becomes ineffective.

■ BRONCHIOLITIS

This is an infantile equivalent of asthma. It is a winter disease, caused by a particular virus. It often occurs in epidemics.

* Initially the baby is snuffly, with a slight cough indistinguishable from a common cold.
* Wheezing begins and worsens over a few hours.
* Breathing produces a crackling sound, also felt through the chest.
* Breathlessness interferes with feeding.
* Breathing becomes rapid, often with grunting.
* When severe, blue lips and pale skin.

First aid: run hot water in bath-tub or shower and hold child in the steam to improve breathing. Call emergency service, if child is lethargic, and transport child to hospital quickly.

Children whose parents smoke are three times more likely to enter hospital in their first year with a breathing problem or infection of the airways than infants of non-smokers.

CHEST

■ LUNG INFECTION
A severe lung infection or pneumonia can rapidly progress to difficulty in breathing.
* Wet cough, with colored mucus.
* High temperature.
* Flaring nostrils.
* Rapid breathing.
* Pain over the affected part of the chest.
* Blue lips and tongue.
* Sometimes bloodstained mucus.
* Confusion.

This is more likely in the elderly or in those who are debilitated for other reasons.

POSSIBLE

■ HEART FAILURE
Predominantly a disease occurring later in life. There is often a history of heart trouble, perhaps heart attack, high blood pressure.
* Early symptoms are tiredness, breathlessness on exertion.
* Swelling of ankles
* Breathlessness worse on attempting to lie flat.
* You need to stack up pillows in order to sleep.
* In more advanced cases you may wake from sleep with a feeling of suffocation.
* Copious, frothy, pinkish mucus.
* Relief gained from sitting upright for a few minutes.

This situation needs urgent medical help.

■ ACUTE OR CHRONIC BRONCHITIS
An infection can be the minor, extra stress that pushes the individual with chronic bronchitis into respiratory failure. The already limited effort that someone can put into breathing becomes too little to expel waste carbon dioxide, or to take in fresh oxygen. The result is the equivalent of suffocation over a short period.
* Severe headache.
* Warm, blue hands; rapid pulse; twitching of muscles.
* Agitation, confusion worsening to coma.

This situation needs urgent attention with immediate oxygen administration.

■ PNEUMOTHORAX
See page 227.

■ ANXIETY
Extreme nervousness can produce rapid breathing and a feeling of breathlessness (hyperventilation) in otherwise healthy people.

RARE

■ ALLERGIC ALVEOLITIS
The alveoli are the sacs in the lung where carbon dioxide is exchanged for oxygen. An allergic reaction causes inflammation in these sacs. The subsequent swelling interferes with gas transfer. It is caused by allergies to natural fibers, molds and grain dusts.
* Breathlessness, wheezing within a few hours of exposure.
* Fever, cough, feeling sick and joint pains.
* Symptoms take a few days to disappear. The chronic condition shows:
* Recurrent difficulty in breathing.

* Clubbed (highly curved) fingernails *(see illustration on page 296)*.Treatment is to avoid exposure to the cause of the allergy.

BREATHLESSNESS OVER DAYS, WEEKS OR MONTHS

This type of breathlessness does not have particularly prominent secondary symptoms, at least not at first. And there are no hard and fast distinctions between all the conditions which share these symptoms, so read this section right through before drawing any conclusions.

Breathlessness that sets in over only a few days or weeks clearly needs medical evaluation.

Breathlessness that appears more gradually can be more puzzling. It should be related to your usual level of exercise. If your principal form of physical activity is opening the garage door, do not be too surprised at your breathlessness if you have to change a tire. Remember also that your ability to cope with sudden effort can decline completely unnoticed as long as you are still able to perform your regular activities. For example: shopping trips and gentle strolls may present no problem, but you may be alarmed at how breathless you become climbing stairs. This does not in itself suggest disease; it means you are not fit.

But there is a pitfall in this: while it is natural to limit exertion to the level you know you can tolerate, that level may actually be abnormally low. The best guide is to compare yourself with others of your age and general fitness. If you are the one who has to rest half-way round a golf course you may have a problem.

Bear this in mind before you jump to conclusions. Ask yourself a few questions. How long since you last did any exercise that made you sweat? Have you gained weight recently? Do you smoke heavily?

Honest answers to these questions may be helpful.

There are other, everyday circumstances in which breathlessness is normal. Excitement, fear and anger all generate a high breathing rate and may make you feel breathless. Only after you have excluded all these possibilities is it reasonable to wonder whether your breathlessness is a symptom of illness:

PROBABLE

HEART FAILURE

CHEST

POSSIBLE
PREGNANCY
ANEMIA
LUNG EFFUSION
LUNG CANCER

RARE
SKELETAL ABNORMALITIES
PNEUMONCONIOSIS
MOUNTAIN SICKNESS
FIBROSING ALVEOLITIS

PROBABLE

■ HEART FAILURE
Mainly a problem for older people. The symptoms of heart failure can mistakenly be put down to aging unless a dramatic or sudden deterioration occurs. There will often be a history of high blood pressure, angina or heart attack. Early symptoms are:
* Tiredness, decreased tolerance of exercise.
* Swelling of ankles.
* Loss of appetite.
* Later, breathlessness while lying flat in bed.
* You sleep stacked up on pillows.
* Breathlessness wakes you at night, with a frothy cough; symptoms pass off after you have sat upright for a while.

In the elderly, tiredness alone can be the only symptom of heart failure. Treatment is currently undergoing a great change for the better, so that most people can be helped considerably.

POSSIBLE

■ PREGNANCY
A common feature of middle to late pregnancy, when the womb is enlarged and presses against the diaphragm

■ ANEMIA
Red blood cells carry oxygen around the body, so that if the volume of blood in one's body drops significantly, breathlessness results, together with:
* Tiredness, easy fatigue.
* Pallor on the under-surfaces of eyelids, nail beds.

Symptoms of the disorder which causes the anemia may also be apparent, for example blood loss, poor diet. Simple tests should quickly confirm the diagnosis.

■ LUNG EFFUSION
The lungs react to irritation in the same way that the skin reacts to a minor burn. Tissue fluid seeps out, collecting in a pool at the base of the lungs. If this pool grows large enough, it compresses the lung above, reducing its ability to function and causing breathlessness. There are no specific symptoms to indicate an effusion: it has to be detected by medical examination or chest X-ray. There is nearly always some predisposing condition. The commonest are severe heart failure, pneumonia, pulmonary embolus and lung cancer. These cause symptoms considered under *HEART FAILURE, page 208, and on pages 214, 218 and 223.*

■ LUNG CANCER
A tumor may block off a major airway, thereby putting out of action all or part of a lung, and causing breathlessness. This is not a common way for a growth to show itself. More frequent is a cough with blood or chest pain. Considered in detail on *page 223.*

RARE

■ SKELETAL ABNORMALITIES
Gross distortions of the chest wall cause the ribs to squash the lungs and heart so that their expansion is restricted. These deformities, called *KYPHOSIS or KYPHO-SCOLIOSIS, are discussed on page 288.*

■ PNEUMOCONIOSIS
A group of occupational lung diseases caused by years of exposure to dust. Common ones are silicosis, pneumoconiosis, asbestosis and byssinosis. The symptoms are:
* Progressive breathlessness on exertion.
* Cough.

Dust control and masks reduce the risks for workers in hazardous industries.

■ MOUNTAIN SICKNESS
The direct effect of the lack of oxygen at altitudes of about 3,000 meters or higher. The young and fit are at risk just as much as the unfit or elderly; in fact, possibly more at risk because the young will be climbing faster. This is a dangerous condition. Early symptoms are:
* Breathlessness.
* Headache, tiredness.

If ignored these will progress to:
* Profuse bloodstained cough.
* Nausea, confusion.
* Coma.

All cases must descend to lower altitudes; serious cases may also require resuscitation.

■ FIBROSING ALVEOLITIS
The final stage of *ALLERGIC ALVEOLITIS (see page 208)*, or sometimes of unknown origin.
* Chronic breathlessness.
* Clubbed fingernails *(see page 296).*
* Cough, blue lips and fingers.

BREATHLESSNESS AND WHEEZE

Excluding acute chest infection, considered *on page 223*, this extremely common combination points to narrowing of airways, producing obstructed air flow. Often there is an allergic factor: many asthmatics, sensitive to dust and fumes, exhibit these symptoms for hours, even days on end.

PROBABLE
ASTHMA
CHRONIC BRONCHITIS
EMPHYSEMA

POSSIBLE
OCCUPATIONAL ASTHMA

CHEST

RARE

MEDICATION REACTION
ASPERGILLOSIS

PROBABLE

■ ASTHMA

This is an increasing problem. The classic symptoms are:
* Recurrent breathlessness.
* Wheeze and cough.
* In children, persistent night-time cough.
* Common colds that regularly go to the chest.

Physicians are often disinclined to label a child as asthmatic until there is no doubt: it can be a disservice to the child. Effective treatment is available. *See also page 220.*

■ CHRONIC BRONCHITIS (COPD)

Believed to result from years of exposure to fumes, chemicals and smoke, of which cigarette smoke is the main avoidable cause. The prime features are the gradual increase of:
* Increasingly persistent cough.
* Wheeze.
* Breathlessness.
* Large amounts of mucus ("smoker's cough").

Chronic bronchitis does not have the same reputation as lung cancer, yet quality of life can be considerably reduced. Perpetual breathlessness, in severe cases, is every bit as miserable as the final stages of cancer.

■ EMPHYSEMA

Whereas normal lungs look like sponges with millions of tiny bubbles, in emphysemic lungs, large holes replace many of the small bubbles. This is much less efficient as a means of gas exchange, hence the breathlessness. Emphysema and chronic bronchitis nearly always co-exist, the symptoms emerging over several years.
* Breathlessness and wheeze on exertion.
* A barrel chest.
* Lips pursed to breathe out.
* Eventual cyanosis (blueness) of hands and tongue.

The damage to the structure of the lungs cannot be reversed.

Treatment aims to prevent further damage by discouraging smoking, preventing exposure to fumes and treating associated bronchitis.

POSSIBLE

■ OCCUPATIONAL ASTHMA

This includes many conditions associated with specific industries, in particular those producing flax, sisal, hemp or cotton. Bysinnosis is one of the commonest of these problems. It produces an asthma-like condition through allergy to cotton dust.
* A hazard in cotton mills.
* "Monday morning breathlessness" on re-exposure to cotton dust.
* Wheeze, breathlessness.

RARE

■ MEDICATION REACTION
The medications in widest use that can produce this reaction are beta-blockers, used to control high blood pressure or angina; aspirin and similar anti-rheumatic medications, and a few anti-cancer medications such as methotrexate, may also be responsible.

■ ASPERGILLOSIS
An infection caused by a fungus called aspergillus, commonly found in rotting and decaying vegetation. For most people, aspergillus is harmless. If the lungs are damaged by previous infection (such as tuberculosis) or asthma, the fungus may cause the following symptoms:
* Recurrent wheeze, cough.
* Feverish episodes.
The diagnosis is determined by blood tests and allergy testing.

BREATHLESSNESS AND COUGH

PROBABLE
CHEST INFECTION

POSSIBLE
CHRONIC BRONCHITIS
EMPHYSEMA
PNEUMONIA

RARE
BRONCHIECTASIS
LUNG CANCER
TUBERCULOSIS

PROBABLE

■ CHEST INFECTION
Recognized by the combination of:
* Cough with yellow or green mucus.
* Fever, feel unwell.
* Breathlessness plus wheeze.
All these appear in only a couple of days, often preceded by a sore throat and a common cold.
Antibiotic treatment is usual for these common and not very serious infections.

POSSIBLE

■ CHRONIC BRONCHITIS
The strict medical definition is:
* A cough productive of mucus for at least three months of the year for at least two consecutive years.
It is well known that smokers and workers in dusty environments risk developing the condition, but it also has an association with cold damp climates. The excessive production of mucus amounts to an exaggeration of the lungs' defence mechanism against infection and dust: the gooey mucus "traps" the foreign matter, which the lungs then try to expel by coughing. Individuals are at risk of frequent chest infections and, in the long

CHEST

run, progressive shortness of breath.

Though the disease cannot be reversed, further deterioration can be delayed by giving up smoking and by avoiding dust and fumes.

■ EMPHYSEMA

Often co-exists with chronic bronchitis, but can only be diagnosed by chest X-ray in combination with lung function tests. However, it is suggested by:
* A barrel chest.
* Lips pursed to breathe out.
* At worst, cyanosis (blueness) of lips and nail beds.

■ PNEUMONIA

A serious chest infection, usually of rapid onset with:
* High fever, chills.
* Rapid breathing and cough.
* Mucus may be rust-colored or obviously contain blood.
* Aching, or severe sharp pain, in the chest.

Occasionally, especially in the elderly or people with medical problems, pneumonia exhibits less clear-cut symptoms, and is suggested by abrupt weakness, fever and confusion. Aggressive antibiotic therapy is needed.

RARE

■ BRONCHIECTASIS

In this disease, once far more common than it is today, the lung structure breaks down, making the lungs susceptible to pockets of chronic infection.
* Initially, frequent chest infections.
* Constant production of large amounts of colored mucus.
* Mucus often bloodstained.
* As it worsens, breathlessness, clubbed (highly curved) fingernails.
* Poor growth in children; fatigue.

■ LUNG CANCER

This diagnosis must be considered not only for a cough with breathlessness but for any persistent breathing problem. Adult smokers are particularly vulnerable. *See page* 223.

■ TUBERCULOSIS

Developing drug-resistant strains have made this disease more common than it was five or ten years ago. Most vulnerable are drug addicts, people who live in prisons and shelters, people who are immuno-compromised (AIDS patients and the elderly).The usual features are:
* Sickness, weight loss.
* Cough, often bloodstained.
* Breathlessness resulting from complications.

Treatment, though prolonged, cures the disease.

BREATHLESSNESS AND FEELING TIRED/EXHAUSTED

Though lung disease is usually the cause of breathlessness, it can arise from subtle changes in the condition of the heart, blood or metabolism. Fatigue will then be a prominent symptom, before breathlessness is noticeable. Breathlessness in these situations may result from an imbalance between acid and alkaline chemicals in the body. Diabetes and kidney failure generate excess acid which the body tries to reduce by blowing off more carbon dioxide with heavy deep breathing.

Remember that prolonged or severe breathlessness, for any reason, will eventually cause fatigue simply through exhaustion and a chronic lack of oxygen.

PROBABLE
ANEMIA
HEART FAILURE

POSSIBLE
HEART DISEASE

RARE
DIABETIC COMPLICATIONS
KIDNEY FAILURE

PROBABLE

■ ANEMIA
Red blood cells carry oxygen around the body so that if the volume of blood drops significantly breathlessness ensues, together with:
* Tiredness, easy fatigue.
* Pallor, particularly the under-surfaces of eyelids, nail beds.

Symptoms of the disorder which causes the anemia may be evident, for example blood loss, poor diet. Simple investigations indicate the diagnosis. *See pages 417-424.*

■ HEART FAILURE
Breathlessness is a frequent symptom in the middle-aged; in the elderly an early indication of heart failure can be unusual tiredness. Once this is recognized, look for other symptoms of heart failure:
* Swollen ankles.
* Breathlessness when lying flat.

See page 208.

POSSIBLE

■ HEART DISEASE
Disturbance of heartbeat with rhythms either too fast or too slow, felt as a flutter in the chest, or as palpitations. These are inefficient rhythms producing breathlessness with fatigue. *See pages 193-203.*

Other heart diseases, for instance valve problems, cause breathlessness by decreasing the efficiency of the heart. In general, these disorders can only be detected by medical examination.

CHEST

RARE

■ DIABETIC COMPLICATIONS

Diabetes is the condition that produces a high blood sugar level. The early symptoms are:
* Passing large amounts of urine.
* Thirst.
* Weight loss.

In young people, onset tends to be rapid, over a couple of weeks. In older people it may go unnoticed, apart from slightly increased urine output and a vague sense of tiredness.

Diabetes is caused by a lack of insulin, needed by the body's cells to make use of sugar. Thus, there are high levels of sugar in the bloodstream, yet the cells are unable to use it. But life must go on: the cells' metabolism turns to alternative means of generating energy. The trouble with these is their tendency to produce large amounts of acidic waste products. The body tries to compensate by blowing off large amounts of carbon dioxide, hence heavy breathing.

Meanwhile, sugar in the bloodstream spills out through the kidneys, dragging water with it. The final result is the dangerous state called diabetic ketoacidosis, and is a major medical emergency.
* Dehydration, dry mouth, intense thirst.
* Deep, sighing breathing.
* Sweet smell on breath.
* Confusion, nausea.

Rapid treatment is required to save the person's life. Known diabetics may develop acidosis during other stressful illnesses.

■ KIDNEY FAILURE

Early symptoms are only:
* Increased passage of urine.
* Tiredness.

Blood tests at this stage allow diagnosis and consequent changes in diet which may give years of reasonable health. If eventually the kidneys fail there is an array of symptoms, including:
* Tiredness, developing into confusion.
* Deep, gasping breathing.
* Dry, furred tongue.
* Nausea, hiccups.
* Itching, anemia.

The development of kidney transplantation has revolutionized the treatment of this condition.

BREATHLESSNESS AND CHEST PAIN

Symptoms of this kind are often caused by serious disruption of the output from the heart, or by lung malfunction. If breathlessness is the most prominent symptom, *see ASPHYXIA, page 225, or BREATHLESSNESS, RAPID ONSET, page 206*, as well as reading this section. If chest pain is most prominent, look at the sections on heart beat. In view of the importance of these symptoms, some of the information found there is repeated here.

PROBABLE
CHEST INFECTION
HEART ATTACK
PLEURISY
PNEUMOTHORAX

POSSIBLE
PNEUMONIA
PULMONARY EMBOLUS
LUNG CANCER
IRREGULAR HEARTBEAT

RARE
PERICARDIAL EFFUSION
HEART TAMPONADE

PROBABLE

■ CHEST INFECTION
The gradual appearance of fever, cough and mucus is often accompanied by a slight ache over both lungs. *See page 208.*

■ HEART ATTACK
See also page 229.

In a middle-aged or older person person, suspect a heart attack if there is:
* Sudden central chest pain.
* Sweating.
* Pain radiating up to the jaws or into the left arm.
* Breathlessness.

These are the classic symptoms, but in quite a few cases the heart attack is "silent", meaning that chest pain is not the most obvious feature or may be absent. Instead, a heart attack may be suspected on the basis of:
* Sudden general tiredness.
* Breathlessness as a new symptom.
* Sudden worsening of existing breathlessness.
* Symptoms of heart failure: swollen ankles, breathlessness when lying flat, breathlessness during the night, tiredness.

Recently, there have been major advances in treatment so that early recognition of the problem means a much-improved chance of recovery. It is, therefore, essential to establish the diagnosis as soon as possible. Heart attacks are most common in old people, but are possible at any age; so always take dramatic chest pain seriously.

■ PLEURISY
The thin membranes that surround the lungs become inflamed for a variety of reasons, particularly infection. There will be knife-like pain over a small area of the chest.
* Pain worse on breathing in.
* Breathlessness as a consequence of avoiding deep breathing.

Pleurisy commonly accompanies a chest infection. In this case, it sets in gradually over a few hours.

Treatment aims both to relieve the pain and to cure the underlying condition.

■ PNEUMOTHORAX
Sudden pain and collapse of part of a lung, sometimes the whole lung on one side. Quite common and needs urgent evaluation. The pain may be disabling.

CHEST

POSSIBLE

■ PNEUMONIA
Suggested by a combination of:
* High fever.
* Rapid breathing.
* Painful cough.

See also page 214.

■ PULMONARY EMBOLUS
A blood clot which lodges in the blood supply to a lung. Sudden breathlessness follows the reduction in the lung's efficiency. Pain in the chest is not always a symptom, but will certainly be felt if the affected part of the lung begins to die from lack of oxygen. A particular risk after a heart attack, major surgery or thrombosis in leg.

■ LUNG CANCER
This diagnosis should always be borne in mind when unusual breathlessness and chest pain are the symptoms in elderly individuals, particularly those who smoke. *See page 224.*

■ IRREGULAR HEART BEAT
Very rapid or very slow heart rates can cause chest pain, with breathlessness a result of low output from the heart. *See sections on heartbeat, pages 193-203.*

RARE

■ PERICARDIAL EFFUSION
The heart is surrounded by a lining which can become inflamed. This is known as pericarditis. The fluid released from inflammation collects around the heart, interfering with its ability to pump blood effectively. Most often, this condition follows a heart attack. Viral infections, trauma and kidney failure are other causes.
* At first, the sharp central chest pain of pericarditis.
* Pain seems to radiate to shoulders.
* Often relieved by bending forward; worse lying down.
* Breathlessness, worsening as fluid builds up.

This is not an easy diagnosis, but may be the reason for breathlessness after certain diseases. X-rays and ECGs help confirm the diagnosis.

■ HEART TAMPONADE
This is the most severe effect of a pericardial effusion. The condition may begin with pericarditis *(this page)* or perhaps an injury to the heart, such as a stab wound. Fluid or blood gathers around the heart until it is squashed and unable to pump. There are no straightforward or obvious symptoms apart from rapidly increasing breathlessness after the illness or injury which caused the pericarditis; occasionally swollen veins in the neck may also be observed.

Diagnosis is by ECG recording and chest X-ray. Treatment is to drain off the fluid.

CHEST SYMPTOMS, COUGH INTRODUCTION

Cough is generally a reflex action of irritated lungs or voice box, or lungs trying to expel mucus or a foreign body. Most coughs are easily recognizable for the minor problem they are, but sometimes need to be taken more seriously because of duration, pain or associated symptoms. In the very young and the elderly, coughs can be a sign of more serious illness and need more attention.

DRY COUGH WITHOUT MUCUS

Few of us pass a year without suffering this sort of cough. It nearly always reflects minor irritation of the lungs rather than more serious disease. It passes in a week or so of using simple remedies, such as tylenol or plenty of fluid and avoiding a dry atmosphere.

If there are other symptoms of illness, such as raised temperature lasting more than 48 hours, or if the cough becomes chronic, it would be sensible to see a physician.

PROBABLE

COMMON COLD OR UPPER RESPIRATORY INFECTION (URI)
IRRITANT ATMOSPHERE
POST NASAL DRIP

POSSIBLE

LARYNGITIS
TRACHEITIS
ASTHMA
HABIT
WHOOPING COUGH

RARE

LUNG CANCER
ASBESTOSIS, ALLERGY, FIBROSING ALVEOLITIS
MEDICATION SIDE-EFFECT
DISEASE OF LARYNX

PROBABLE

■ COMMON COLD OR URI

Cough, commonly accompanied by other common cold symptoms such as:
* Rapid onset of sneezing, congestion and aches.
* Usually cures itself.

■ IRRITANT ATMOSPHERE

* Dry, dusty conditions.
* Cough is relieved in a more humid atmosphere.
* Not otherwise ill.

Chest

■ POST NASAL DRIP
Secretions from the nose or from the sinuses run to the back of throat and provoke cough. Treatment is aimed at the underlying condition, the commonest being chronic sinusitis, hay fever and (in children) adenoid trouble.

POSSIBLE

■ LARYNGITIS
A common winter illness causing many of the symptoms of the common cold but also:
* Raw feeling in the throat.
* Hoarseness or loss of voice.
* Often develops into chest infection.

■ TRACHEITIS
Rather similar to laryngitis, but:
* Raw feeling more in lower neck/upper chest.
* Often "goes to the chest".
* Rasping feeling behind breastbone.

■ ASTHMA
One of the commonest causes of chronic cough at all ages. The diagnosis, often difficult to make because cough can be caused by so many factors, is suggested by:
* Recurrent wheeze and breathlessness, particularly after exertion. However:
* A frequent, dry, night-time cough may be the first symptom, especially in children.
* Close relative(s) are very often asthmatic, too.
* Associated with eczema and hay fever.

■ HABIT
* Not otherwise unwell.
* Worsens if attention given, goes when distracted.
* Worse if nervous.

■ WHOOPING COUGH
* Causes paroxysms of cough to the point of breathlessness, followed by a whoop as air is breathed rapidly. Mainly a disease of childhood, now increasingly rare, thanks to immunization.
* In adults, repeated, milder paroxysms can occur for weeks.
* Typically in epidemics.

RARE

■ LUNG CANCER
See page 223.

■ ASBESTOSIS, ALLERGIC, FIBROSING ALVEOLITIS
These are chronic conditions of progressive cough, breathlessness and wheezing.
* Associated with working in dusty industries such as coal, silica, cotton, farming.
* Cough, breathlessness, wheeze progressive over months and years.
* Finger clubbing *(see illustration page 296)*. The precise cause is unknown.

■ MEDICATION SIDE-EFFECT
An unpredictable side effect of ACE inhibitors, used to treat high blood pressure.

■ TUMOR OR INFECTION OF LARYNX
* Persistent hoarseness, pain in neck, enlarged glands in neck. *See page 126.*

Three other conditions — MEDIASTINAL COMPRESSION, IRRITATION OF THE DIAPHRAGM and POLYARTERITIS NODOSA — have cough as a symptom.

The first occurs when organs inside the chest are squeezed by tumors. The second is caused by a liver abscess or an abscess beneath the diaphragm and the third is a disease causing generalized inflammation of the blood vessels.

These conditions are not only exceptionally rare but have an array of other symptoms — including breathlessness and progressive weight-loss (cancer); rashes and joint pains (polyarteritis nodosa); sweats and breathlessness (abscess). Among these, cough is relatively minor.

All of these symptoms require early medical attention.

COUGH PLUS MUCUS

Most likely to be caused by a minor infection of the lungs, which in most people will settle rapidly. Those with other serious conditions such as heart disease or diabetes may need antibiotics to control the infection.

CHEST

PROBABLE
COMMON COLD — UPPER RESPIRATORY INFECTION (URI)
BRONCHITIS
CHEST INFECTION

POSSIBLE
CHRONIC BRONCHITIS
EMPHYSEMA
PNEUMONIA

RARE
BRONCHIECTASIS
TUBERCULOSIS
LUNG ABSCESS
INHALED FOREIGN BODY
PNEUMOCONIOSIS
CYSTIC FIBROSIS
AIDS

PROBABLE

■ COMMON COLD OR URI
* After first few days, a "wet" cough with colored mucus, but otherwise feeling well.

■ BRONCHITIS
* Cough, mucus and wheeze.
* Feeling mildly unwell.
* Some breathlessness.

■ CHEST INFECTION
* Cough, copious mucus, fever.
* Sweats and feeling unwell.
* Onset over a day or two.
* May be accompanied by pleurisy — a knife-like pain under the ribs when breathing in.

CHEST

POSSIBLE

■ CHRONIC BRONCHITIS
* Cough, mucus and wheeze for weeks on end, possibly for most of the year. A disease especially of smokers, long-term exposure to dusty atmospheres and of people who live in damp, northern climates. Don't dismiss the morning "smoker's cough"; this is your lungs telling you that they are being damaged by fumes — their reaction is to push out large amounts of mucus.
* Frequent episodes of bronchitis, summer and winter.
* Chronic cough.
* Breathlessness eventually becomes a constant feature.

It is essential to give up smoking.

■ EMPHYSEMA
* A late development of chronic bronchitis or asthma, giving breathlessness and constant wheezing.
* Ability to breathe deeply decreases.
* Barrel-shaped chest may be a later sign.

Chest X-ray and lung function tests needed to confirm diagnosis.

■ PNEUMONIA
A serious infection of part or all of one lung. You feel very ill.
* Rapid onset.
* Breathlessness or fast breathing.
* General aching, tiredness, cough.
* Sweats — sometimes drenching, especially at night.
* Pain over affected part of lung.

RARE

■ BRONCHIECTASIS
A disease in which the structure of the lungs breaks down, reducing their efficiency.
* Gradual appearance of chronic cough, with copious mucus.
* Bad breath.

Chest X-ray needed to confirm diagnosis.

■ TUBERCULOSIS
* Chronic fatigue, feeling sick, weight loss, loss of appetite *(see page 473)*.
* Groups especially at risk are: the poor, those with overcrowded housing, alcoholics, drug addicts, people with AIDS.

■ LUNG ABSCESS
See under COUGH PLUS BLOODY MUCUS.

■ INHALED FOREIGN BODY
* Typically in children. A child can (unnoticed) inhale a peanut or similar small object. A coughing fit probably follows. Chest infection plus typical symptoms *(see page 223)* then develops, and never really clears. If these symptoms are neglected, the child becomes listless and run-down after several weeks. Inhaling a foreign body sometimes creates stridor; *see ASPHYXIA, page 225.*

Chest X-ray needed to confirm diagnosis.

■ PNEUMOCONIOSIS
A group of diseases in which the lungs become stiffer and stiffer,

unable to expand properly.
* Associated with dusty industries such as coal, silica, cotton and farming.
* Cough, breathlessness, wheeze progressive over months and years.
* Finger clubbing: *see page 296.*

■ CYSTIC FIBROSIS
A childhood disease, caused by inherited genetic abnormality.
* Repeated chest infections, failure to grow.
* Diarrhea, weight loss.

■ AIDS
Groups especially at risk are intravenous drug users, prostitutes and their clients, homosexuals and bisexuals.
* Weeks of sickness, weight loss, fatigue, fevers, swollen glands.

Diagnosis confirmed by blood tests. Sputum culture will show unusual organisms.

COUGH PLUS BLOODY MUCUS

This is an "alert" signal. Never ignore it. In older people (50 plus) and especially in smokers it calls for careful investigation. In younger people there is more likely to be a relatively innocent cause. Even so, they should have an immediate check-up.

Remember that many cases of cough plus bloody mucus are eventually diagnosed as "cause unknown"— the symptom simply goes away.

PROBABLE
CHEST INFECTION

POSSIBLE
PNEUMONIA
LUNG CANCER
BRONCHIECTASIS
CAUSE UNKNOWN

RARE
HEART FAILURE
MITRAL STENOSIS

PROBABLE

■ CHEST INFECTION
* Yellowish or greenish mucus which contains streaks or blobs of blood, possibly red, possibly rust-colored. Not an uncommon symptom.
* Mildly unwell with raised temperature and aches.

POSSIBLE

■ PNEUMONIA
See page 214. The infection causes so much inflammation that blood oozes into the lungs where it mixes with mucus.

■ LUNG CANCER
There is now little doubt that smoking causes most cases of this, one of the commonest cancers. Smokers in particular, and especially smokers in the 50-plus

age range, should be alert to the early warning signs because the sooner the disease is diagnosed, the better the results of treatment, and the outlook of treatment is slowly improving.

None of these symptoms on their own is absolutely diagnostic of lung cancer, indeed they often prove to be false alarms. However, this is a situation when over-caution is to be encouraged, particularly if you are in the risk group. Combinations of two or more symptoms should arouse increased suspicion.

* A persistent cough, whether dry or with mucus. Smokers get used to smokers' coughs, making it all the more important to be aware if the cough worsens. An early lung tumor causes this symptom by irritating the lining of the air passages.

* Frequent or unusually persistent chest infections. This can mean that a small tumor is acting as a focus for repeated infection.

* Coughing blood. Even small amounts mixed with sputum should be investigated and all the more so if the cough produces pure blood. A small tumor can have this effect by oozing blood from its surface.

* Breathlessness — because a tumor has caused collapse of part of a lung.

* Persistent pain or ache in the chest, due to inflammation from a tumor.

* Loss of appetite and weight. For reasons not clearly understood, many cancers cause loss of weight and appetite before the cancer has otherwise shown itself.

Ninety five per cent of lung cancer cases are due to smoking. It is increasingly recognized that the remaining five per cent may largely be caused by passive smoking.

■ BRONCHIECTASIS

See page 222.

■ CAUSE UNKNOWN

* Despite thorough investigation, in some cases the cause remains unknown.

RARE

■ HEART FAILURE

* Gradual onset of breathlessness, swollen ankles, inability to lie flat.

* Frothy pink sputum, rather than pure blood.

■ MITRAL STENOSIS

* History of rheumatic fever — *see page 448.*

* Gradual development of breathlessness, fatigue, dilated veins on cheekbones, giving a "flushed" appearance, breathlessness when lying flat.

COUGH, BLOODY MUCUS and CHEST PAIN

Pain in the lungs points to inflammation or injury of the pleura the thin outer layer that covers the lungs. Inflammation of the pleura frequently accompanies chest infections, when it is called pleurisy.

PROBABLE
CHEST INFECTION

POSSIBLE
PNEUMONIA
PULMONARY EMBOLUS
CHEST INJURY

RARE
LUNG CANCER WITH BONE SPREAD

PROBABLE

■ CHEST INFECTION
See page 223.

POSSIBLE

■ PNEUMONIA
See page 214.

The mucus is typically rust-colored (that is, bloodstained) rather than containing pure blood and is otherwise green or yellow due to the underlying infection.

■ PULMONARY EMBOLUS
This is a blood clot blocking blood flow to part of a lung. Symptoms may range from mild, knife-like chest pain to collapse.
* Increased risk after surgery, in the obese, in those recovering from a heart attack, in women on the contraceptive pill and during pregnancy.
* Coughing blood.
* Pain worse on breathing in.
* If the embolus is large, faintness and sweating, collapse.
* The cause may be a leg thrombosis if the calf is swollen and painful. *See page 310.*

■ CHEST INJURY
Caused by an injury severe enough to damage the lungs directly, or to break a rib, which then punctures a lung.
* Knife-like pains.
* Worse on breathing in.

RARE

■ LUNG CANCER WITH SECONDARY SPREAD TO BONES
In the later stages of lung cancer, a patient might experience this combination of symptoms.

Cancer of the lung can spread to other parts of the body, for example the bones. If a rib is involved, there will be persistent chest pain, especially at night; a specific tender spot on the rib; and other signs of the disease; *see page 223.*

ASPHYXIA (SUFFOCATION)

Obstruction to the flow of air through the mouth, down the trachea or into the lungs. Always look for some simple reversable cause, typically something stuck in the throat. The symptoms of asphyxia are:
* Rapid or abrupt onset.
* Sudden cough, choking and spluttering.

* Rapid cyanosis (bluish coloring) of lips, tongue.
* Panic.
* Stridor, a low- to middle-pitched sound from the larynx, mainly on breathing in. It is also caused by viral infection and is common in children: the child may wake with loud, frightening breathing noises — a highly distinctive coarse wheezing intake of breath, plus cough and fever. Steam inhalation relieves the symptoms.

If you suspect something trapped in the throat, try to dislodge it and use the Heimlich's Maneuver *(see page 204)*. Then call for help. Then, if you know how, give artificial respiration until help arrives. Usually these situations call for emergency attention as quickly as possible.

PROBABLE
FOREIGN BODY
SWELLING OF LARYNX
LARYNGO-TRACHEITIS

POSSIBLE
PNEUMOTHORAX
PULMONARY EMBOLUS

RARE
EPIGLOTTITIS
DIPHTHERIA
TRACHEO-ESOPHAGEAL FISTULA
TUMORS AND CYSTS

PROBABLE

■ FOREIGN BODY
A piece of meat or a similar chunk of firm food is the usual culprit in adults. In children, food can be to blame, but consider also small toys, pen tops, beads, peanuts. The prime signs are:
* Choking.
* Acute stridor: noisy, hoarse, "wheezing" intake of breath.
* Clutching at throat.

First aid: try to dislodge any easily accessible foreign body, or else perform *HEIMLICH'S MANEUVER, see page 204.*

If the foreign body gets past the larynx and makes its way down into the lungs, the coughing and stridor will pass off. In the lungs it will act as a focus for chronic infection, or even a lung abscess, so get medical attention. Cough and recurrent infection after a choking fit should be viewed with suspicion because of this possibility.

■ SWELLING OF LARYNX
An acute, severe allergic reaction causes widespread swelling of soft tissues, including the larynx.

Commonest after insect stings or injections. Some people are hypersensitive to specific foods: nuts are commonly to blame.
* Swelling of lips, limbs and throat
* Acute wheezing.
* Collapse.

■ LARYNGO-TRACHEITIS
A simple laryngitis may occasionally develop into severe swelling. Children's airways are

narrow and will become obstructed with slight swelling of the soft tissues.
* Hoarseness developing into stridor *(see page 226)*.
* Labored breathing, cyanosis (bluish tinge to skin, especially lips).

POSSIBLE

■ PNEUMOTHORAX
Lungs are like balloons in some ways, and, like a balloon, sometimes part of a lung bursts and collapses. Small collapses go unnoticed. Large ones will cause noticeable symptoms and if air continues to leak out from the puncture into the chest, rapid breathlessness will become a problem.
* Sudden, knife-like chest pain.
* Worse breathing in.
* Breathlessness worsening over a few minutes.

Treatment of a large pneumothorax will require emergency treatment: a needle will be inserted through the chest wall to let out the air compressed inside the chest. The lung gradually re-inflates over a few days with the help of a chest drain — a tube leading out of the lung.

■ PULMONARY EMBOLUS
A blood clot obstructing blood flow through the lung.
* Sudden chest pain, often knife-like.
* Coughing blood. *See page 218.*

RARE

■ EPIGLOTTITIS
The epiglottis, the upper part of the windpipe, lies just out of sight at the very back of the throat. Infection can cause it to swell until it obstructs the back of the throat. This illness occurs in young children, whose airways are still narrow.
* Begins as a simple sore throat.
* Child develops a very high temperature.
* Begins to drool saliva because swallowing is painful.
* Labored breathing, cyanosis.

If you suspect that your child has epiglottitis it is important *not* to try to peer down the throat as that can cause complete obstruction. An examination should only be performed in hospital where an emergency tracheotomy can be undertaken.

■ DIPHTHERIA
A terrible illness which routine vaccination has virtually eliminated from developed countries. A membrane forms at the back of the throat which obstructs breathing. In addition, the germ responsible produces toxic substances that affect the heart and nervous system.
* Begins as a simple sore throat.
* A grey membrane forms at the back of the throat.
* Dramatic enlargement of lymph nodes in the neck.
*Breathlessness, cyanosis.

Although there is specific treatment, diphtheria is still a most serious illness.

CHEST

■ TRACHEO-ESOPHAGEAL FISTULA
An abnormality of new-born babies. In the womb, the airways and the esophagus develop next to each other. If the trachea opens into the esophagus rather than the back of the mouth, food may travel straight from the esophagus into the lungs.
* Cough, choking each time the baby feeds.
* Chest infection develops rapidly.

Once recognized, the problem is cured by surgery.

■ TUMORS AND CYSTS
Although these diseases of the larynx or thyroid gland grow quite slowly, they can rapidly increase in size if they start to bleed. The swelling causes obstruction.

The diagnosis might be considered in an adult who is known to have a growth and who suddenly becomes breathless.

CHEST PAIN

Though chest pain is commonly and understandably taken as a sign of heart disease, there are many other causes to be considered, not all of them involving the heart. So many vital structures pass through the chest that the list of possibilities is long. There are the esophagus, the great vessels coming from the heart, the windpipe and the airways going down into the lungs. Pain may stem from the ribs themselves, the muscles between the ribs or from the nerves. The lungs can ache and inflammation from within the abdomen may cause pain in the chest. Chest pain can also come from the neck. Some chest pains are psychological in origin. Finally there are pains which remain totally unexplained, even after extensive investigation.

However, sudden severe chest pain must be taken seriously and needs urgent medical assessment to exclude a heart attack. Recent advances in the treatment of heart attacks require medical attention be given as soon as possible.

This section is divided as follows:

A heart attack.
Sudden chest pain.
Persistent or recurrent chest pain.

A HEART ATTACK

Everyone should be aware of the classic symptoms of a heart attack because early treatment is vital.
* Sudden, severe central chest pain.
* Can occur at rest.
* Worse on exertion.
* Pain is crushing, vice-like, gripping.
* May radiate up to the jaws or down the arms, usually the left.
* Nausea
* Breathlessness.
* Sweating.
* Cyanosis (blueness) of lips.

A heart attack occurs when the blood supply to part of the heart is blocked off. Pain comes from a lack of oxygen to the heart muscle.

Treatment aims to limit the amount of damage to the heart that occurs during the attack, but this calls for treatment within hours. This makes it all the more important to get an early diagnosis in hospital.

Not all heart attacks will show all of the features above: pain is not always a prominent symptom, especially in the elderly; sometimes there is just:
* Sudden onset of tiredness.
* Irregular pulse.
* Heart failure, with breathlessness and swollen ankles.

In these circumstances, much can still be done to help.

Keep this picture in mind when referring to the sections dealing with other causes of chest pain.

SUDDEN CHEST PAIN, POSSIBLY A HEART ATTACK

Diagnostic possibilities are different at different ages. Heart disease would not be the first diagnosis for a young person, whereas in an older person it is often difficult to rule out heart disease completely, so tests will commonly be ordered even if the symptoms are not completely typical. It is generally safest to regard severe chest pain in an adult as a heart problem until proven otherwise.

Physicians will make additional judgements based on the individual's overall condition, including skin color, pulse, blood pressure or signs of heart disease such as fluid on the lungs or abnormal heart rhythms. Electrocardiogram monitoring of the heart will be started and blood tests ordered.

PROBABLE
HEART ATTACK

POSSIBLE
ESOPHAGITIS
NERVE IRRITATION
PEPTIC ULCER
PNEUMOTHORAX

RARE
PULMONARY EMBOLUS
DISSECTING AORTIC ANEURYSM
PERICARDITIS
PANCREATITIS

PROBABLE

■ HEART ATTACK
See this page. Should be suspected on the basis of
* Sudden onset of severe central chest pain.
* Onset at rest.
* Prolonged and crushing in nature.
* Sweating and nausea.

CHEST

POSSIBLE

■ ESOPHAGITIS
Inflammation of the esophagus can be extremely painful, with many features resembling a heart attack:
* Central chest pain.
* Spreads up to neck, down arms.
* Sweating.

Can be difficult to distinguish from heart pain. There may be a previous history of:
* Indigestion, belching.
* Burning pain after food.
* Taking medications which irritate the esophagus such as aspirin.
* Relief with antacids.

However, if occurring for the first time in the middle-aged or elderly, heart disease must be carefully considered.

■ NERVE IRRITATION
Nerves run in bands between the ribs, encircling the chest. It is quite common for one of these nerves to become irritated, causing pain.
* Sharp chest pain.
* Radiates from the back towards the front of the chest.
* Worse on movement.
* No breathlessness or sweating.
* Pain comes and goes from minute to minute.
* Often one small part of the chest wall is tender.

This condition can be dramatic when it appears but is entirely benign, needing no more than painkillers and rest.

■ PEPTIC ULCER
Ulceration in the stomach or upper small bowel (duodenum). The pain from a peptic ulcer tends to be:
* Confined to the upper abdomen.
* Burning in nature.
* Worse at night.
* Appears to radiate into the back.
* Preceded by weeks or months of indigestion.
* Possibly blood in vomit.
* Upper abdominal pain on pressure.

Treatment is totally different from that for a heart attack, consisting of intensive anti-acid treatment.

One in ten people will have an ulcer at some time in their lives. This condition used to be commonest in men; now it is almost as common in women. Smoking, family history and taking certain painkillers all increase the risk of developing a peptic ulcer.

■ PNEUMOTHORAX
Sudden collapse of part of a lung.
* Sudden, knife-like chest pain.
* Localized usually to the side of the chest, not central.
* Breathlessness is a possibility.

Often in young adults.

RARE

■ PULMONARY EMBOLUS
A blood clot lodging in the lungs causing:
* Sudden pressure in chest.
* Discomfort rather than pain.
* Pain, if present, is knife-like.
* Breathlessness.

* Sudden cough with bloodstained mucus.

Pulmonary embolus is associated with thrombosis of leg veins, giving a painful swollen calf. It can occur after surgical operations.

■ DISSECTING AORTIC ANEURYSM

The aorta is the great artery which carries blood away from the heart. If diseased, the walls can weaken, bulge and eventually start to leak. In the days or weeks before this stage there may be warning signs such as:

* Vague upper chest pain.
* Pulsation (feeling of strong, throbbing pulse) in the upper chest.
* Breathlessness through obstruction of part of the lung.
* Hoarseness.

If the aneurysm begins to leak there will be:

* Pain similar to heart attack.
* Possibly vomiting blood.
* Collapse through blood loss.

This condition is very difficult to distinguish from a heart attack by examination alone. The diagnosis is usually made on the result of a chest X-ray. Surgery is possible, depending on the site of the leakage. Frequently fatal.

■ PERICARDITIS

Inflammation of the lining around the heart giving rise to:

* Sharp central chest pain.
* Worse on movement.
* Worse on breathing.

Pericarditis may arise by a viral infection. It can usually be treated and a full recovery is possible.

The heart

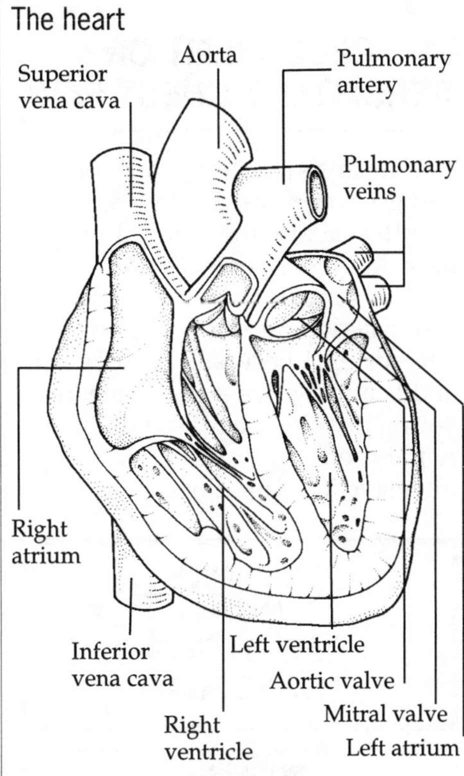

■ PANCREATITIS

The pancreas lies at the back of the upper abdomen. It is the gland that produces insulin and other substances that digest food. If the pancreas becomes inflamed, these substances are released and start to "digest" the internal organs with which they come into contact. Inflammation of the pancreas is most common in alcoholics or in those with gallstones. The very severe pain of pancreatitis can appear to spread up into the chest.

* Pain radiates into the back.
* Nausea and vomiting.

There will be upper abdominal tenderness on examination. This is a serious condition which calls for intensive treatment in hospital.

RECURRENT OR PERSISTENT CHEST PAIN

This means symptoms that come and go over days, weeks or months. Again, the possibilities depend on the person's age, previous medical history and any associated features of disease.

Recurrent chest pain is common and is not always explainable. In young people, the reason often remains obscure, even after intensive investigation.

PROBABLE
ANGINA
HIATUS HERNIA
MUSCLE STRAIN

POSSIBLE
CHONDRITIS
DA COSTA'S SYNDROME
HEART RHYTHM DISORDERS
LUNG DISEASE
GALL BLADDER DISEASE

RARE
AORTIC VALVE DISEASE
SEVERE ANEMIA
AORTIC ANEURYSM
PERICARDITIS

PROBABLE

■ ANGINA
Angina is pain arising from the heart. The reason is nearly always coronary artery disease: that is, narrowing of the blood vessels that carry blood to the heart itself. This causes a *partial* blockage of blood flow, and gives no symptoms until you exert yourself. Then, the heart's increased demand for blood cannot be met, resulting in angina:
* Central chest pain.
* Often radiates to neck or down left arm.
* Comes on with exertion.
* Goes after only a few minutes of rest.
* Worse in cold weather, after meals, emotional stress.

It is common to investigate angina with a stress test and X-rays which highlight the blood flow around the heart, a technique known as angiography. The information gathered from this test will help the doctor to decide whether to replace the blood vessels to the heart, done in an operation known as coronary artery bypass grafting.

Angina is an important warning sign of heart disease, but in itself it is not dangerous and is *not* a warning of an imminent heart attack.

■ HIATUS HERNIA
A common condition in which part of the stomach moves up into the chest. As a result the diaphragm — which normally creates a valve-type mechanism — allows gastric acid to cause pain in the upper part of the stomach and the esophagus .

Symptoms may be noticed for the first time during pregnancy, or be made worse by it, or if you are obese.

* Pain worse on lying flat or bending over.
* Pain which is burning or searing in nature.
* May appear to radiate up to the neck.
* Burping or belching.
* Relieved by antacids and other medications.

Treatment varies from simply avoiding tight clothing and raising the head of the bed, to a range of medications or, very rarely, an operation to tighten up the muscles.

■ MUSCLE STRAIN

Muscles such as the pectorals can be strained by lifting or other injury and produce recurrent pain.
* Muscle is sore.
* Worse on movement.

POSSIBLE

■ CHONDRITIS

Where the ribs meet the breastbone there are joints made up of cartilage which can become inflamed. This may occur after injury, sometimes a result of a viral inspection, or often no reason is found.
* Onset over a few hours.
* Aching on either side of the breastbone.
* Individual joints may be swollen and tender.
* Worse on breathing, or with changes of posture.
* Sometimes a mild fever.

This condition is not dangerous, but may be extremely painful and alarming at the start and can last for several weeks.

■ DA COSTA'S SYNDROME

A psychological problem of anxiety about having heart disease showing itself as:
* Recurrent pains over the heart.
* Breathlessness out of proportion to effort.
* Nervousness.
* Palpitations.

There is no doubt that individuals are genuinely distressed by their symptoms, which are treated by psychological support once heart disease has been ruled out.

■ HEART RHYTHM DISORDERS

Very rapid or very slow heart rates can bring on angina, even in individuals with no other heart disease.
* Palpitations.
* Breathlessness.
* Abrupt onset, abrupt finish.

For details, *see pages 193-203.*

■ LUNG DISEASE

Many disorders can give rise to chest pain which may be mistaken for heart disease, including severe infections and cancer.

See pages 219-25.

■ GALL BLADDER DISEASE

Lying high up in the right side of the abdomen, a diseased gall bladder can give rise to pain which appears to be in the chest. It is commonest in middle-aged women. There is usually little difficulty in distinguishing this as a cause.
* Pain builds up over a few minutes.
* Lasts for several hours.
* Pain and tenderness mainly

under the ribs on the right side.
* May appear to radiate into the chest or to the tip of the shoulder.
* Nausea, vomiting is common.
* Restlessness.

A first attack may be puzzling, but usually a pattern emerges: pain provoked by certain foods, especially fatty ones, with episodes of nagging pain in between major attacks. The usual reason is gallstones, for which there is a variety of treatments, mainly surgical.

RARE

■ AORTIC VALVE DISEASE

This valve controls blood flow between the heart and the aorta, the major artery from the heart. The valve can become stiff and inefficient; this is known as aortic stenosis, usually a result of aging, though rheumatic heart disease was once a common cause.

Occasionally, children are born with an abnormal valve. As the valve is so stiff, it has to beat harder to force blood out and this puts a strain on it. For years there may be no symptoms, but with increasing stiffness there will be some combination of:
* Angina.
* Heart rhythm irregularities.
* Breathlessness.
* Fainting on exertion.

The condition produces a characteristic heart murmur that a doctor can detect. The treatment is by heart valve replacement, though other treatments are used in childhood or in the elderly and infirm.

■ SEVERE ANEMIA

It is unusual for anemia to become so severe without other symptoms, but it does happen occasionally, especially with pernicious anemia. This starves the heart of oxygen, and angina is the result.
* Pale skin or yellowish tinge in pernicious anemia.
* Sore tongue.
* Tiredness, breathlessness.

Most forms of anemia respond rapidly to treatment.

■ AORTIC ANEURYSM

In the days or weeks before this ruptures, there may be intermittent chest pain. *See page 231.*

■ PERICARDITIS

May account for several days of chest pain. *See page 231.*

HEIMLICH'S MANEUVER

* Stand behind the person choking.
* Extend your arms in a hug around their upper abdomen.
* With clenched fists make a hard, fast squeeze just under the breast bone.

The maneuver forces a blast of air out of the lungs, sufficient to dislodge something stuck in the upper airway. For full details see any modern manual of first aid.

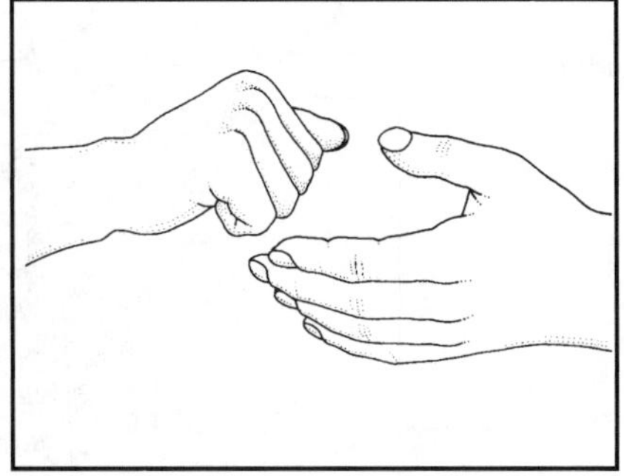

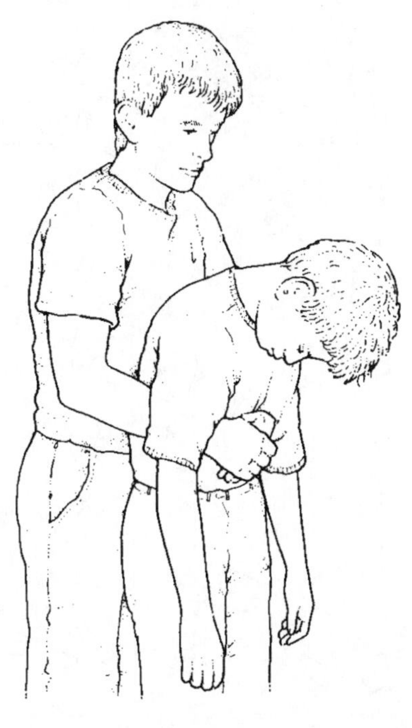

The Skin and Hair

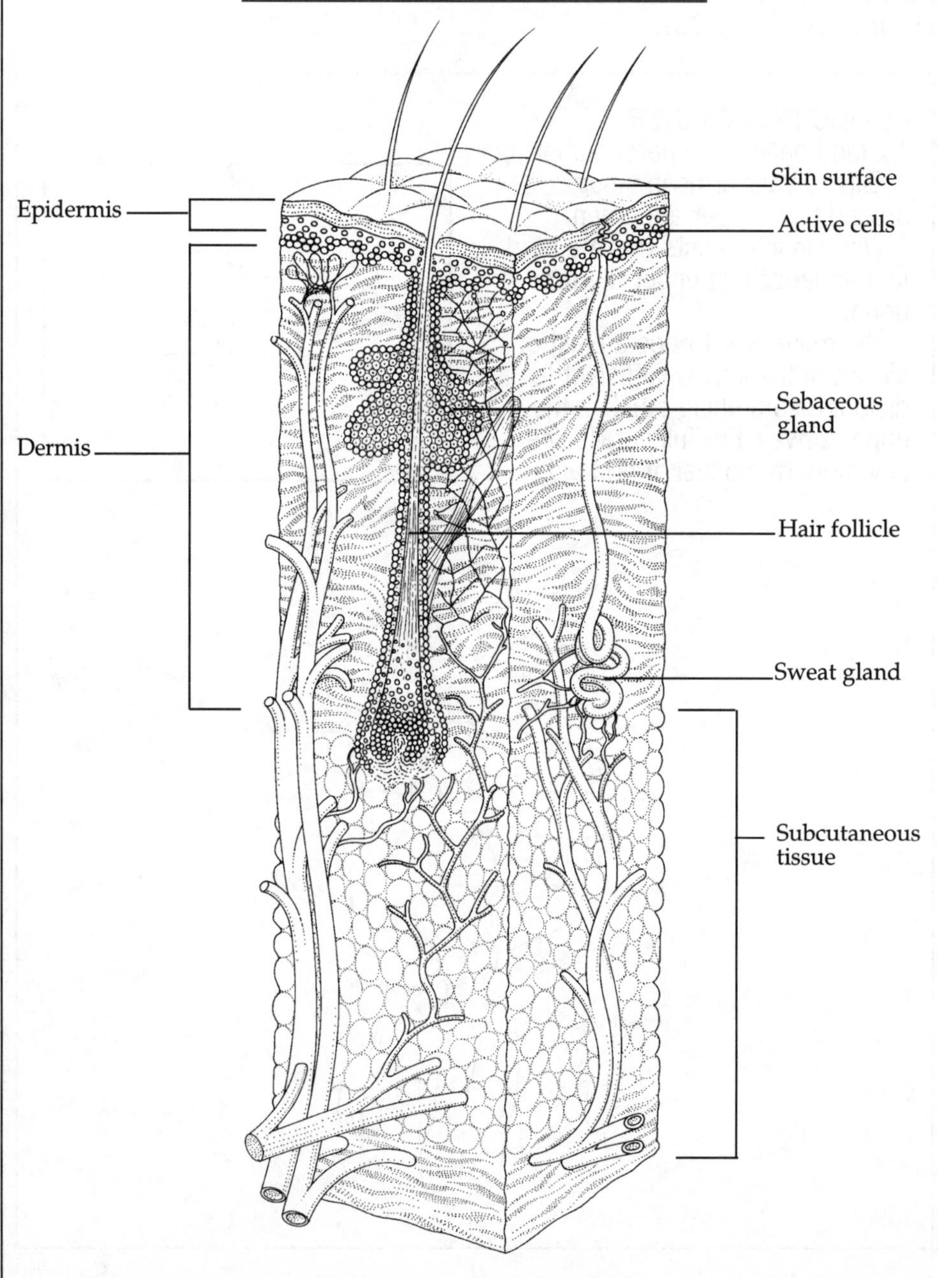

THE SKIN INTRODUCTION

When it comes to diagnosis, your skin (largest of the body's organs) has the advantage that it can be seen and felt; and the changes it undergoes due to illness in other parts of the body or diseases of the skin itself will be fairly obvious.

Most people think skin changes are very unpleasant, but don't let that stop you from showing them to your physician as they may be essential clues to diagnosis.

RASHES

Are divided into four categories, with cross-references to pages where they are covered in detail.

1. **RASHES DEVELOPING BLISTERS**

2. **RASHES OF RED/PURPLE OR BLACK/DARK SPOTS**
See BLEEDING 'UNDER' THE SKIN, page 253.

3. **RASHES EXTENDING OVER MOST OF THE BODY**

4. **RASHES IN A LOCALIZED AREA**
See section covering that part of body.

■ CHICKEN POX
See page 242.

■ ECZEMA
■ HERPES SIMPLEX
■ HERPES ZOSTER
■ IMPETIGO
See page 239.

■ PUSTULAR PSORIASIS
See under PSORIASIS, page 242.

■ POISON IVY
See page 258.

■ DERMATITIS HERPETIFORMIS
See page 240.

■ MEDICATION REACTIONS
See page 247 under REDNESS — GENERAL.

■ ECZEMA
See page 239.

■ GERMAN MEASLES
Rubella. See page 139.

■ MEASLES
See pages 444-5.

■ PORPHYRIA CUTANEA TARDA
See page 240.

■ PSORIASIS
See page 242.

■ SCALDED SKIN SYNDROME
See page 240.

■ TINEA VERSICOLOR
See page 248.

■ URTICARIA
See page 257.

■ VITAMIN A DEFICIENCY
See HARD SKIN, page 256.

THE SKIN

■ VITILIGO
■ VIRAL INFECTIONS
See page 248, and PAPILLOMA or WART, page 251.
(Smallpox is now considered to be eradicated worldwide.)

■ ROCKY MOUNTAIN SPOTTED FEVER
■ LYME DISEASE
See page 247.

PIMPLES

Most people have a number of blackheads at any one time and they are not necessarily a sign of any skin abnormality.

They develop whenever the skin's pores become blocked. Some of them may become whiteheads (pimples), or even *Acne vulgaris*, commonly known as acne or teenage pimples. The exact cause of acne is unclear to doctors. The changes seen on the skin are the effects of infection and inflammation.

Over-activity of the sebaceous, or oil-producing, glands in the skin is one factor. Undoubtedly, hormones also play a part. Diet plays less of a role than was once thought.

■ ACNE VULGARIS (PIMPLES)
* Starts at puberty.
* Blackheads — spots of black matter — can be seen blocking the entrance to sebaceous glands. Also known as comedones.
* Most commonly affects face, upper chest and back.
* Skin may appear greasy.
* Skin bacteria infect the matter in the blocked duct causing local redness, pain and swelling (papules).
* Pus develops, forming pustules (whiteheads).
* This process can continue for years.

If untreated, it can scar the skin. Modern treatments may not cure it, but they can improve matters considerably. Anyone with severe acne should be offered antibiotic treatment, either as tablets or in a lotion to apply to the skin.

BLISTERS

Collections of fluid trapped between different layers of skin. They come in different shapes and sizes.

PROBABLE
INJURY
ECZEMA
HERPES SIMPLEX
IMPETIGO
POISON IVY

POSSIBLE
CHICKEN POX
SHINGLES
ERYTHEMA MULTIFORME

RARE
PEMPHIGOID
PUSTULAR PSORIASIS
DERMATITIS HERPETIFORMIS
PEMPHIGUS VULGARIS
PORPHYRIA CUTANEA TARDA
EPIDERMOLYSIS BULLOSA
SCALDED SKIN SYNDROME

PROBABLE

■ INJURY
Extremes of heat or cold; friction; caustic chemicals; certain plants (e.g. poison ivy); some animals; jelly fish; insect bites: all can cause blisters.
* Localized to the site of injury.
* Surrounding skin may be reddened.

■ ECZEMA
* Often most marked in the skin "flexures", for example the creases at the elbows, or behind the knees.
* Itching.
* Redness.
* Raised red areas.
* Vesicles.
* Weeping.
* Scaling.
* Crusting.

■ HERPES SIMPLEX
This can cause blisters anywhere on the body. the commonest form is that known as a "cold sore", affecting the lips. After the first infection, recurrences may occur at times of debility or after exposure to hot sun or cold.
* Skin is locally irritable.
* Then reddening and painful.
* Small lumps appear to form vesicles.
* The vesicles burst and crust over.
* The whole cycle takes 10 to 14 days to subside

See also LIPS — CRACKED etc, page 84.

■ IMPETIGO
A skin infection which is passed on easily by contact.
* Redness.
* Blisters form.
* Bursting and dirty brown/black crusting occurs.
* Common around mouth, face and ears.

See also page 84.

■ POISON IVY
See page 258.

POSSIBLE

■ CHICKEN POX
See page 242.

■ SHINGLES
Herpes zoster. Arises when the chicken pox virus is reactivated after lying dormant for years in the nerves of the area affected.
* Initially, an itchy, localized area of skin on one half of the body.
* Pain develops.
* Reddening occurs; small lumps appear.
* Small blisters form.
* Crusting, followed by healing, sometimes taking up to a month.
* Pain (post-herpetic neuralgia) may continue after healing and be difficult to treat.

The Skin

■ <u>ERYTHEMA MULTIFORME</u>
See page 87. Large and small blisters may occur with this disease, which arises from an infection or a reaction to medication.

RARE

■ <u>PEMPHIGOID</u>
In the elderly.
* Sudden onset of blisters on limbs and trunk. They may arise from reddened or swollen skin.
* Blisters may be filled with blood-stained fluid.
* Unlike the blisters of pemphigus, these are intensely itchy.

■ <u>PSORIASIS (PUSTULAR)</u>
See page 242.

■ <u>DERMATITIS HERPETIFORMIS</u>
An auto-immune disease.
* Itchy rash on the outer aspect of elbows, knees and buttocks.
* Multiple small blisters appear in these areas.
* Almost always associated with celiac disease *(see page 146)*. As the celiac disease improves with treatment, so will the skin condition.

Treated with dapsone and a special diet; *see under METHEMOGLOBINEMIA, page 245.*

■ <u>PEMPHIGUS VULGARIS</u>
A serious condition commonly affecting people between 40 and 60 years old.
* Widespread large blisters (skin and mucous membranes), often starting in the mouth.
* Skin may blister after simple pressure.
* Blisters burst, leaving weeping, reddened and painful skin, which may become infected.

Cannot be cured, but treatment with steroids and antibiotics will improve symptoms.

■ <u>PORPHYRIA CUTANEA TARDA</u>
* Associated with liver damage — often alcohol induced.
* Exposed skin blisters, scars and becomes pigmented.
* Excess hair may grow on face and eyebrows.

Treatment includes giving up alcohol.

■ <u>EPIDERMOLYSIS BULLOSA</u>
Several different types of this inherited disease exist. Blisters develop after minimal injury — typically minor friction — and become infected.

■ <u>SCALDED SKIN SYNDROME</u>
Caused by infection in children, and medication allergies in adults.
* Sudden onset of malaise.
* Raised temperature.
* Widespread redness.
* Multiple blisters .
* Blisters join, causing large areas of skin to lift off, like a severe scald.

May be fatal.

SCARRED OR PITTED SKIN

In theory, any repeated inflammation or disease process will leave the skin scarred and pitted. In practice, the commonest culprit is acne, the universal plague of adolescence; *see page 238.* The worst cases leave permanent marks on the face and shoulders.

SCALY SKIN

True scaling is limited to just a few conditions and diseases.

Excluding the commonest of them, dandruff *(see page 265)*, this leaves:

PROBABLE
FUNGAL INFECTIONS
ECZEMA

POSSIBLE
PSORIASIS

RARE
PELLAGRA
ICHTHYOSIS

PROBABLE

■ FUNGAL INFECTIONS
See page 252.

■ ECZEMA
See page 239.

POSSIBLE

■ PSORIASIS
See page 242.

RARE

■ PELLAGRA
Vitamin B3 (niacin) deficiency.
* Dementia.
* Severe diarrhea.
* Scaly changes (dermatitis) of exposed skin.

■ ICHTHYOSIS
See page 262.

SCABS

If the skin surface is damaged and fluid (serum, pus, blood) leaks out (either directly or into blisters which subsequently burst) then golden brown or black crusts — scabs — form on the surface or at the edges of the damaged skin. *See also BLISTERS, pages 238-40.*

The Skin

PROBABLE
IMPETIGO
ECZEMA
INJURY
HERPES SIMPLEX

POSSIBLE
CHICKEN POX
HERPES ZOSTER

RARE
PEMPHIGUS VULGARIS
PSORIASIS
DERMATITIS ARTEFACTA

PROBABLE

■ IMPETIGO
■ ECZEMA
■ INJURY
■ HERPES SIMPLEX
See page 239.

POSSIBLE

■ CHICKEN POX
An infectious disease caused by the same virus that causes shingles *(see HERPES ZOSTER)*.
* Crops of spots at different stages.
* Spots are red, raised, form vesicles then pustules (vesicles filled with pus).
* Pustules burst and crust over.
* Fever.
* Feel sick.

■ HERPES ZOSTER
See page 239.

RARE

■ PEMPHIGUS
See page 240.

■ PSORIASIS
A skin disorder of unknown cause.
* Multiple red patches of varying size.
* The red areas are covered with thick silver scales.
* If the scales are scraped off, the underlying skin may bleed.
* May occur on any part of the body, but frequently on knees, elbows and scalp.
* Some individuals develop arthritis *(see page 301)* in association with the psoriasis.

Pustular psoriasis is an uncommon form of the condition in which pus-filled blisters (pustules) develop on the affected skin. When these break down some crusting may occur.

■ DERMATITIS ARTEFACTA
Some people suffering from psychological disorders deliberately harm themselves, for example by burning, scratching or even applying caustic fluids. The resulting injuries may well include extensive scabs and crusts, for which there is no clear explanation.

Sometimes child abusers cause similar injuries to children. To specialists' eyes these patterns can appear quite distinctive.

PEELING OR FLAKING SKIN

Occurs in association with many skin diseases, but typically BLISTERS and RASHES, whose other symptoms are just as, if not more, noticeable, and which are listed under those headings.

Peeling skin is also the eventual and unfortunate outcome of sunburn.

Some skin diseases benefit from sunlight: psoriasis and vitamin deficiencies are obvious examples. However, it is now established beyond doubt that sun exposure predisposes to skin cancer. You increase your risk of developing skin cancer if:

– You have fair skin and sunbathe (redheads with freckles should avoid the sun);

– You expose yourself to the sun around the middle of the day;

– If you develop any redness of the skin. This means you are burnt. Burnt skin means a higher risk of skin cancer.

At the start of summer and when on vacation:

- Increase your exposure to the sun very gradually.
- Wear T-shirts and hats.
- Use a high-factor sun protection cream.
- Cover children well.
- Re-apply sun blocks after bathing.
- Avoid the midday sun.

Protective creams *are* effective and should be used. Children's skin is very sensitive; never let them burn.

SKIN APPEARS PALE

See pages 417-24.

SKIN APPEARS BLUISH

See pages 424-5.

SKIN APPEARS BLACKENED

See DISCOLORATION OF THE SKIN, page 244.

YELLOW SKIN

See YELLOWISH SKIN — JAUNDICE, page 244.

LOCALIZED YELLOW AREAS IN THE SKIN

■ XANTHOMATA

Localized, well-defined deposits of fatty material just below the skin surface. May occasionally be a sign of excess lipids (fats) in the blood, which in turn may predispose to arterial disease. Most commonly seen around the eyes, when the deposits are called xanthelasma.

■ GOUTY TOPHI

See GOUT, page 278.

YELLOWISH SKIN — JAUNDICE

See page 247; also pages 154, 155, 173, 434.

DISCOLORATION OF THE SKIN

Meaning any abnormal change in the color of your skin. This can happen because of a local problem, or because of a general ("systemic") disease of one or more of the body's organs or systems. There are several conditions where changed skin color is a major feature.

Well-known types are listed here by the type of color change and by whether the change is local or general. Obviously, color changes will usually be more obvious in people with light skins than in those with dark skins.

Not listed here are spots and rashes, covered on *pages 237-8*.

BLACK — LOCAL

■ MOLE
Common in adults; they vary in size. Typically brown/black in color. Some have hairs growing from them. They are harmless, but see immediately below.

■ MALIGNANT MELANOMA
A general term for the several different forms of skin cancers, commonest in fair-skinned individuals who have had lengthy, frequent exposure to the sun. They are increasingly common, very probably because more people expose themselves to the sun and use tanning beds. Some malignant melanomas are extremely aggressive.

Malignant melanomas start as small black areas and are often difficult to tell from moles. Even a vague suspicion that you may have one is reason enough to show it to a physician without delay: early diagnosis improves the chances of successful treatment. Once treated, you may need to be followed up for several years. The warning signs are:

* Bleeding.
* Itching.
* Color change.
* Pain.
* Change in size or shape.
* Appearance of smaller lesions nearby.
* Ulceration.

Any one of these warning signs should prompt you to visit your physician.

■ ACANTHOSIS NIGRICANS
Black linear pigmentation in the armpit, the groin, on the face and neck. Most commonly occurs in association with an underlying malignant tumor. Rare, and untreatable.

■ DRY GANGRENE
See also ITCHING OR NUMBNESS OF THE FINGERS AND TOES, page 321.
Gradual loss of blood supply to a toe or a foot, or any extremity, may cause this condition. The affected part becomes withered and black and may drop off — typically a frost-bitten toe.

BLUE — LOCAL

■ CYANOSIS
See BLUISH SKIN, page 424.

■ MONGOLIAN BLUE SPOT
A blue/black area typically seen on the buttocks and sacral region in West Indian and Asian children. May often be mistaken for a bruise; can be several centimeters across.

■ BLUE NEVUS
Similar to *MONGOLIAN BLUE SPOT*, above, but occurs elsewhere on the body. May be very small.

■ LIVIDO RETICULARIS
An exaggeration of the body's normal response to heat and cold: white areas of skin surrounded by a "chicken wire" pattern of bluish blood vessels.

BLUE — GENERAL

■ CYANOSIS *See page 424.*

■ AMIODARONE
This medication, for treating heart irregularities, may rarely cause a bluish-grey, discoloration of the skin.

■ METHEMOGLOBINEMIA
Can occur through exposure to certain medications, for example dapsone, for treating leprosy or dermatitis herpetiformis, or certain chemicals. Some people inherit the condition, which affects the oxygen-carrying capacity of the hemoglobin in red blood cells.

■ OCHRONOSIS
Affects cartilage and other connective tissue, for example the whites of the eyes. The cartilage underlying the skin looks bluish or blue-black, whereas normally the overlying skin color would predominate. Caused by an abnormality of amino-acid metabolism called alkaptonuria.

BROWN — LOCAL

■ PREGNANCY
As pregnancy progresses, the nipples, the genitalia and a line down the center of the abdomen become progressively darker - turning from pinkish to brownish — *See also CHLOASMA, below.*

■ CHLOASMA
A brownish pigmentation of the face that occurs in some pregnant women.

■ VENOUS ULCERATION
Long-standing varicose veins in the legs *(see page 310)* cause brownish pigmentation of the lower legs and feet. Sometimes there is ulceration, too, particularly on the inner side of the ankle.

■ ERYTHEMA ABIGNE
A reddish-brown irregular discoloration which appears after long exposure of skin to heat. May be noticed on the shins of an elderly person who spends hours in a chair close to a fire or heater. May also be caused by use of a heating pad.

■ SEBORRHEIC WART
A flattish, brownish wart, slightly raised above the surrounding skin. Sometimes they occur in considerable numbers. Also

The Skin

known as senile warts because they appear during middle age and later. Harmless.

■ CAFE-AU-LAIT SPOTS
Like large freckles; may be multiple. Occasionally associated with "neurofibromatosis".

■ ADRENAL INSUFFICIENCY
Caused by long-standing underactivity of the adrenal glands.
* Brownish/dark pigmentation of skin, especially skin creases, nipples, genitalia, old scars and gums (in the last, may appear grey).
* Weakness, fatigue.
* Weight loss, loss of appetite.
* Craving for salt.
* Nausea, vomiting, diarrhea.
* Low blood pressure.
* Hair loss — occasionally.
* Vitiligo — occasionally.
See page 248.

BROWN — GENERAL
■ FRECKLES
May occur naturally or may appear in increased numbers after exposure to the sun. May grow darker than usual and may coalesce, if exposed to sun. Mostly on face, shoulders and arms, but may cover the entire body. Commonest on redheads.

Avoid the sun if you have freckles; *see PEELING OR FLAKING SKIN, page 243.*

■ HEMOCHROMATOSIS
Also called bronze diabetes. An abnormality of metabolism of iron from birth, causes:
* Diabetes mellitus *(page 484)*.
* Bronze colored skin.
* Cirrhosis of liver.
* Joint inflammation.
* Heart abnormalities.
* Shrunken testicles, reduced sex drive.

ORANGE — GENERAL
■ CAROTENEMIA
Eating too much food containing carotene, typically carrots and tomato juice, causes an orange discoloration of skin. Carotene is the active ingredient of some "sun-tan" tablets.

PINK — LOCAL
■ SALMON PATCH NEVUS
A salmon-pink birthmark. Can occur anywhere, but often on the neck. Some persist, but most disappear after a few years.

PURPLE — LOCAL
■ PORT-WINE STAIN
A permanent birth mark caused by an abnormality of the capillary blood vessels producing an often extensive discolored area on the face and neck. Can be disguised with make-up. New laser treatment may be helpful.

■ KAPOSI'S SARCOMA
Bluish-red areas appear on the skin. This is a malignant tumor that used to be seen mainly in Africa, but is now encountered all over the world as one of the complications of AIDS.

PURPLE — GENERAL
Likely to be cyanosis; *see page 424. See also BLUE — GENERAL, page 245.*

REDNESS — LOCAL
Described as erythema.

■ FLUSHING
As a response to heat, or embarrassment; and in association with the menopause, *page 328*.

■ ERYTHEMA ABIGNE
See BROWN, page 246.

■ PALMAR ERYTHEMA
Redness of the palms of the hands. Seen in alcoholics and in others suffering from liver disease.

■ ERYTHRASMA
Reddish-brown discoloration of the skin, particularly near skin folds (breasts, armpits, groin). The skin is dry and the areas are irregular and slightly scaly. Caused by bacterial infection.

■ LYME DISEASE
Disease carried by small ticks. Becoming more common. Often no evidence of tick bite.
* Red expanding patches on skin that clear in the center.
* Fever.
* Joint pains.
* Muscle pains.
* Stiff neck.
* Headache. Tends to improve but then can cause:
* Heart rhythm problems.
* Fatigue.
* Nerve damage.
* Arthritis.

■ ROCKY MOUNTAIN SPOTTED FEVER
Infection carried by ticks, commonest in the summer.
* Fever.
* History of tick bite.
* Headache.
* Rash starts on wrists and ankles; spreads to arms, legs, palms and soles of feet.
* Muscle aches.
* Belly pain.
* Nausea.

Early treatment with antibiotics is essential. When removing ticks, do not squeeze the body of the tick. This may inject the infection into your bloodstream. Pull on the head of the tick with tweezers to remove it.

■ PAGET'S DISEASE OF THE NIPPLE
Localized redness with scaling and inflammation, mimicking eczema. If you notice such changes on the nipple or areola (the pink area around the nipple), see your physician immediately so that the possibility of breast cancer can be excluded. *See also pages 336-8.*

REDNESS — GENERAL

■ VIRAL INFECTION
Many viruses will cause non-specific reddening of the skin. As soon as the infection subsides, so does the rash.

■ MEDICATION REACTION
A diffuse reddening of the skin associated with taking new tablets or other medication. The reddening may be patchy or blotchy, or widespread. Itching (medical term, pruritus) often accompanies these reactions. Penicillin, sulphonamides and aspirin commonly cause this reaction.

THE SKIN

YELLOWNESS — GENERAL
This is never a local condition.

■ JAUNDICE
Yellowish whites of the eyes, and yellow skin gradually progressing to a deeper, browner color. There may also be itching (with resulting scratch marks), pale stools and dark urine.

■ UREMIA
See page 260.

■ MEPACRINE
This anti-malarial medication can cause yellowing of the skin.

WHITENESS OR PALENESS — LOCAL

■ VITILIGO
Destruction of pigment-producing cells (melanocytes) in the skin, giving white patches. In the dark-skinned, these can be quite disfiguring. *See also ADRENAL INSUFFICIENCY, page 246.*

■ HALO NEVUS
Some moles *(see BLACK, page 244)* become pale and the area round them loses pigment. Mole and surrounding area are known as halo nevi. Vitiligo *(above)* may also develop.

■ TINEA VERSICOLOR
A fungal infection of the skin.
* Initially, areas of irregular brown coloration.
* Predominantly upper body, arms and neck.
* Later, these patches lose their pigment, giving pale areas.

Treatable with anti-fungal creams.

■ POST-INFLAMMATORY
Any inflamed or damaged skin — say from a graze, a burn, a herpes sore — may lose its usual color after healing. Normal pigmentation may return after a few months.

■ LEPROSY
See page 319.

■ ARTERIAL BLOCKAGE
See PERIPHERAL VASCULAR DISEASE, page 318.

■ PHLEGMASIA ALBA DOLENS
This means blockage of the principal veins draining blood from the leg. Typically after being bed-ridden.
* Initially feel sick.
* Pain in groin and thigh.
* Leg-swelling follows.
* Leg is pale and feels cold.

■ RAYNAUD'S PHENOMENON AND DISEASE
See page 488.

WHITENESS OR PALENESS — GENERAL

■ ANEMIA
See page 419.

■ LEUKEMIA
See pages 424 and 490.

■ ALBINISM
An inherited abnormality of metabolism that results in absence of pigment in body tissues.
* Fair skin.
* White hair.
* Pink irises of the eyes.
* Problems with sight.

■ PHENYLKETONURIA
Caused by an error of metabolism resulting in an accumulation of chemicals which affect the brain. Children are screened at birth. Treatment involves avoiding foods containing phenylalanine.
* Blond hair.
* Blue eyes.
* Mental deficiency and aggression if untreated.

■ HYPOPITUITARISM
See page 265.

■ SHOCK/FEELING FAINT
See page 408.

LINEAR MARKS ON THE SKIN

These are the most likely causes of colored lines on the skin.

■ LYMPHANGITIS
Infection in a limb can track up the lymphatic pathways to the lymph glands. May be seen on the arm and forearm after a simple injury, even a cat scratch to the hand, for example.
* Site of wound may be apparent.
* A red line extends directly from the region of the wound, continuing up towards the armpit or groin.
* Tender lymph nodes may be felt in the armpit or groin.

Antibiotic treatment is essential, to stop the infection.

■ SCABIES
Fine grey lines a few millimetres long. *See page 259.*

■ ACANTHOSIS NIGRICANS
See page 244.

■ POISON IVY
See page 258.

■ WARTS
Can sometimes occur in lines.

WHITE PATCHES

PROBABLE
VITILIGO

POSSIBLE
HALO NEVUS
TINEA VERSICOLOR
POST- INFLAMMATORY

RARE
LICHEN SCLEROSIS ET ATROPHICUS
LEPROSY
MORPHEA
RAYNAUD'S PHENOMENON AND DISEASE

PROBABLE

■ VITILIGO
See page 248.

The Skin

POSSIBLE

■ HALO NEVUS
■ TINEA VERSICOLOR
■ POST-INFLAMMATORY
See page 248.

RARE

■ LICHEN SCLEROSIS ET ATROPHICUS
See page 259.

■ LEPROSY
See page 319.

■ MORPHEA
See page 256.

■ RAYNAUD'S PHENOMENON AND DISEASE
See page 488.

MINIATURE RED SPOTS

There are two causes worth considering:

■ CHERRY HEMANGIOMA
* Tiny and bright red, often raised above the surrounding skin surface.
* Present on the chest and abdomen.

Commonest in elderly people. Of little significance.

■ SPIDER NEVI
These are red marks with several tiny blood vessels radiating from the center. They can appear in children and in adults. Multiple nevi may be a feature of pregnancy, and of liver disease; also of hereditary hemorrhagic telangiectasia; *see page 87.*

SORES OR ULCERS

Are described elsewhere in the book in relation to the part of the body on which they occur.

VESICLES

Are small blisters. *See page 238.*

HIVES

A term describing raised marks on the skin. *See URTICARIA, page 257.*

WARTS

See LUMPS IN THE SKIN, below.

LUMPS IN THE SKIN

It is best to play safe and report any lump in the skin to a physician: most are innocent, but some need expert evaluation to rule out the possibility of malignant disease.

The earlier the diagnosis and treatment, the better the outlook.

If a lump is pigmented, bleeding, irregular, ulcerated or growing rapidly, all the more reason to see a physician without delay.

See sections for specific parts of the body for lumps in the skin not included here.

PROBABLE
SEBACEOUS CYST
DERMOID CYST
PAPILLOMA
WART
PLANTAR WART

POSSIBLE
LIPOMA
PYOGENIC GRANULOMA
GANGLION
MOLLUSCUM CONTAGIOSUM
VASCULAR MALFORMATIONS
BASAL CELL CARCINOMA

RARE
SQUAMOUS CELL CARCINOMA
MALIGNANT MELANOMA
SECONDARY TUMOR
LYMPHOMA

PROBABLE

■ SEBACEOUS CYST
A harmless lump caused by build-up of sebaceous material — solidified, waxy, body fluid — in a sweat gland near the surface of the skin. May start as an unsqueezed zit: which, if it does not become infected, can develop, over many years, into a sebaceous cyst. No relation to cancer.

* Smooth; not tender.
* Frequently multiple on scalp, neck or scrotum.
* Size ranges from a few millimeters to several centimeters.

■ DERMOID CYSTS
These are cysts which develop from birth on the head and neck, and are commonest at the outside end of the eyebrow. They may also occur as benign tumors elsewhere on the body.

■ PAPILLOMA
Harmless, small growth of skin.

■ WART
Caused by a viral infection of the skin. Small, often multiple, pain-free thickening of skin with rough skin on the surface, growing above the level of the normal skin.

■ PLANTAR WART
A wart on the base of the foot. Because the foot is weight-bearing, the wart is pushed into the sole of the foot and can be painful to walk on.

POSSIBLE

■ LIPOMA
A benign, fatty tumor that may appear as a smooth, often soft, lump in or beneath the skin.

■ PYOGENIC GRANULOMA
Possibly caused by minor injury. A soft, red, fleshy benign tumor which bleeds easily when knocked. Often sited near a finger– or toenail.

THE SKIN

■ GANGLION
A local degeneration of fibrous tissue. Appears as a small, firm lump, near tendons or joints. Commonly seen on the back of the wrist. Can be left alone or removed surgically.

■ MOLLUSCUM CONTAGIOSUM
Caused by a virus.
* Groups of small pink lumps.
* Often on trunk or face.
* Each lump has a depression in the middle.

They clear up on their own but can be removed.

■ VASCULAR MALFORMATIONS
There are many different types: spider nevus, salmon patch (also known as strawberry nevus), port wine stain, Campbell de Morgan spots, hereditary hemorrhagic telangiectasis are examples. These are rarely seen as lumps, but a cavernous hemangioma may develop as a lump. It may be extensive, covering part of the face. Often present at birth. Normally clears by about six years.

■ BASAL CELL CARCINOMA
Skin cancer. *See page 104.*

RARE

■ SQUAMOUS CELL CARCINOMA
A malignant tumor, commonest in the elderly.
* Often on the head or neck.
* May be a an irregular lump.
* May bleed.
* May ulcerate.
* Local lymph nodes may be enlarged.

■ MALIGNANT MELANOMA
See page 244.

■ SECONDARY TUMOR
Technical term, metastasis. This is cancer that has spread from a primary site to create tumors elsewhere in the body. Irregular, hard, fleshy nodule(s) or plaque(s) seen or felt in the skin of someone known to have a primary cancer raise the suspicion of metastases. It is rare for skin metastases to be the first symptom you notice of internal primary cancer, but it is possible.

■ LYMPHOMA
One particular type of lymphoma starts in the skin. It is noted as an irregular thickening. Diagnosis can only be made by taking a sample and examining it under the microscope. *See also page 490.*

SKIN TENDS TO CRACK

This is a feature of inflammation or infection of the skin. The most common causes are fungal infection and eczema.

■ FUNGAL INFECTION
Different fungal infections may affect all parts of the body, but commonly hands, feet *(see also ATHLETE'S FOOT, page 320)* and groin.
* Dry, reddened, itchy, painful areas of skin.
* Skin gets soft and rubs off.
* Sometimes, associated blisters.
* Some fissuring, cracking and thickening of the skin.

* There may be an unpleasant smell.

Easily treated with anti-fungal creams and ointments.

■ ECZEMA

The term is often used interchangeably with dermatitis. May be confused with fungal infections, and vice-versa.

* Diffuse patchy redness.
* Red lumps.
* Weeping, crusting.
* Cracking, scaling.

See page 239.

MOLES

See page 244.

BUBBLES FROM A SKIN WOUND

Bubbles and fluid oozing from a wound, or surrounding skin that feels "crackly" when pressure is applied, suggests a very severe infection known as "gas gangrene". Pain and discoloration of the skin will almost always be present. Get medical help immediately.

BLEEDING "UNDER" THE SKIN

Medical term, purpura. In fact, the skin has several layers and the term properly describes blood leaking into surrounding surface tissue. The cause is either an injury which did not pierce the skin surface; or an abnormality of blood vessels, or of blood.

When blood leaks into surrounding tissue, it is broken down and undergoes several changes of color, from red/purple/black to brown, green and yellow.

The significance of purpura ranges from the minimal to an indication of life-threatening disorders.

PROBABLE
BRUISE
SENILE PURPURA

POSSIBLE
MEDICATION-RELATED
HENOCH SCHÖNLEIN PURPURA
MENINGOCOCCAL SEPTICEMIA

RARE
BLOOD DISORDERS
SCURVY
EHLERS-DANLOS SYNDROME
DISSEMINATED INTRAVASCULAR COAGULATION

PROBABLE

■ BRUISE

Bruises can be caused by a blow (hitting your thumb with a hammer) or by pressure. Squeezing a child's arm hard will

THE SKIN

produce bruising. Blood leaks out of the tiny blood vessels, called capillaries, and seeps into the tissues. A bruise that causes swelling may be called a hematoma by your physician.

■ SENILE PURPURA
* Blotchy, well outlined purple patches.
* Often seen on legs or arms.
* Part of the aging process.

POSSIBLE

■ MEDICATION-RELATED
May be associated with taking steroids.
* Well-demarcated red and purple blotches.
Stop the medication and see your physician if purpura develops.

■ HENOCH SCHÖNLEIN PURPURA
Cause unknown. In adults and children.
* Red/purple spots under the skin.
* Hives.
* Painful joints.
* Abdominal pain.
* Bloody diarrhea.
* Blood in the urine.
Normally resolves on its own, although steroids may be advised. Complications may affect kidneys.

■ MENINGOCOCCAL SEPTICEMIA
See also MENINGITIS, pages 444 and 452. A life-threatening condition occurring with or without meningitis. Affects pre-school children most severely.
* Sudden onset of spotty red/purple rash, which may be extensive or minimal.
* Very sick.
* Fever.
* Rapid deterioration and collapse.
* Death may occur within hours.
If suspected, and certainly if the child has had contact with another case of meningitis, go to the hospital emergency room immediately.

RARE

■ BLOOD DISORDERS
Blood disorders such as leukemia or aplastic anemia often show themselves with sudden onset of widespread bruising. *See also page 417.*

■ SCURVY
See page 427.

■ EHLERS-DANLOS SYNDROME
An inherited disease in which the body cannot make normal supporting tissue.
* Markedly "double-jointed" joints.
* Skin scars easily.
* Bruising is common.
* Skin is soft and velvety in texture.

BOILS AND CARBUNCLES

■ A BOIL
Is an abscess in a hair follicle.
* Prime sites are the neck, armpit and buttocks.

* Local redness.
* Swelling.
* Pain.
* Develops a point and discharges yellow/green pus.

■ CARBUNCLE
Is a collection of boils that may interconnect under the skin.

Recurrent boils or carbuncles suggest the possibility of underlying disease, particularly diabetes mellitus, *see page 484.* Urine can be tested for sugar as a quick screening method. Another cause of recurrent boils may be poor personal hygiene. Occasionally, the diagnosis of acne vulgaris *(see page 238)* may have been missed.

Boils and carbuncles will usually come to a head, discharge their fluid naturally and disappear. They can be very painful and opening them up, to drain, can relieve the pain and speed healing. Do not be tempted to do this at home. See your physician or nurse practitioner to have a boil opened and drained.

Antibiotics can often clear boils either before they become too painful or before they discharge.

CORNS AND CALLUSES

Both words describe harmless thickening of the skin, which develops as a protective measure.

■ A CORN
Typically appears on the upper surface of the little toe, where the toe rubs against shoes.

■ A CALLUS
Is a thickening of the skin of the hands or feet. People who go habitually barefoot develop calluses on the pressure-bearing areas of the sole.

Manual workers develop calluses on the palms of the hands, typically at the base of the fingers.

FLAB

Apart from obvious folds of fatty tissue that go with obesity, flab is sometimes used to describe skin which has lost elasticity: you can pick it up in folds, and it fails to return immediately to its original contours. There are three main causes:

■ AGING
With age, skin loses its elasticity. Wrinkles, skin creases and sagging jaw lines are part of the process — and provide plenty of work for cosmetic surgeons.

■ DEHYDRATION
The body needs a certain amount of water in order to function properly. Severe lack of fluid can be caused by reduced intake (for example when someone is in a coma). Fluid loss can occur with diarrhea or vomiting.

The result is flabby skin, which will not unwrinkle when pinched.

The Skin

■ MASSIVE WEIGHT LOSS
If you are obese and manage to lose a large proportion of your weight very rapidly, you may be unjustly repaid with a new problem. The skin needs time to compensate for the loss of fat; meanwhile, folds of flabby skin develop, particularly on the abdomen, buttocks, thighs and upper arms. Cosmetic surgery may be helpful in some cases.

HARD SKIN, LOCAL OR GENERAL

The obvious diagnosis is a corn or callus, covered separately on *page 255*. Here are the less self-evident causes.

PROBABLE
KELOID

POSSIBLE
LYMPHEDEMA
POST-PHLEBITIC LIMB
MYXEDEMA

RARE
VITAMIN A DEFICIENCY
MORPHEA
SCLERODERMA
CANCER

PROBABLE

■ KELOID
Describes excessive scarring after cuts or injury and is seen most commonly in African-americans. The site of the injury hardens, with an overgrowth of hard scar tissue above the level of the surrounding skin. Severe cases sometimes require treatment for the scar tissue, either by steroid injection or by surgery. There is no guarantee that this will lead to a more satisfactory appearance.

POSSIBLE

■ LYMPHEDEMA
■ POST-PHLEBITIC LIMB
See SWOLLEN ANKLE, page 310.

■ MYXEDEMA
Puffy swelling of the skin, particularly on hands, feet and ankles and around eyes. May be seen with hypothyroidism, *page 461.*

RARE

■ VITAMIN A DEFICIENCY
* Night blindness.
* Abnormality of the cornea leading to inflammation, scarring and blindness.
* Rough, dry skin.

■ MORPHEA
A localized variant of scleroderma, *see page 257.*
* Well-defined, pale areas.

* The skin in these areas is smooth and hard.
* Loss of hair at these sites may occur.
* Ulceration may occur.

■ SCLERODERMA
An auto-immune disease.
* Hard, rigid skin develops.
* Tiny red spots (telangiectasia) are evident.
* Skin becomes shiny and smooth.
* Hands become stiff.
* Joints may become stiff.
* Skin of face is affected, making the mouth appear small.
* Face lacks expression.
* Raynaud's phenomenon *(see page 488)* develops.
* Swallowing is impaired and weight loss follows.

See also PROBLEMS WITH SWALLOWING PLUS WEIGHT LOSS, page 122.

■ CANCER
Secondary or metastatic cancer deposits (having spread from a primary site elsewhere) can arise in the skin, giving small areas which are hard to the touch. They may be single or multiple.

AN ITCHY RASH

PROBABLE
ECZEMA
URTICARIA (HIVES)
POISON IVY
SCABIES
LICE
INSECT BITES
FUNGAL INFECTION

POSSIBLE
PITYRIASIS ROSEA
LICHEN SIMPLEX
PRURITUS ANI
VULVAL ITCH
MEDICATION REACTION

RARE
NODULAR PRURIGO
LICHEN SCLEROSIS ET ATROPHICUS

PROBABLE

■ ECZEMA
See page 239.

■ URTICARIA
Commonly called hives. A type of allergic reaction, triggered by various agents. Typically, urticaria appears suddenly and dramatically. The hives may come and go quite quickly, clearing in one area, only to reappear in another.
* Red, blotchy areas with puffy, paler patches in the middle.
* Some swelling.
* Itchy, often intensely so.

There are several types, grouped according to cause or appearance. One form, dermatographia, is particularly severe: just stroking the skin firmly raises a wheal or picture on the skin.

The most common form is allergic urticaria. Common causes include: plants, chemicals, food, medicine colorants.

The Skin

■ POISON IVY (OR OAK)
Itchy, blistering rash. Often occurs in patches or lines. Caused by reaction to an oil of the plant which is easily transferred from one part of the skin to another. Leaves, roots, stalk and smoke (if plant is burned) can cause the rash. Thorough washing of hands and garden tools can minimize exposure.

After exposure, wash with soap, in the tub or shower and launder clothes. Steroid cream may relieve mild attacks. Steroids by mouth may be needed for severe or persistent attacks.

■ SCABIES
■ LICE
■ INSECT BITES
Can occur as an itchy rash, or with no obvious rash. *See pages 259-60.*

■ FUNGAL INFECTION
See page 252.

POSSIBLE

■ PITYRIASIS ROSEA
Commonest in young people, and may occur with a viral infection.
* A single, itchy red lesion may appear anywhere on the trunk — the herald patch.
* After a few days, scattered patches of pinkish elevated areas develop. They characteristically lie along the line of the ribs.
* The rash persists for about six weeks.

Usually no treatment is required. Calamine lotion or, in severe cases, antihistamine medications, may help.

■ LICHEN SIMPLEX
You scratch an itchy place. The itchiness goes for a while, but as soon it comes back, you scratch again. A vicious cycle of scratching and itching develops, causing local inflammation. The inflammation causes thickening of the skin, with furrows or lines developing in the chronic case.

■ JOCK ITCH
■ PRURITUS ANI
■ VULVAL ITCH
These conditions are often characterized by itching plus rash.
See pages 160 and 360.

■ MEDICATION REACTION
If you are allergic to a medication, the classic reaction is:
* Widespread rash, but predominating on trunk.
* Patchy reddening.
* Some local swelling.
* Intense itching.

Reactions to medications can start, even after long-term use.

RARE

■ NODULAR PRURIGO
* Multiple warty areas.
* Intensely itchy.

Cause unknown, but possibly initiated by scratching.

■ LICHEN SCLEROSIS ET ATROPHICUS
* Involves skin around the vulva.
* White, pale skin.
* Clearly delineated.
* Reddened areas within the affected skin.
* Itchy.

When seen on children this may wrongly be attributed to abuse.

ITCHING - WITHOUT A RASH

Covered here is persistent, severe itching that has become a nuisance. The medical term is pruritus.

Close inspection with a magnifying glass may reveal either of the common causes — scabies and lice. Scratch marks are the obvious evidence of severe itching, and they also show where the symptom is at its worst. Excluded here are an itching scalp caused by dandruff, covered separately on *page 265*; and itching in the anal area, covered on *page 161*.

PROBABLE
SCABIES
LICE
INSECT BITES, INCLUDING FLEAS
FIBERGLASS
SENILE PRURITUS
PINWORM

POSSIBLE
PREGNANCY
LIVER DISEASE
JAUNDICE
MEDICATIONS
PSYCHOLOGICAL

RARE
DERMATITIS HERPETIFORMIS
UREMIA
BLOOD DISORDERS

PROBABLE

■ SCABIES
Infestation with the scabies mite, which burrows under the skin.
* Severe itching is noted.
* Mite burrows may be seen as short grey lines.
* Burrows are often between fingers or front of wrists.
* Eventually, raised, reddened areas may appear all over the body.
* Scabs may develop because of scratching.

See your physician for a prescription medication to apply to the skin.

■ LICE
There are three main types: head lice, body lice and pubic lice.
* Persistent itching.
* Local lymph nodes may enlarge.
* Eggs may be seen on the hairs near the skin – these are "nits", or you may see lice themselves.
* Spread by direct contact with other infected hairs or skin.
* The pubic louse may cause itching in the anal or vulval regions.

■ INSECT BITES, INCLUDING FLEAS
* Itching at the site of the bite.
* Reddened, hard nodules at the site of the bite appear later.

The Skin

Fleas are commonly the culprits; commonest in homes with cats and dogs.

■ FIBERGLASS
Glass fibers can become invisibly embedded in skin, causing itching. Protective clothing should be worn, for instance, when laying insulation.

■ SENILE PRURITUS
The elderly sometimes complain of itching for which no cause can be found: it may be the result of the aging process.

■ THREADWORM
See WORMS, page 153.
* Itching and irritation around the anus.

Most children have this common complaint at some time. Treatment is simple, and available either directly from the chemist or from a physician.

POSSIBLE

■ PREGNANCY
Many women complain of itching in the last months of pregnancy. Local causes such as fungus infection (candida) need to be excluded.

■ LIVER DISEASE
■ JAUNDICE
Any condition, and typically liver disease, which causes *JAUNDICE*, may also cause intense itching. The itching may arise before the yellow skin color is noticed.

■ MEDICATIONS
Some medications, for instance, penicillin and aspirin, can cause severe allergic reactions, with itching. And some of the narcotic medications, including cocaine and heroin, may cause itching, sometimes related to impurities.

■ PSYCHOLOGICAL
Itching without any cause found after full examination and investigation may be a sign of underlying psychological problems.

RARE

■ DERMATITIS HERPETIFORMIS
See page 240.

■ UREMIA
High levels of urea in the blood are one of the end results of renal (kidney) failure. A number of symptoms may be present:
* Dry, coated tongue.
* Breath smelling of urine.
* Hiccups.
* Nausea and vomiting.
* Dry, yellow-brown skin with a whitish "frost".
* Marked itching.
* Anemia.

■ BLOOD DISORDERS
A number of blood and related diseases may cause severe itching. They include: *Polycythemia rubra vera*; lymphoma; Hodgkin's disease; leukemias.

PRURITUS

The medical term for itching. *See pages 257-60.*

SKIN FEELS SWEATY

See page 471, also 408. If associated with coldness, look at ITCHING OR NUMBNESS etc, page 320.

DRY SKIN

Simple explanations are: exposure to sun, wind and airconditioning. Some people need to use moisturizers daily.

PROBABLE
ECZEMA
FUNGAL INFECTIONS

POSSIBLE
HEAT (SUN) STROKE
HYPOTHYROIDISM

RARE
UREMIA
VITAMIN A DEFICIENCY
ICHTHYOSIS

PROBABLE

■ ECZEMA
See page 239. When not in a phase of acute inflammation, patches of skin affected by eczema may feel dry and rough to the touch.

■ FUNGAL INFECTIONS
See page 252.

POSSIBLE

■ HEAT (SUN) STROKE
Prolonged physical work in hot conditions or staying too long in the sun puts anyone, even the fit athlete, at risk of heat stroke.

Commonest in the very young and the elderly. Symptoms may develop rapidly.
* Dry skin, hot to the touch.
* High temperature.
* Weakness.
* Thirst.
* Headache.
* Confusion.

If untreated, can be fatal. It is important to protect yourself against the sun:
• wear hat, shirt; apply sun block; maintain a high fluid intake (no alcohol);
• keep cool by taking frequent showers or swimming;
avoid exposure to the midday sun.

If you suspect this condition, seek medical help urgently.

■ HYPOTHYROIDISM
See page 460.

THE SKIN

RARE

■ UREMIA
See page 260.

■ VITAMIN A DEFICIENCY
See page 256.

■ ICHTHYOSIS
A group of inherited disorders of the skin, in which the skin is thickened, dry and flaky. Often the inner aspect of skin overlying joints (typically armpits and elbow creases) is spared.

Very occasionally, these changes, appearing in later life, may be associated with underlying malignant disease.

BODY ODOR

This is possibly the vaguest and most subjective symptom of all. Physicians and dentists see many people who believe that they smell bad, or that some part of them smells, even though no one else has commented.

Some people seem to be abnormally sensitive to smells. And some people, notably small children, have a virtually non-existent sense of smell.

Serious underlying disease is *very* rarely the reason for offensive body odor. Other than body odor caused by stale sweat, body odor usually comes down to three relatively common possibilities:

■ ATHLETE'S FOOT
A fungal infection of the feet with reddened, itchy, painful areas between the toes, fissuring and cracking. The feet and shoes give off a characteristic cheesy odor, which is sometimes strong enough for others to smell, even if the shoes are on.

■ BAD BREATH
See page 89.

■ OFFENSIVE DISCHARGES
For example, vaginal discharge... and one rare possibility:

■ FISH ODOR SYNDROME
One of several rare metabolic diseases.

The first two are easily remedied by self-help and common sense use of over-the-counter medications.

Vaginal discharge may be due to poor hygiene, a long forgotten tampon or infection. Try two or three days of vinegar and water douching and check for a foreign object. If it does not clear, or if there is itching or burning, see your physician.

Fish odor syndrome needs specialist treatment and advice on odor-concealment.

LIFELESS HAIR

Loss of "body" or "life" in the hair is to some extent inevitable with advancing years. It is also seen in association with the medical conditions that cause baldness. Severe stress, such as that caused by major, prolonged illness, can also affect the quality and thickness of hair. Vitamin and iron and zinc deficiency and severe undernourishment will also affect hair quality.

LOSS OF HAIR OR BALDNESS

Normal baldness (also described as alopecia) — part of the male aging process — is characterized by:
* Recession of the hairline at the forehead and temples.
* Thinning of the hair on the crown. It becomes dry and lifeless; loses "body".
* A gradual meeting of the hairless areas so that hair remains only on the sides and back of the head.

Women do not have a hereditary tendency to baldness. Although dramatic hair loss may be experienced by women *(see page 264)* total baldness is not seen.

Female hair does, however, thin with age. While some thinning is inevitable, occasionally families notice a marked trend towards thin hair, again associated with aging, passed from mother to daughter.

Stages of male baldness

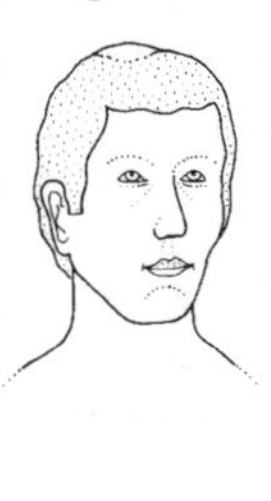

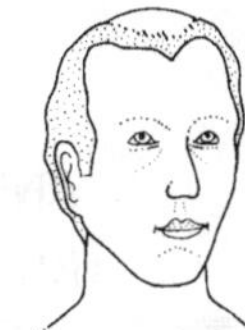

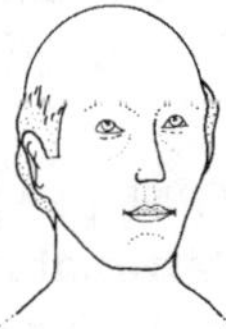

Abnormal hair loss can of course be a sign (in women as well is in men) of scalp disease, or more generalized disease. Most such cases, as this section shows, are fairly easy to distinguish from normal baldness.

PROBABLE

ECZEMA OR DERMATITIS
ALOPECIA AREATA
CHILDBIRTH

POSSIBLE

INJURY
PSORIASIS
IRON DEFICIENCY
HYPOTHYROIDISM
POST-MENOPAUSAL CHANGE
RINGWORM
TELOGEN ALOPECIA
MEDICATION

Hair

RARE

AIDS
HYPOPITUITARISM
ANOGEN ALOPECIA
TRAUMATIC ALOPECIA

PROBABLE

■ ECZEMA OR DERMATITIS
Any skin inflammation may cause loss of hair in the areas affected.
* Complete patches of hair loss.
* Skin is inflamed, weeping and crusting.
* Scales may be seen.
* There may be dermatitis or eczema elsewhere on the body.

■ ALOPECIA AREATA
The commonest cause of patchy baldness.
* Local areas of total baldness.
* Normal skin.
* Several patches may occur together.
* Regrowth normally occurs spontaneously after a few months.
This is often seen at a time of stress, such as bereavement.

■ CHILDBIRTH
Many women notice changes in hair substance and texture before and after childbirth: it tends to be generally thinner and finer.
After childbirth, or even in pregnancy, it is not unusual for there to be dramatic hair loss. Large quantities of hair seen in the tub or shower at this time are not unusual. Normally hair growth recovers with time. In rare cases, the original texture of the hair is never restored.

POSSIBLE

■ INJURY
Burns, skin loss or even deep cuts can damage hair-bearing skin, so that hair may never re-grow.
Generally speaking, hair does not grow on scar tissue. The only solution is to hide such areas by expert combing and styling.

■ PSORIASIS
* Hair loss in areas of psoriasis on the scalp.
* Silvery, scaly red patches seen in scalp.
* Other signs of psoriasis seen elsewhere on body; *see page 242.*

■ IRON DEFICIENCY
* Generalized hair loss or thinning.
* May improve after taking iron supplements.
See also IRON DEFICIENCY ANEMIA, page 422.

■ HYPOTHYROIDISM
See page 460.
* Hair is sparse.
* Hair may be dry and thin.

■ POST-MENOPAUSAL CHANGE
Hair texture may change in and around the menopause due to alterations in hormone balance. The role of hormone replacement therapy in protecting against or reversing the effects of the menopause is a subject of continuing research.

■ RINGWORM
Medical term *tinea capitis*. A fungal infection of the skin of the scalp.

HAIR

* Circular bald patches.
* Scaling of the skin.
* Brittle hair stumps remain.
Treated with anti-fungal creams.

■ MEDICATION
Antithyroid, blood thinning and anti-cancer medications can lead to hair loss. Excess vitamin A may also be a cause.

■ TELOGEN ALOPECIA
A term describing diffuse loss of hair which is in the resting stage of its life-cycle. A number of causes have been identified, unrelated to local scalp disease, including: childbirth *(see page 264)* emotional stress; any illness with fever; loss of blood; any major illness.

Except in some *very* rare cases, the hair commonly grows again after a few months.

RARE

■ AIDS
Hair loss may be noted in the later stages of AIDS.

■ HYPOPITUITARISM
Under-activity of the pituitary gland may show itself in many ways, including:
* Absence of sexual function (absence of libido).
* Absence of menstruation in females.
* Pale skin.
* Hair loss.
* Visual defects.
* Weight gain and fatigue.
See also page 418.

Site of pituitary gland

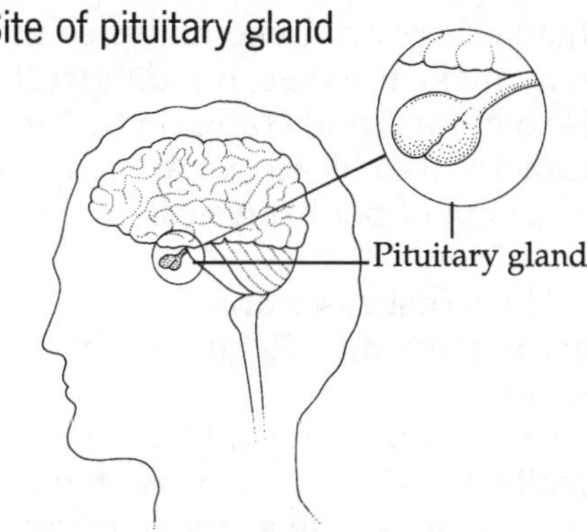

■ ANOGEN ALOPECIA
Some medications affect hair during their growth phase, notably anti-cancer medications given as courses of chemotherapy.

Vitamin A toxicity is another example. After stopping the medication, hair will eventually grow again, but the texture of the hair may be quite different from what it was before.

■ TRAUMATIC ALOPECIA
The habit of pulling and twisting hair can produce patchy hair loss. Traction alopecia is the result of certain hairstyles (pony tails and braids).

DANDRUFF

The causes of this almost universal condition are unclear. For most people, dandruff arises from time to time because of the skin's natural tendency to flake — to shed its topmost layer — so that it can be renewed from below. If you have dry skin and dry hair, you may suffer more from dandruff than others do. General ill-health may make it worse, but dandruff is so natural and common that it is unhelpful to try to explain it away as a sign of poor physical condition.

The worst cases are accompanied by itching of the scalp.

Use of anti-dandruff shampoos really does help. Persist with the treatment as long as the dandruff remains. If this does not improve the situation, see your physician. He or she can prescribe a variety of treatments, ranging from strong, tar-based shampoos to special shampoos containing ketoconazole. This is extremely effective. Steroid scalp lotions may also be helpful in some circumstances.

UNWANTED BODY HAIR

It is one of nature's many ironies that while baldness is almost universally an unwanted male symptom, unwanted body hair is almost exclusively a female symptom. Covered here is hirsutism in its specific sense of a male pattern of hair distribution on a woman.

PROBABLE
NORMAL PATTERN

POSSIBLE
POLYCYSTIC OVARIES
MENOPAUSE

RARE
MEDICATIONS
ACROMEGALY
HYPERADRENALISM
TURNER'S SYNDROME
CONGENITAL ADRENAL HYPERPLASIA

PROBABLE

■ NORMAL PATTERN
Patterns of hair growth on face, limbs and body vary according to country or region of origin. Individuals should compare themselves with others from a similar ethnic background before deciding that they have abnormally hairy bodies. For example, Japanese and Chinese women have very little body hair, whereas Mediterranean people may have much more.

POSSIBLE

■ POLYCYSTIC OVARIES
Otherwise known as the Stein-Leventhal syndrome.
* Hairiness.
* Obesity.
* Often absent menstruation.
* Ovaries have multiple cysts.

■ MENOPAUSE
Women going through the menopause may note increased amounts of hair, typically fine hair that appears on the face.

Site of adrenal gland

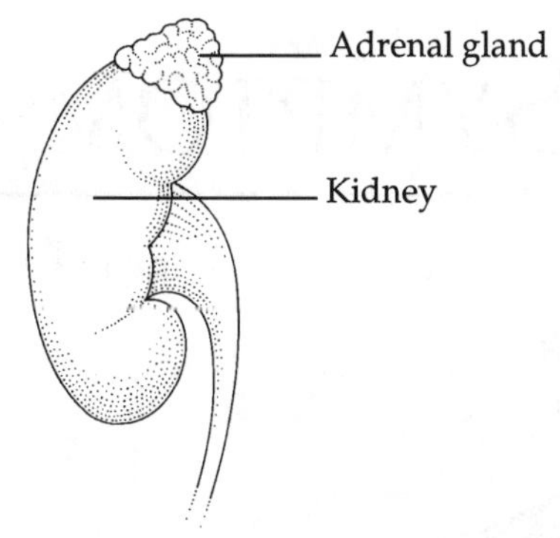

RARE

■ MEDICATIONS
A number of medications may increase either fine hair on the face or body hair elsewhere. They include:
* Some steroid preparations.
* Hormone treatments, including the pill.
* Minoxidil, used to treat raised blood pressure, but now also used as a hair restorer.
* Some anti-epileptic medications.

■ ACROMEGALY
In addition to its other features (*see page 275*) women with acromegaly may have increased body hair.

■ HYPERADRENALISM
May be caused by a disorder of the adrenal gland, or by taking steroids.
* Round, "moon" face.
* Fat deposited on back (buffalo-hump).
* Fat deposited on body (not legs).
* Muscle fatigue.
* Easily bruised skin.
* Stretch marks.
* Bone pain.
Women also note:
* Increased body hair.
* Menstruation stops.
* Enlarged clitoris.
Men may suffer from:
* Impotence.
* Acne.

■ TURNER'S SYNDROME
A chromosomal abnormality. The individual is genetically male, but has female characteristics, including:
* Short stature.
* No secondary sexual characteristics.
* Very short neck.
* Broad chest with widely separated nipples.
* Deafness.
* Hairiness.

■ CONGENITAL ADRENAL HYPERPLASIA
Excessive growth of the adrenal glands from birth.
* Mild hirsutism.
* Enlarged clitoris.
* Fused labia.
May appear at a later age with:
* Acne.
* Early false puberty.
* Enlarged clitoris.
* Absent or scanty menstruation.

SKELETAL AND MUSCULAR SYMPTOMS

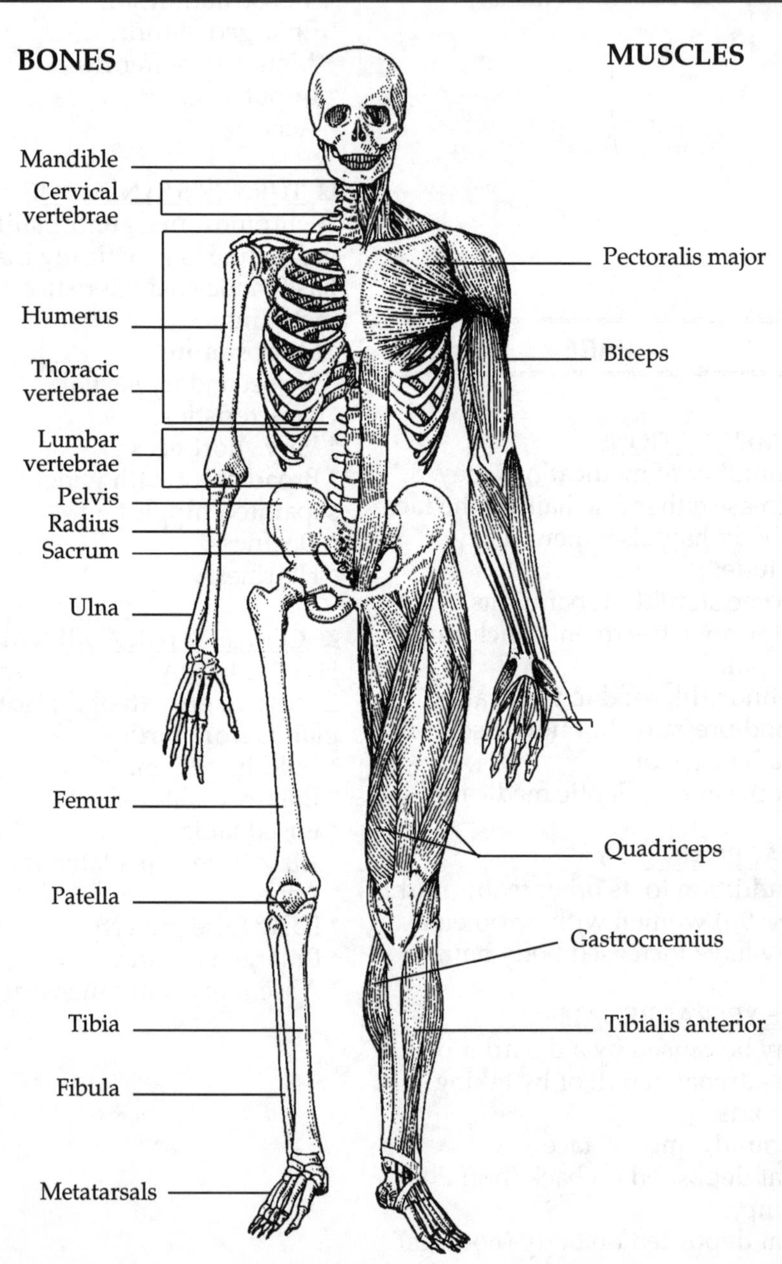

THE BONES, JOINTS AND MUSCLES – INTRODUCTION

This section covers the body's bones and muscles and joints. Joints are where bones come together; the "straps" that keep bones in place at a joint are called ligaments. Muscles are attached to bone by tendons, and as muscles contract and relax they provide movement.

The symptoms of some diseases affecting bones, joints and muscles are unique to them alone. It is also true that few firm diagnoses are made in this area by physicians, without additional information from X-rays, blood tests or other tests. Further tests may be needed after diagnosis and treatment to check progress.

In this section the usual order of symptoms has been varied in order to begin with some key general symptoms of muscles and bones occurring elsewhere in the body. We then move to specific bone, joint and muscle symptoms as experienced in different parts of the body, working from the shoulders downwards. Finally, under the heading FINGERS AND TOES, are grouped symptoms affecting the outer reaches, or extremities, of the body, which are vulnerable in certain special ways.

WASTING AND LOSS OF POWER IN THE MUSCLES

Muscular wasting, or atrophy, results from either damage to the nerve or blood supply to a muscle; lack of use because of illness or injury; or primary muscle disease.

PROBABLE

INJURY
GENERAL BODY WASTING

POSSIBLE

CARPAL TUNNEL SYNDROME
INJURY OF A NERVE OR NERVES
DIABETES
ALCOHOLIC NEUROPATHY
RHEUMATOID ARTHRITIS

RARE

MOTOR NEURONE DISEASE
MUSCULAR DYSTROPHY
TUBERCULOSIS
SUBACUTE COMBINED DEGENERATION OF THE SPINAL CORD

Muscles

PROBABLE

■ INJURY
The body's normal protective response to immobilization of the affected part. One of the best examples of this is a damaged knee. The knee is held slightly bent, and you try to prevent movement for a few days. By the end of a week, you may well see some wasting of the quadriceps muscle at the front of the thigh.

The weaker the muscle, the less safe the joint feels, and a vicious cycle of disuse and further wasting then continues. This is why careful medical assessment and controlled exercises to maintain muscle bulk are important for all such injuries.

■ GENERAL BODY WASTING
Bed-bound patients can develop generalized disuse atrophy (wasting) of muscles. This can be made worse by the underlying condition. Muscles also get smaller with aging.

POSSIBLE

■ CARPAL TUNNEL SYNDROME
See page 293.

■ INJURY OF A NERVE OR NERVES
See page 319.

■ DIABETES
See DIABETIC NEUROPATHY, page 317.

■ ALCOHOLIC NEUROPATHY
See page 318.

■ RHEUMATOID ARTHRITIS
See page 279.

RARE

■ MOTOR NEURONE DISEASE
A disease of the nervous system. There are several forms, but the main features are:
* Progressive onset of muscular weakness, accompanied by muscle wasting.
* Small muscles of the hand are affected first.
* "Flickering" contractions of parts of muscles.

The disease progresses relentlessly, ultimately affecting speech, swallowing and breathing muscles.

■ MUSCULAR DYSTROPHY
This is a primary muscle disease, which starts during the first few years of life.
* Wasting and weakness of back and pelvic muscles; affects both sides of the body.
* Failure of function affecting both sides of the body leads to a "waddling" gait while still mobile.
* Gradual degeneration leading to inability to walk and general immobility.
* Immobility leads to the muscles shortening, and deformity becomes inevitable.

The outlook is poor.

■ TUBERCULOSIS
See page 447.

■ SUBACUTE COMBINED DEGENERATION OF THE SPINAL CORD
See page 320.

CRAMPS, ACHES AND PAINS IN THE MUSCLES

Most are of little significance. If they die away within a few days they should not be taken seriously, unless they keep returning.

PROBABLE
SIMPLE CRAMP
VIRAL OR BACTERIAL INFECTION
INJURY

POSSIBLE
INTERMITTENT CLAUDICATION
BIOCHEMICAL IMBALANCE
FIBROMYALGIA

RARE
MEDICATIONS
DERMATOMYOSITIS
POLYMYOSITIS
POLYMYALGIA RHEUMATICA
TETANUS

PROBABLE

■ SIMPLE CRAMP
* Sudden onset of muscle spasm, often while asleep.
* Muscle, often the calf, feels hard due to contraction.
* Relieved by massage.
* Often residual discomfort for a few hours.

■ VIRAL OR BACTERIAL INFECTION
Fleeting muscular pains are commonly associated with the flu and other infectious diseases. Most settle within a day or two. No specific treatment is required, apart from that for the underlying infection.

■ INJURY
A direct blow to a muscle can cause painful local swelling and bruising. Indirect injury, for instance straining to lift a heavy object, can make muscle fibres stretch and tear. Repetition of the movement reproduces the pain. Treatment for both is painkillers and resting the affected muscle.

POSSIBLE

■ INTERMITTENT CLAUDICATION
See PERIPHERAL VASCULAR DISEASE, page 318.

■ BIOCHEMICAL IMBALANCE
Loss of salt, typically after strenuous exercise, can cause painful cramps.

■ FIBROMYALGIA
Many painful muscle trigger points can occur in the neck, shoulders, upper and lower back and legs.
* Trouble sleeping.
* Sore muscles.

Muscles

RARE

■ MEDICATIONS
A number of medications are known to cause muscle pains. These include lithium, alcohol, amphetamines and suxamethonium (used for general anesthesia).

■ DERMATOMYOSITIS
A disease associated with disordered immunity. May be associated with cancer. Develops from the age of 40 years onwards.
* Inflammation and pains in multiple muscle groups.
* Muscular weakness.
* Dermatitis.
* Edema (swelling).

■ POLYMYOSITIS
Can be associated with many diseases, including collagen disorders and lung cancer. May improve and then get worse.
* Progressive, painful inflammation of muscles — worse when used.
* Affects muscles in a variable manner, but those affected are weak.
* Fever.
* Feel sick.
* Fast heart rate.

■ POLYMYALGIA RHEUMATICA
A disease of the elderly.
* Painful, stiff upper limb muscles.
* Feel sick.
* Fever.

■ TETANUS
Caused by the organism *Clostridia tetani* and acquired by contamination of open wounds. The damage is done by a very powerful toxin that attacks the nervous system. Symptoms may take two weeks to develop.
* Local muscular weakness near site of infection.
* Facial muscles go into spasm: the individual appears to be forcing a grin.
* Muscles of the body go into spasm at the slightest stimulus.
* Fever

Tetanus still claims victims, even when cared for in intensive care. Immunization is the essential precaution, and needs to be repeated every 10 years. To help you remember your immunization, choose every 10th birthday after your tenth, e.g. at 20, 30, etc.

POOR OR ABSENT MUSCLE CONTROL

See THE BRAIN AND NERVOUS SYSTEM, pages 377-409, especially CONVULSIONS, page 387 and PARALYSIS, pages 404-5.

INVOLUNTARY TWITCHING OR TREMBLING MUSCLES

See pages 437-40.

UNUSUALLY WEAK MUSCLE

Muscle weakness without muscle wasting is rare. However, two conditions are worth considering. Both are very rare.

■ HYPERADRENALISM
Caused by an excess of corticosteroids, and often the result of doctors giving steroids to treat other diseases such as rheumatoid arthritis.
* Weight gain, except for limbs.
* Moon face.
* Hump at the back of the neck.
* Muscle weakness.
* Purple lines (strie) on belly, back and upper thighs.
* Osteoporosis.
* Diabetes.
* High blood pressure.
* Hair grows on body.
* Occasional psychiatric disorders.

■ PRIMARY ALDOSTERONISM
A very rare disease, caused by excess secretion of aldosterone by the adrenal gland.
* Muscle weakness.
* Excessive thirst.
* Excessive urine output.
* High blood pressure.

PAINFUL BONES

Pain in bones can be either localized — to part of one or more bones — or generalized.

PROBABLE
INJURY
OSTEOARTHRITIS
OSTEOPOROSIS

POSSIBLE
SECONDARY BONE CANCER

RARE
RICKETS AND OSTEOMALACIA
TUBERCULOSIS
INFLAMMATORY ARTHRITIS
PRIMARY BONE CANCER

PROBABLE

■ INJURY
Is it broken?

Signs of a break (fracture) are:
* Pain at the site of injury.
* Possibly deformity — the limb looks bent.
* Loss of function — typically inability to bear weight.

Depending on the site and force of the injury, skin, nerves and blood vessels may be involved.

Obviously, urgent medical care is needed.

Persistent pain following an injury, particularly when accompanied by swelling, should raise the suspicion of a fracture. Seek medical help.

Lesser injury may not cause a break, but can still cause pain and loss of function.

See also SUBPERIOSTEAL HEMATOMA, this page.

■ OSTEOARTHRITIS
See page 285.

■ OSTEOPOROSIS
See page 286.

POSSIBLE

■ SECONDARY CANCER
Localized bone pain can be caused by a secondary (metastatic) cancer in the bones. So if an individual has a *known* cancer elsewhere in the body, this possibility needs considering. In someone without cancer, this would be a rare diagnosis.

RARE

■ RICKETS AND OSTEOMALACIA
See page 287.

■ TUBERCULOSIS
See page 289.

■ INFLAMMATORY ARTHRITIS
A term for joint inflammation, e.g. rheumatoid arthritis or ankylosing spondylitis, *pages 279 and 286.*

■ PRIMARY BONE CANCER
See under CANCER OF BONE OR CARTILAGE, 275.

BONES, SWOLLEN OR MISSHAPEN

PROBABLE
CALLUS
SUBPERIOSTEAL HEMATOMA

POSSIBLE
ACUTE OSTEOMYELITIS
CHRONIC OSTEOMYELITIS
RICKETS
MALUNION OF FRACTURE
PAGET'S DISEASE OF BONE

RARE
ACROMEGALY
BENIGN TUMOR
CANCER OF BONE OR CARTILAGE
TUBERCULOSIS

PROBABLE

■ CALLUS
Lump felt on bone; new bone formed after a fracture.
* Lump felt on bone.
* Previous, definite bone fracture.
* Forms within a few weeks.
* The larger the bone, the greater the amount of callus.
* Pain-free when bone is fully healed.

■ SUBPERIOSTEAL HEMATOMA
A direct injury to bone, typically the shin, but no fracture.

* Clear history of local injury.
* Swelling (bruising) noted almost immediately.
* Painful for several weeks after the injury.
* A hard lump still apparent weeks or months afterwards.
* Common in those who play contact sports.

POSSIBLE

■ ACUTE OSTEOMYELITIS
A bone infection which, if suspected, requires immediate treatment. Infection may start elsewhere in the body. The bone is affected by bacteria carried in the bloodstream.
* Persistent fever.
* Sudden onset of pain in bone with swelling, which may not be obvious.
* Redness and swelling of the soft tissues, over the affected bone.
* Extreme pain on movement.
* Chills.
* Feel sick.

■ CHRONIC OSTEOMYELITIS
May occur after untreated or inadequately treated acute osteomyelitis; or after a compound fracture (where there is a fracture and a cut down to the bone).
* Thickening of bone.
* Wound (sinus) discharging pus.
* Local pain.
* Inflammation around wound.

■ RICKETS
See page 287.

■ MALUNION OF FRACTURE
Means a poorly joined break. Sometimes this occurs despite careful realignment or setting of the broken bone. It may give the appearance of deformity or swelling.

■ PAGET'S DISEASE OF BONE
See page 437.

RARE

■ ACROMEGALY
General enlargement of the skeleton caused by excessive growth hormone from the pituitary gland. Jaws and hands appear especially large.

■ BENIGN TUMOR OF BONE AND CARTILAGE
Both bone and cartilage in any part of the body may give rise to benign tumors which present as:
* Pain-free hard lumps.
* Smooth surfaces.
* Slow-growing.

■ CANCER OF BONE OR CARTILAGE
Individuals with known cancer of other organs of the body (for example breast or lung) may develop secondary tumors (metastatic deposits) in the bones.
* Chronically and progressively painful.
* Pain may be very localized.
* A lump may *not* be present.

Other symptoms of advanced cancer may be present, but sometimes bone secondaries are the first indication of an as-yet undiagnosed cancer. This is why localized pain in a bone without a history of injury should be followed up with your physician.

Primary malignant bone tumors are rarer than secondary tumors. They may form at any age, and there are several different types.

■ TUBERCULOSIS
See page 289.

BONES BREAKING EASILY

Meaning fractures occurring without an obvious history of injury. They divide into two types: those which are the result of disease (pathological) and those in apparently normal bones (spontaneous or stress fractures).

Spontaneous or stress fractures may occur because of repeated injury, as when athletes train; or after repeated compression, for instance repetitive lifting affecting the spine.
* Local pain.
* Local swelling.
* Relieved by rest over a few days.
* Pain recurs when activity is repeated.
* May not be seen on an X-ray and may be diagnosed by bone scan.

Typical sites include the small bones of the foot (metatarsals); upper arm bone (humerus); upper thigh bone (neck of femur); knee cap (patella); and spine.

In pathological fractures, the bone is abnormally weak because of either local abnormality (for example, malignant tumors, tuberculosis, osteomyelitis) or general weakness of the bone (for example, osteoporosis, osteomalacia, brittle bone disease or rheumatoid arthritis) present from birth. Also, if a bone is unused, it becomes thinner and is more likely to break.

PROBABLE
OSTEOPOROSIS

POSSIBLE
PAGET'S DISEASE OF BONE
OSTEOMALACIA
DISUSED BONE

RARE
OSTEOMYELITIS
BENIGN BONE TUMORS
BONE CANCER
BRITTLE BONE DISEASE
MARBLE BONES
RHEUMATOID ARTHRITIS

PROBABLE

■ OSTEOPOROSIS
Gradual thinning of the bone, particularly in elderly white females, may result in broken bones without significant injury. A fracture of the neck of the femur (the hip) is very common. The symptoms are:
* Pain in the groin/hip (after a fall).
* Apparent shortening of the leg.
* Inability to bear weight on the affected side.
* The foot on the affected side may be turned outwards.

Most commonly treated with an operation to realign and fix the broken bone or hip joint.

POSSIBLE

■ PAGET'S DISEASE OF BONE
See page 437.

■ OSTEOMALACIA
See RICKETS AND OSTEOMALACIA, page 287.

■ DISUSED BONE
Bone requires regular use to maintain its normal structure. If unused because of paralysis (for instance by a stroke, multiple sclerosis or spina bifida), the bones become weak and may even break when the individual is being carried, or turned in bed.
So, bone pain in any bedridden or partially paralysed individual may be caused by a fracture.

RARE

■ OSTEOMYELITIS
■ BENIGN BONE TUMORS
■ BONE CANCER
See page 275.

■ BRITTLE BONE DISEASE
There are two main types of this disease, *osteogenesis imperfecta congenita*, where fractures develop in the womb and at birth; and *osteogenesis imperfecta tarda*, a milder variant with fractures later in life. This is a hereditary disorder which prevents bones and other tissue forming properly.
The symptoms are:
* Bones fracture with minimal injury.
* Whites of the eyes appear blue.

THE SKELETON

The skeleton

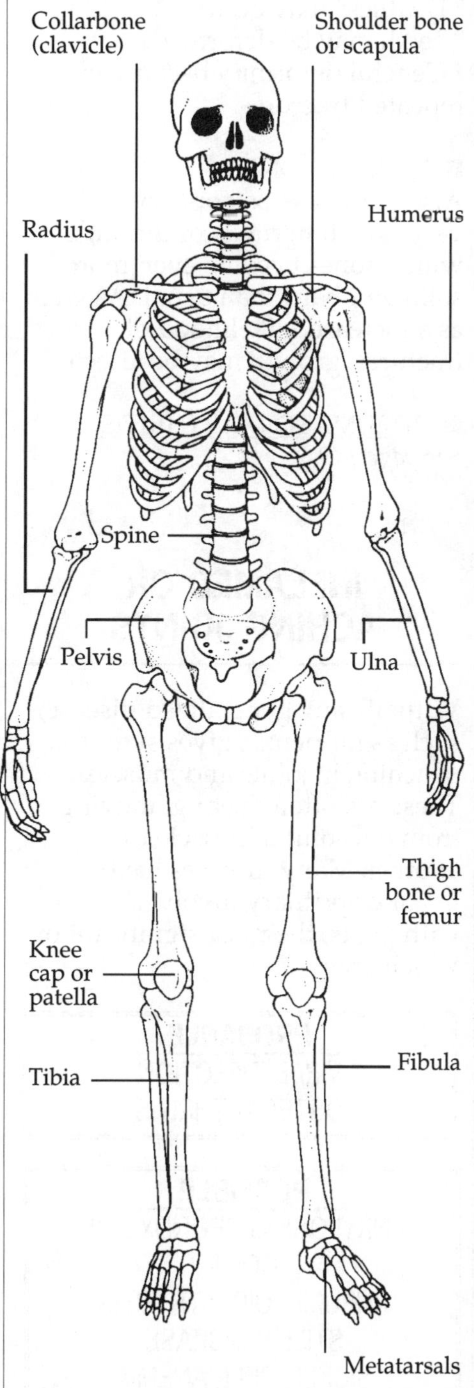

* Ligaments may be lax (allowing excess mobility of joints).
* Deafness may occur.
* Teeth may be deformed.
* General deformity because of repeated fractures.

■ MARBLE BONES
Also known as osteopetrosis. A very rare, inherited condition, in which bones become even more solid and hard than usual. As well as a increased likelihood of fractures, growth may be affected.

■ RHEUMATOID ARTHRITIS
See page 279.

INFLAMED OR ACHING JOINTS

Virtually any generalized disease, such as influenza, gives symptoms of aching in joints and muscles. These are often fleeting, moving from one joint or muscle to another. Many diseases have major or primary involvement with joints, the most significant of which are:

PROBABLE
VIRAL INFECTION
OSTEOARTHRITIS

POSSIBLE
ANKYLOSING SPONDYLITIS
GOUT
RHEUMATOID ARTHRITIS
STILL'S DISEASE
SICKLE CELL ANEMIA

RARE
REITER'S SYNDROME
PSORIATIC ARTHRITIS
GONOCOCCAL ARTHRITIS
SYSTEMIC LUPUS ERYTHEMATOSIS (SLE)
RHEUMATIC FEVER
HEMOPHILIA
SYPHILIS

PROBABLE

■ VIRAL INFECTION
Any viral infection, such as the common cold or influenza, will give vague joint pains.
* General sickness.
* Fever.
* Cough, runny nose.
* Muscle pain.
* Joint pain.
* Normally cures itself in a few days.

■ OSTEOARTHRITIS
See page 285.

POSSIBLE

■ ANKYLOSING SPONDYLITIS
See page 287.

■ GOUT
Caused by excess uric acid in the blood.
* One joint affected to begin with; most commonly, first affects the big toe joint.
* Sudden onset.

* Joint is hot, shiny, red and excruciatingly painful.
* There may be fever. Attacks recur and involve other joints:
* Gouty lumps form in the skin, particularly on the ears and adjacent to joints.

The high levels of uric acid, if untreated, can cause kidney stones and kidney failure. Blood tests are needed to confirm the diagnosis, and medication to control the symptoms.

■ RHEUMATOID ARTHRITIS

The commonest type of chronic, generalized inflammatory joint disease. It is actually a connective tissue disease and it may run in the family. Symptoms are caused by persistent inflammation of the synovial membrane, which lines joint capsules. Commonest in young women. This is a disease of flare-ups and quiet periods; treatment involves medication and reduction of inflammation. At later stages, in severe cases, surgery may be necessary to improve function because of deformity of joints.

An immunoglobulin called rheumatoid factor is commonly present in the blood of affected individuals. Features include:
* Painful swelling of joints (often symmetrical).
* Early morning stiffness.
* Progressive joint deformity. (See also sections on specific joints.)
* Progressive loss of function.
* Lumps may appear in skin and around joints.
* Osteoporosis may develop.
* Anemia.
* Muscle wasting.

■ STILL'S DISEASE

This is rheumatoid arthritis (above), occurring in childhood.

■ SICKLE CELL DISEASE

An inherited disease found in people of African origin. The red blood cells become sickle-shaped and so carry smaller amounts of oxygen. These sickle cells are less pliable than normal cells and so block up capillaries (small blood vessels) causing damage to organs because of lack of oxygen and poor blood supply. Some individuals are less affected — they are described as having sickle cell trait. Those with full-blown disease have recurrent attacks of severe pains, in limbs and abdomen — sickle crises.

Features of the disease include:
* Anemia.
* Increased likelihood of infection.
* Joint pains.
* Fever.
* Jaundice.
* Abdominal pains.

Treatment is mainly aimed at relieving the symptoms. Blood transfusions, administering oxygen and strong painkillers are main types of therapy

RARE

■ REITER'S SYNDROME

Its cause is unknown but usually there will be the following three symptoms:
* Urethritis or diarrhea — developing up to a month after sexual intercourse — not caused by bacteria.

THE SKELETON

* Conjunctivitis — up to three weeks after the urethritis.
* Arthritis — up to two weeks after the conjunctivitis. This is mild, and occurs in more than one small- to middle-sized joint.

■ PSORIATIC ARTHRITIS
Occasionally, arthritis can be a complication of psoriasis, a skin disease.
* Various joints, in different parts of the body, are affected.
* The joints at the ends of the fingers may be the only ones involved.
* Possibly nail pitting.

■ GONOCOCCAL ARTHRITIS
One of many complications of the sexually transmitted disease gonorrhea. In males the main symptom is:
* Urethral discharge.
In females up to 75 percent may have no symptoms. Those that do may have:
* Pain on passing urine.
* Vaginal discharge.

May develop in one or more joints with symptoms of infectious arthritis. *See page 293.*

■ SYSTEMIC LUPUS ERYTHEMATOSIS (SLE)
See page 448.

■ RHEUMATIC FEVER
See page 448.

■ HEMOPHILIA
See page 427.

■ SYPHILIS
See page 448.

Distal interphalangeal joint

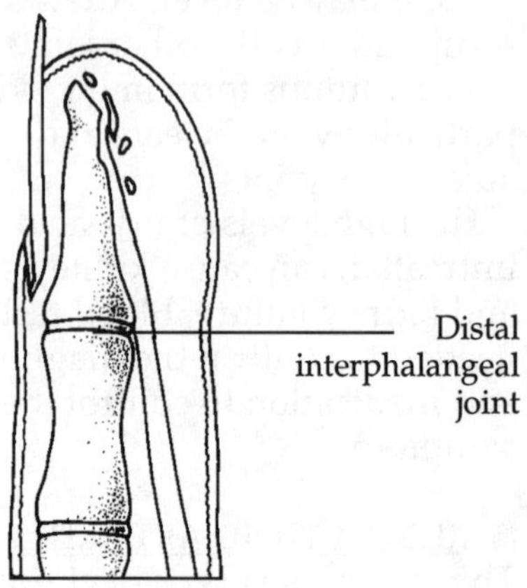

SWOLLEN JOINT WITH NODULES

PROBABLE
BURSA
OSTEOARTHRITIS

POSSIBLE
RHEUMATOID ARTHRITIS
GOUT

RARE
CHARCOT'S JOINTS

PROBABLE

■ BURSA
Many joints have sacs, like empty balloons, overlying their surfaces. These help lubricate the

movement of the muscles and joints. If damaged, these fill with fluid and enlarge. They feel like smooth, fluid-filled swellings and may be uncomfortable and irritating.

■ OSTEOARTHRITIS
See page 285.

POSSIBLE

■ RHEUMATOID ARTHRITIS
See page 279.

■ GOUT
See page 278.

RARE

■ CHARCOT'S JOINTS
Joints that have lost the sense of pain and position. If the joint is damaged, it can become progressively more deformed, as degeneration occurs rapidly. The joint looks as if it should be very painful, possibly with extreme swelling and deformity. Fluid, bony protuberances and loose pieces of bone may easily be felt in and around the joint. Dislocation is not uncommon. The commoner causes include anything that can damage the peripheral nerve system, including diabetes and alcohol.

PAINFUL JOINTS

See INFLAMED OR ACHING JOINTS, page 278.

STIFF JOINTS

See INFLAMED OR ACHING JOINTS, page 278.

PAINFUL SHOULDER

PROBABLE
FROZEN SHOULDER
OSTEOARTHRITIS

POSSIBLE
PAINFUL ARC SYNDROME
ROTATOR CUFF TEAR
ACROMIOCLAVICULAR INJURY
DISLOCATION OF THE SHOULDER
RHEUMATOID ATHRITIS
FRACTURED COLLARBONE (CLAVICLE)
FRACTURED HUMERUS

RARE
RUPTURED BICEPS TENDON
POLYMYALGIA RHEUMATICA
OSTEOMYELITIS
INTERNAL BLEEDING
SECONDARY BONE CANCER

PROBABLE

■ FROZEN SHOULDER
Commonest in later middle age.
* Injury to shoulder joint may or may not have occurred.
* Subsequently progressive pain and stiffness.
* Pain starts at shoulder tip and runs down outer arm to hand.

* Can be very disabling.
* Tends to cure itself.
Called "frozen shoulder" because someone with this condition tends to hold their shoulder very still, due to the pain.

■ OSTEOARTHRITIS
See page 285.

POSSIBLE

■ PAINFUL ARC SYNDROME BURSITIS
Most common in a middle-aged or later middle-aged person.
* Pain at shoulder tip.
* Variable in intensity; worse at night.
* Limited shoulder movement.
* Local area of tenderness — can be identified with one fingertip.
* Pain worse over part of the "arc" made by raising the arm from the side.

■ ROTATOR CUFF TEAR
Tendons lying at the upper part of the shoulder can tear or rupture without warning. Tends to occur with pre-existing wear and tear changes, and so typical of the elderly.
* May be associated with a fall or lifting.
* Sudden onset of pain.
* Arm cannot be moved outwards.

■ ACROMIOCLAVICULAR INJURY.
The joint between the collarbone and the shoulder blade is separated by direct injury, usually in contact sports.
* Painful movement of shoulder.
* Tender point in front of shoulder.

■ DISLOCATION OF THE SHOULDER
A common injury in "contact" sports. The two components of the shoulder joint (scapula and humerus) are separated. Forceful injury makes the humeral head slip down and forwards.
* Pain on movement.
* Loss of shoulder contour.
* Humeral head may be felt below the outer end of the clavicle.
* Arm is held out from the body at elbow.

■ RHEUMATOID ARTHRITIS
See page 279.

■ FRACTURED COLLARBONE (CLAVICLE)
The collarbone may break as a result of direct or indirect injury.
* Pain at the point of the break.
* Pain on arm movement: often the individual holds the affected arm with the opposite hand to prevent movement.
* Deformity at fracture site.

■ FRACTURED HUMERUS
The bone of the upper arm. The upper end of the humerus can break in a number of ways, but the damage is almost always the result of a direct blow or a fall.
* Pain when attempting to move shoulder or arm.
* Often, substantial tracks of bruising down arm.
* Variable amount of deformity — dependent on the degree of displacement.

RARE

■ RUPTURED BICEPS TENDON
In the elderly. The top end of the biceps muscle runs over the top of the humeral head. Changes due to wear and tear can make it rupture.
* Sudden onset of pain at shoulder tip.
* Flexing arm against resistance allows upper end of biceps (now unattached) to bunch up and become visible in the upper arm.

■ POLYMYALGIA RHEUMATICA
See page 272.

■ OSTEOMYELITIS
See page 275.

■ INTERNAL BLEEDING
Anyone who develops pain at a shoulder tip after abdominal injury, when lying flat, must be urgently investigated for internal abdominal bleeding. It is thought that blood from the bleeding point tracks up to the diaphragm, from where pain is referred to the shoulder, which shares the same nerve supply.

■ SECONDARY BONE CANCER
Cancer can sometimees spread from a primary site (such as the lung or breast) to other parts of the body via the bloodstream. The cancer may settle in bones, particularly the upper arm bone (humerus) or the shoulder blade (scapula).

CANNOT STRAIGHTEN BACK

See PAINFUL BACK, page 284.

ROUND OR HUNCHED SHOULDERS

See KYPHOSIS and SCOLIOSIS, covered under *A LUMP ON THE BACK, page 288.*

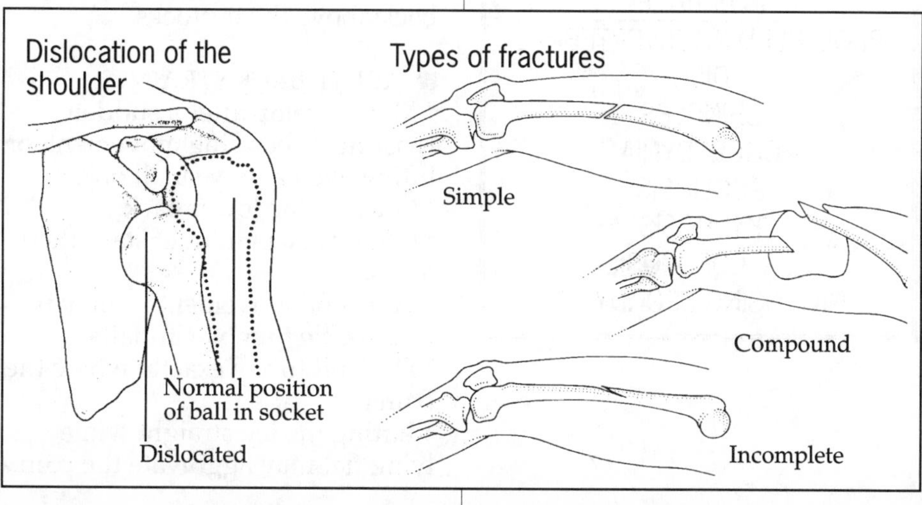

PAINFUL BACK

The back is taken here as the area from the neck down to the tailbone (the coccyx). All of us will have at least one episode of back pain during our lives caused by either injury or disease.

Back pain lasting more than two to three weeks and which does not respond to simple painkillers must be reported to a physician.

Pain may prevent you from straightening up, but may also be felt when in a "normal" upright posture.

PROBABLE
MUSCULAR
MYOFASCIAL PAIN
ACUTE BACK STRAIN
CHRONIC BACK STRAIN
OSTEOARTHRITIS
SCIATICA
CERVICAL SPONDYLOSIS

POSSIBLE
PROLAPSED INTERVERTEBRAL DISC
SHINGLES
COCCYDYNIA
SCOLIOSIS
KYPHOSIS
OSTEOPOROSIS
ANKYLOSING SPONDYLITIS

RARE
CANCER OF THE SPINE
BENIGN TUMOR
RICKETS AND OSTEOMALACIA
TUBERCULOSIS
GASTRO-INTESTINAL DISEASE

PROBABLE

■ MUSCULAR
Tearing or bruising of muscles or ligaments.
* Distinct history of injury — typically a blow, pulling or pushing.
* Dull ache initially, but the pain increases.
* Pain is local.
* Worse on movement, typically coughing or deep breathing.
* Resolves after a few days.
May need strong pain killers.

■ MYOFASCIAL PAIN
* Tender local areas of muscle spasm.
* Usually around neck and shoulder blades, and in the lower back above the buttocks.

■ ACUTE BACK STRAIN
* May develop after a sudden twisting or bending movement, or lifting even a very small object.
* Often in the lower back.
* Often very painful at start, then less so.
* Worse on movement — may be impossible to move initially.
* Difficult to say exactly where the pain is.
* Lifting the leg straight while lying flat may aggravate the pain.

* Normally responds to bed rest and pain killers.

A physical therapist, osteopath or chiropractor may be able to help.

■ CHRONIC BACK STRAIN
Low back pain that recurs. The individual has had similar episodes over a number of years and will be aware of the types of activity that cause it and relieve it. Symptoms can be made worse by obesity.
* Similar symptoms to acute back strain, but may be less intense.

■ OSTEOARTHRITIS
The wear and tear disease. Involves weight-bearing joints such as hips and low lumbar spine, but any joint can be affected.
* Low back pain comes and goes.
* Worse after standing and at the end of the day.
* Relieved by rest.
* *However*, it is possible that discomfort remains even whilst lying in bed.
* Gradually, as the joint becomes stiffer, pain decreases, and some mobility is lost.

■ SCIATICA
Really a symptom itself, rather than a diagnosis, and a common one for many who suffer from bad backs. Caused by pressure on the sciatic nerve, which has its origins in the lower back. Can, rarely, be caused by actual damage to lumbo-sacral nerves, lumbar spine and the sciatic nerves. Persistent sciatica needs investigation as it can indicate serious underlying disease.
* Pain originates in low back or buttock.
* Pain radiates down the back of the thigh to the back and outer aspect of the calf and foot.
* Tingling or altered sensation may also be noted in the leg.
* Symptoms can be made worse by raising and straightening the leg.

■ CERVICAL SPONDYLOSIS
See page 136.

POSSIBLE

■ PROLAPSED INTERVERTEBRAL DISC
Often known as a "slipped disc" (as are acute and chronic back strains and sciatica). The fibrous disc that acts as a buffer between the vertebre has a gelatinous center. Age or injury can cause this centre to bulge out, applying pressure on the nerves which emerge between the vertebre and supply sensation to the body.
* Minor episodes of backache are an early warning.
* Sudden onset of severe back pain when bending or stooping: you may be unable to stand.
* Sciatica (above) may be present.
* Coughing and straining make the pain worse.
* Numbness or tingling may develop in a leg or foot.
* Very occasionally, a slipped disc may cause difficult urination. This is a medical emergency.

The symptoms may subside in a few days or weeks; although a few may persist.

The Skeleton

Prolapsed intervertebral disc

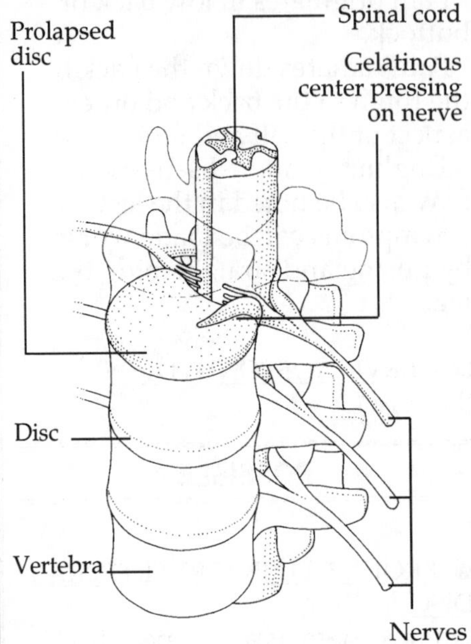

Numbness or tingling

If you have numbness or tingling in the feet or legs or in the genital region, and/or your ability to pass water seems to be affected, seek medical help urgently.

■ SHINGLES

* Initially, skin irritation.
* Red spots develop, often in a band a few inches wide on one side of the body.
* The spots develop into fluid-filled blisters which burst and form crusts.
* Can become very painful.
* If suspected, can be treated with acyclovir, a strong anti-viral treatment, but best given before the spots develop.
* Tends to cure itself in 10 to 14 days.

Shingles is caused by the chicken pox virus. Those who have not had chicken pox can catch it from someone with shingles.

■ COCCYDYNIA

Pain associated with the coccyx or tail bone.
* Persistent pain after a fall.
* Pain aggravated by local pressure.
* Pain aggravated by sitting.

■ SCOLIOSIS

See page 288.

■ KYPHOSIS

See page 288.

■ OSTEOPOROSIS

Thinning of the bones caused by aging. In women, this is especially a post-menopausal (change of life) problem. Prevention of osteoporosis is one of the main reasons for hormone replacement therapy (HRT).
* There may be non-specific pain in the spine.
* Increased susceptibility to stress fractures, which may account for localized pain of sudden onset in vertebra after a fall.
* Occurs in otherwise fit individuals.
* Increasing deformity as age increases.
* Bending and shortening of the spine results in loss of height.

■ ANKYLOSING SPONDYLITIS

An inflammatory disorder, affecting the spine and sacroiliac joints — commonest in young males. It tends to occur in families.
* Intermittent backache at the early

stage.
* Intermittent stiffness.
* Symptoms worst in the early morning.
* As the disease progresses, swelling and stiffness of other joints may develop.
* Occasionally, eyes, heart, lungs and ears may be affected.

RARE

■ CANCER OF THE SPINE (PRIMARY OR SECONDARY)
The spine is a well-recognized site of secondary cancer — meaning a malignant tumor which has spread from another (primary) site. Anyone developing the following should see a physician without delay:
* Localized, continuous pain in the back.
* Unremitting vague pain in the back, often through the night.
* Pain radiating from the back to the limbs.
* The development of pain, weakness or altered sensation in the limbs.

Other symptoms of cancer, including weight loss, feeling sick and loss of appetite may also be evident.

■ BENIGN TUMOR OF THE BACK
Although benign tumors rarely give rise to pain, large ones, or ones adjacent to pressure areas, for example, at the level of the waist band of your pants or skirt, may do so. Even if you think it is benign, report it to a physician.

■ RICKETS AND OSTEOMALACIA
Both represent similar disease processes in children (rickets) and in adults (osteomalacia), and are caused by lack of Vitamin D.
The symptoms of rickets are:
* Skull deformity.
* Knee, ankle and wrist thickening.
* Enlargement of the bony cartilages of the chest.
* Lower limb deformities.
* Rarely, spinal curvature and pain.

The symptoms of osteomalacia are:
* General bone pain.
* Backache.
* Muscle pain.
* Loss of height due to vertebral collapse.
* Stress fractures.

■ GASTRO-INTESTINAL OR ABDOMINAL DISEASE
A number of diseases may cause back symptoms, although very rarely in isolation.

Inflammation of the pancreas and peptic ulcer may cause pain (often centrally in the small of the back). Inflammatory bowel disease such as Crohn's disease or ulcerative colitis can cause back pain, either by referred pain from the diseased bowel or because of the joint inflammation that, rarely, may be associated with them.

■ TUBERCULOSIS
See page 289.

THE SKELETON

A LUMP ON THE BACK

PROBABLE
BENIGN TUMOR OF SKIN STRUCTURES
INFECTION
NORMAL BODY PROMINENCE
HEMATOMA – BRUISE

POSSIBLE
KYPHOSIS
SCOLIOSIS

RARE
SPINA BIFIDA
CANCER
TUBERCULOSIS

PROBABLE

■ BENIGN TUMOR OF SKIN STRUCTURES
Meaning a harmless lump, such as a lipoma or sebaceous cyst, which may occur in the skin anywhere in the body. Common features are:
* Pain-free.
* Slow increase in size.
* Otherwise good health.

■ INFECTION
Commonest in those with acne, greasy skin or poor personal hygiene.
* Often sited on the upper back.
* Painful.
* Red.
* Localized swelling.
* Pus may ooze out.

Any infection may eventually become an abscess — a collection of pus. Often, it may discharge itself, but occasionally surgical drainage may be needed. Sometimes a cellulitis (*page 311)* develops, which requires antibiotics. If recurrent infections occur, then a physician should ensure that diabetes is not the cause.

■ NORMAL BONY PROMINENCES
Occasionally, a previously unnoticed lump may become apparent. This often occurs after a loss of weight.The spine itself is a rather knobbly structure.

■ HEMATOMA – BRUISE
Swelling caused by direct injury with bleeding into the back muscles.

POSSIBLE

■ KYPHOSIS AND SCOLIOSIS
Deformities of the spine causing humps.

Kyphosis:
* Spine is unusually curved.
* Curve of the upper spine is exaggerated when viewed from side.
* Hump-back appearance.
* Some pain.

There are various causes: bad posture; disease; ankylosing spondylitis; rare congenital disease.

Scoliosis is a sideways deformity

of the spine:
* Usually a family history.
* Spine appears to curve more to one side when looked at from behind.
* Some pain.

May be associated with any disease that affects the spine.

RARE

■ SPINA BIFIDA
A congenital abnormality recognized at or soon after birth.

■ CANCER
People with known malignant disease may develop secondary growths in either the skin or skeletal structures of the back. Pain, irregular contour and rapid growth are ominous signs.

Usually, the cancer will have already made itself known.

■ TUBERCULOSIS
Unrecognized tuberculous infection of the spine or other bone(s) can cause sudden collapse of the affected part so that a bony lump can be felt. This may be known as a kyphus (and is a specific type of kyphosis — *see page 288*).
* Develops rapidly.
* Often associated with general sickness and occasional fever.
* Pain is often slight in the early stages, but can then become severe and constant.

BACK PAIN, WOMEN ONLY

PROBABLE
MENSTRUAL PAIN
MIDDLE PAIN

POSSIBLE
PELVIC INFLAMMATORY DISEASE

RARE
CANCER OF THE CERVIX, OVARIES AND WOMB

PROBABLE

■ MENSTRUAL PAIN
Also called dysmenorrhea.
* Low abdominal and back pain associated with menstrual periods.
* Occurs each month and settles.
* Otherwise well.

■ MIDDLE PAIN
* Low back and abdominal pain developing in the middle of the menstrual cycle.
* Believed to be associated with the release of the egg from the ovary.

POSSIBLE

■ PELVIC INFLAMMATORY DISEASE
Infection of the female genital tract. If suspected, requires

treatment to minimize the risk of infertility later.
* Fever.
* Low back and low abdominal pain, ranging from severe to very slight, or even non-existent.
* Vaginal discharge — yellow/ green/brown.
* Discharge is often smelly.
* Possibly sickness and fever.

RARE

■ CANCER OF THE CERVIX, OVARIES AND WOMB
* There may be chronic, constant back or lower abdominal pain.
* Possibly offensive, bloody vaginal discharge (in cases of the uterus and cervix).
* Abdominal swelling: fluid collects in the abdominal cavity.
Other symptoms associated with malignant disease may be present:
* Weight loss.
* Loss of appetite.
* Anemia.
* Sickness.

PAINFUL ELBOW

A number of structures around the elbow can give pain. The elbow joint is made up of three bones: the humerus, the radius and the ulna. A number of muscles and tendons attach near the joint, and nerves pass close by.

A direct blow can, of course, break or bruise the bone: the olecranon (point of the elbow) is the most prominent part and most often damaged. The lower end of the humerus may be broken. The upper end of the radius may be broken indirectly if you fall on an outstretched hand: force is transmitted up the arm to its top end. The symptoms of a fracture are:
* Local pain.
* Local swelling.
* Loss of function– flexing/ extending and twisting the forearm.
* Deformity may not be particularly noticeable.

Bruising can give similar symptoms, but the pain disappears relatively quickly and function returns.

One other elbow problem lies outside our conventional analysis of probable, possible and rare: knocking the "funny bone". The funny bone is not in fact a bone, but a nerve called the ulnar nerve, which runs round the back of the elbow. If you hit it:
* Exquisite pain on the inner elbow (and not knowing whether to laugh or cry).
* Pain and altered feeling (tingling) sensed down the forearm to the hand (mainly on the inner aspect), lasting a few seconds.

PROBABLE
TENNIS ELBOW
GOLFER'S ELBOW

RARE
LOOSE BODIES
INFECTED BURSA

The elbow bones

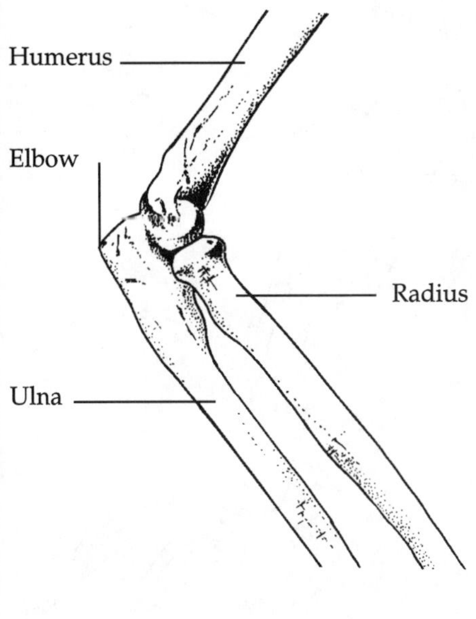

PROBABLE

■ TENNIS ELBOW
■ GOLFER'S ELBOW

These are "repetitive strain injuries", typical of tennis players and golfers, but not exclusive to them.
* Local pain: in tennis elbow, the outside part of the elbow is involved; in golfer's elbow, the inner side.
* Pain worse on certain movements, for instance turning a door handle, shaking hands, lifting, serving at tennis; straightening the elbow with the palm face up; straightening the whole arm above the head when throwing.
* Patients are often middle-aged.

May be treated with rest, or local injection of anesthetic or steroid; occasionally surgery may help. Ultrasound, massage or acupuncture may also be of benefit. An elbow band can help avoid strains.

RARE

■ LOOSE BODIES

Pieces of bone may chip off and lie free in the joint as a result of injury, degeneration (perhaps from osteoarthritis), inflammation (perhaps from rheumatoid arthritis) or some unknown cause.
* Intermittent pain in joint.
* Joint gets stuck.
* Cannot always fully extend or flex the elbow.

If symptoms persist or progress, surgical removal of the loose body may be necessary.

■ INFECTED BURSA

The bursa is a sac, like an empty balloon, that lies under the skin over the olecranon. Injury — a blow or friction — to the olecranon makes the bursa fill with fluid, which can then be seen as a lump on the point of the elbow. This is often pain-free. Occasionally, enlargement is associated with other disease such as gout or rheumatoid arthritis. If the overlying skin is damaged (cut or grazed), then the fluid may become infected needing drainage or antibiotics.

PAINFUL WRIST

PROBABLE
SPRAIN
COLLES' FRACTURE
SCAPHOID FRACTURE
OSTEOARTHRITIS

POSSIBLE
RHEUMATOID ARTHRITIS
CARPAL TUNNEL SYNDROME

RARE
TUBERCULOSIS
INFECTIOUS ARTHRITIS

PROBABLE

■ SPRAIN
Usually the result of a twisting, falling or bending injury.
* Uncomfortable on movement, but no real limitation.
Will settle within a few days.

■ COLLES' FRACTURE
Common in elderly people who fall on to an outstretched hand. The ends of the radius and ulna are broken. Fracture causes unusual deformity of the wrist.
* Pain in wrist.
* Deformity: lump on back of wrist.
* Pain on movement.
* Swelling can be extensive.
Requires realigning and immobilization in a cast.

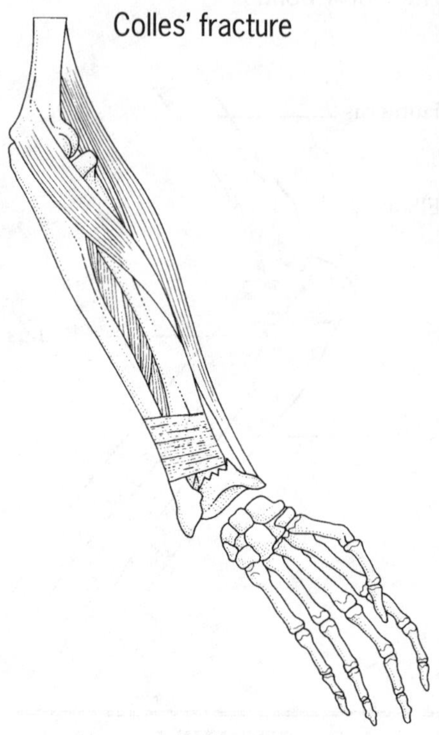
Colles' fracture

■ SCAPHOID FRACTURE
After falling on to an outstretched hand.
* Pain in wrist.
* Swelling.
* Pain on movement.
* Local pain at base of the back of the thumb.
If this fracture is untreated, the scaphoid, a small bone in the wrist, will degenerate, causing early osteoarthritis. Suspected scaphoid fractures must be immobilized initially, and X-rays reviewed after a week or so.

■ OSTEOARTHRITIS
See page 285.

POSSIBLE

■ RHEUMATOID ARTHRITIS
See page 300.

■ CARPAL TUNNEL SYNDROME
Although mainly causing symptoms in the hands and fingers, carpal tunnel syndrome may cause swollen, painful wrists.
* Pressure on nerves passing to the hand through the wrist gives rise to tingling and numbness.
* Common in pregnancy and pre-menstrually, and at menopause or when fluid retention is a symptom. *See also SWOLLEN HANDS, page 294.*

RARE

■ TUBERCULOSIS
See page 289.

■ INFECTIOUS ARTHRITIS
Some infections such as *rubella* or gonorrhea can cause painful joints.

SWOLLEN WRIST

See PAINFUL WRIST, page 292.

A SWELLING AT THE WRIST

PROBABLE
GANGLION
INJURY

POSSIBLE
OSTEOARTHRITIS
RHEUMATOID ARTHRITIS

RARE
TUBERCULOSIS
INFECTIOUS ARTHRITIS

PROBABLE

■ GANGLION
A small, usually pea-sized, fluid-filled swelling adjacent to the wrist joint, capsule or tendon sheath.
* Localized smooth lump, normally on the back of the wrist.
* Cystic.
* Can shine a light through it.
* Mild discomfort; worse if knocked.

May need removal by surgery.

■ INJURY
See PAINFUL WRIST, page 292.

POSSIBLE

■ OSTEOARTHRITIS
See page 285.

■ RHEUMATOID ARTHRITIS
See page 279.

THE SKELETON

RARE

■ TUBERCULOSIS
See page 289.

■ INFECTIOUS ARTHRITIS
See page 293.

UNUSUALLY LARGE HANDS

Will be a feature of *ACROMEGALY, page 275.*

SWOLLEN HANDS

PROBABLE
NORMAL VARIATION
PREGNANCY
INJURY
INFECTION

POSSIBLE
CARPAL TUNNEL SYNDROME
HYPOTHYROIDISM

RARE
AXILLARY VEIN THROMBOSIS
LYMPHEDEMA

PROBABLE

■ NORMAL VARIATION
Intermittent swelling of one hand, or both, is a common, noticeable symptom. You may find it difficult to remove rings, or a wrist strap may make an indentation on the wrist. May be worse in hot weather or, for women, premenstrually.

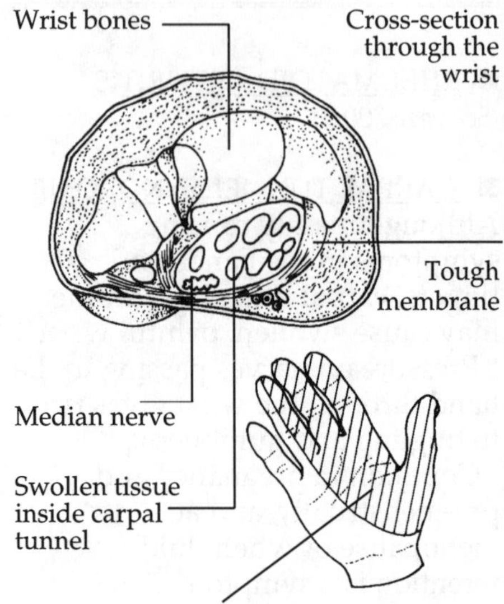

■ PREGNANCY
Particularly in the later stages, the body's normal response is to retain fluid and this tends to make the hands look puffy.

■ INJURY
Swelling would be a normal response to direct physical insult.

■ INFECTION
Infection of the skin or by a wound can cause swelling and pain in the hand. There is usually fever also.

POSSIBLE

■ CARPAL TUNNEL SYNDROME
Certain conditions causing swelling of the tissues of the hand and wrist may also compress the median nerve which supplies sensation and power to part of the hand. Commonest in menopausal women, individuals with arthritis and, in pregnancy; it may also occur with myxedema.
* Pain and tingling in the thumb, index, middle and half the ring finger.
* Waking at night with burning pain, tingling and numbness, as above.
* Weakness of the thumb.
* Difficulty in fine movements, such as sewing or gripping a pen for writing.
* Possibly pain and heaviness in the arm.

Splints may give relief, but in some cases the nerve needs releasing by surgery.

■ HYPOTHYROIDISM
Carpal tunnel syndrome (*above*) can be a symptom of this condition, which is caused by an under-active thyroid gland. (Do not confuse this with *hyper*thyroidism, an over-active gland.) Other symptoms are:
* Skin becomes dry and rough.
* You "feel the cold".
* Voice becomes gruff, features coarsen.
* Weight gain, constipation, slow speech, slow thought.
* Menstrual disorder.

The disorder is easily treated.

For further details, *see HYPOTHYROIDISM, page 460.*

RARE

■ AXILLARY VEIN THROMBOSIS
Blockage of the main vein in the armpit or upper arm. May have no apparent cause, or occurs after vigorous exercise.
* Swelling of entire arm.
* No pain, but there may be a dull ache.
* Superficial veins of arm may appear more prominent because the deep veins are blocked.

Needs medical evaluation.

■ LYMPHEDEMA
Primary or secondary. *See page 311.*

TREMBLING HANDS

See TREMBLING OR SHAKING, page 437.

In addition to the diagnoses listed on *page 438*, a physician might also consider two very rare diagnoses causing tremor of the hands which comes on when an individual wants to carry out a task. This is known as "intention tremor", and is characteristic of Wilson's Disease and Friedrich's ataxia. The first is a metabolic disorder, causing excessive deposits of copper in the brain, eyes and liver. It affects those between 10 and 25 years, and other symptoms include rigidity, abnormal limb movements, eye pigmentation, mental

THE SKELETON

Clubbed fingers

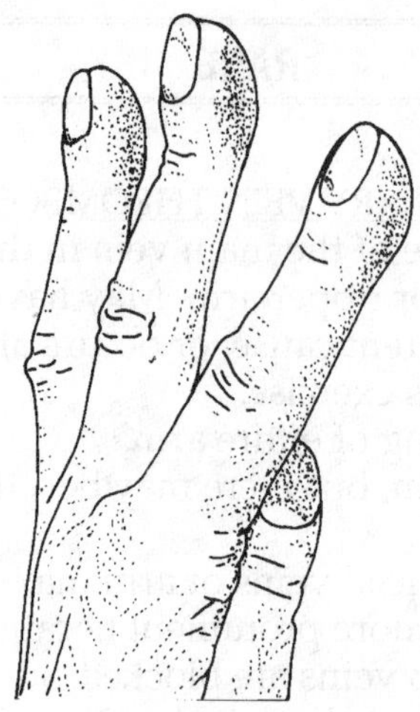

deterioration and ultimately cirrhosis of the liver. Friedrich's ataxia, a hereditary degeneration of the brain and spinal cord, occurs during the first 10 or 20 years of life. Its symptoms include progressive unsteadiness of gait, clumsiness, speech difficulties, loss of sense of position and intention tremor.

CLUBBED OR CURVED FINGERS OR NAILS

This means that:
* The end part of the finger becomes rounded.
* The nails appear larger and more curved lengthways and side to side.
* The angle between the nail bed and the skin on the back of the finger is lost; *see illustration above*.

If the fingers have been clubbed since birth, and there are similar finger-shapes in the family, then the symptom is not significant. But if clubbing develops during life, it may well be associated with other diseases, some of which are listed below. It is rare for clubbing alone to be the first indicator of these diseases. Medical science has not yet explained this phenomenon. Diseases of which clubbed fingers are a symptom:
* Lung diseases such as chronic bronchitis, emphysema, pleurisy, empyema, tuberculosis, cystic fibrosis, lung cancer.
* Heart disease: congenital heart disease, endocarditis.
* Gastro-intestinal disease: Crohns' disease, cystic fibrosis, liver cirrhosis, ulcerative colitis.
* Cancer.

See relevant sections for further details.

PROBLEMS WITH FINGERNAILS

It is said that over 60 diagnoses can be made from examining the nails alone. The appearance of the nail may be a clear sign of certain diseases, and the commonest variations are listed here along with the disease with which they are associated.
* Bitten fingernails: may be no more than a habit, or may point to an underlying tension, even anxiety or depression, particularly if recent.
* Paronychia: an abscess of the fingertip, which becomes red, sore, swollen and throbbing; pus may accumulate. Often needs to

Paronychia

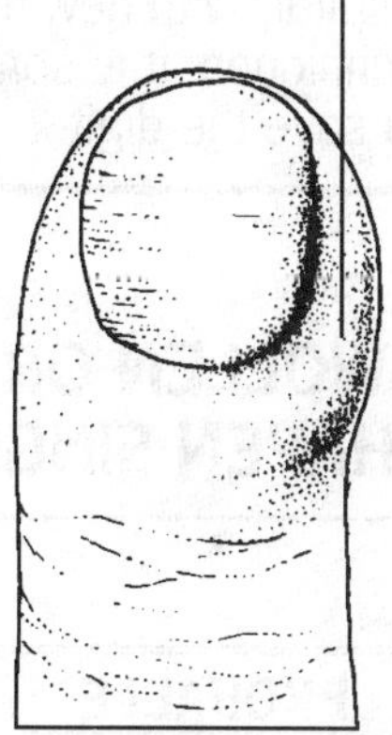

be released by a surgical incision. Antibiotics may be required.
* Horizontal lines: quite common after any illness and may be present for many months.
* Horizontal ridges: often in association with eczema.
* Sub-ungual hematoma: bruising after injury. The classic injury to a nail is a hammer blow, or an object dropped on the toes. Within a few minutes, a blue, then a purplish, then dark brown or black area may appear. The toe feels painful and throbs, because blood, which causes the discoloration, builds up pressure under the nail.

The symptoms are easily relieved by piercing the nail over the hematoma with a heated paper clip or a needle, allowing the blood to escape. There are two reasons for heating the needle: easier penetration of the nail and sterilization.
* Pale nails or leuconychia: in association with pale mucosa and conjunctiva in the eye this symptom suggests anemia.
* Bluish nails: suggests cyanosis. Often accompanies lung or heart disease. Examine also the lips and the ears — breathlessness may be a feature.
* Koilonychia or spoon-shaped nails: iron deficiency, anemia.
* Glomus tumor: an extremely tender, red or violet colored area a few millimeters across under the nail.
* Pitting of the nails: often occurs in association with psoriasis.
* Onycholysis: the nails separate from the nail bed — another feature of psoriasis, or fungus infection, particularly at the end of the nail.
* Fungal infections of the nails give a markedly thickened, irregular and discolored nail. The nail loses its usual color, becoming uniformly cream-colored and opaque. Other fungal infections may be present elsewhere.
* Onychogryphosis: enormous overgrowth and thickening of (mainly) the big toe nail, most commonly seen in the elderly. Advanced cases end up looking like a ram's horn.
* Brittle nails: may be due to excess manicuring and application of polish and polish remover.
* Splinter hemorrhages: longi–tudinal areas of redness that look like small splinters at the tips of the fingernails: may be associated with infection of the heart lining. Heart murmurs, feeling sick, shortness of breath, fever and anemia are other signs.
* Colored lunula or half moons: brown discoloration may be seen in chronic kidney failure, red

discoloration in heart failure.
* White lines: short, white lines are frequently seen across nails. The exact cause is unclear. They may be a sign of a blow to the nail, or may appear after an illness. They are of little significance.

Other diseases associated with nail deformities are:
* Lichen planus: a rare, itchy skin disease that also affects the nails. The whole skin may be affected. The nails (in about 10 percent of cases) become flaky, striated (lined), spoon-shaped, or may be destroyed.
* Alopecia areata: hair loss from the scalp, in patches. The nails may be pitted.
* Nail-patella syndrome: a rare hereditary disease. Rudimentary or absent nails and small or absent patella (kneecap).
* Paronychia congenita: nails are thickened, as is the surrounding skin.
* Dystrophic epidermolysis bullosa: irregularity and thickening of the nails which makes the skin blister easily in response to injury.

EXTREMELY COLD OR FROZEN FINGERS

This symptom occurs with *CHILBLAINS and FROSTBITE: see under ITCHING OR NUMBNESS OF THE FINGERS AND TOES, page 320.*

If a finger or thumb is severed, wrap it in clean material or plastic wrap, surround it with ice, and rush to the nearest hospital. With new microsurgical techniques, it is sometimes possible to save the digit.

SWOLLEN OR MISSHAPEN FINGERS

PROBABLE
PULP SPACE INFECTION
FLEXOR SHEATH INFECTION
TRIGGER FINGER
HEBERDEN'S NODES

POSSIBLE
MALLET FINGER AND THUMB
RHEUMATOID ARTHRITIS
DUPUYTREN'S CONTRACTURE
GOUT

RARE
ISCHEMIC CONTRACTURE
CONGENITAL DEFORMITIES
CONGENITAL CONTRACTURE
MALIGNANT TUMORS
BENIGN TUMORS

Swollen or misshapen fingers

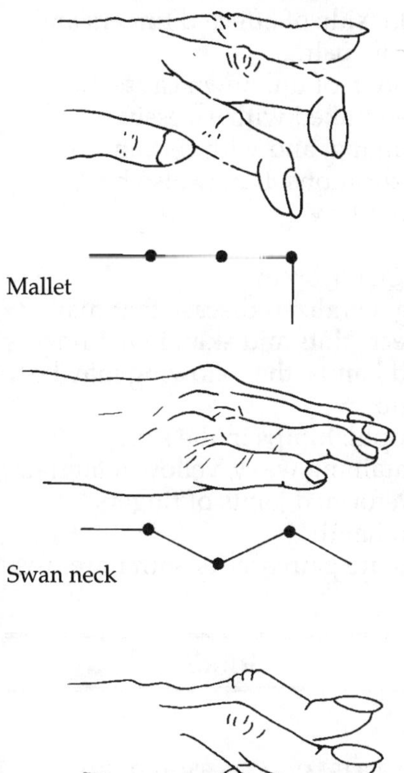

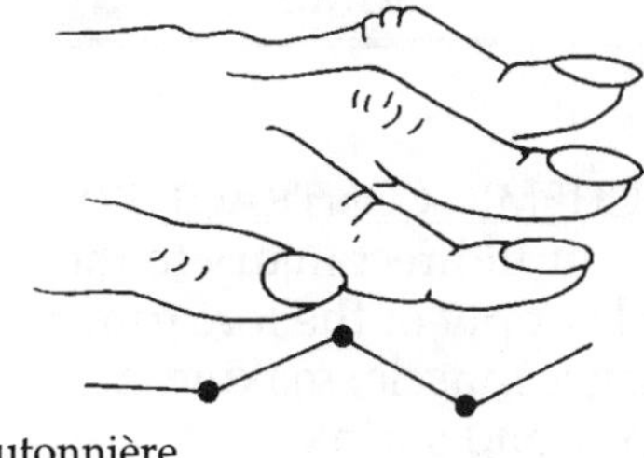

PROBABLE

■ PULP SPACE INFECTION
Infection, typically after a prick from plant or needle in the soft tissue at the finger tip.
* Swelling.
* Pain.
* Redness.
* Throbbing.

May require drainage or antibiotics.

■ FLEXOR SHEATH INFECTION
Infection in the sheath surrounding the tendons that bend the fingers (flexor tendons).
* Entire finger is red and swollen.
* Pain.
* Stiffness.
* Pain worse on movement — finger is held crooked — the most comfortable position.
* Infection (untreated) may spread back into the palm of the hand.

This is an emergency, needing immediate treatment to prevent long-term loss of function and deformity of the hand.

■ TRIGGER FINGER
Thickening or inflammation of part of a flexor tendon in a finger or thumb causes:
* The digit to "stick" when bending or straightening.
* May "unstick" with a snap, spontaneously, or:
* May need to be forced to straighten.
* A small tender nodule may be felt at the base of the digit on the palm.
* This nodule can be felt clicking as the digit is flexed.

Recovery may be spontaneous, but persistent symptoms require local steroid injections or eventually surgery.

■ HEBERDEN'S NODES
Caused by osteoarthritis.
* Distal interphalangeal joints *(see illustration page 280)* are painful.
* Bony overgrowth makes the joints appear enlarged and knobbly.

POSSIBLE

■ MALLET FINGER AND THUMB
Damage to the tendon (extensor) which attaches to the dorsal surface of the terminal phalanx of each digit. The damage may be caused by injury to the end of the digit, or indirectly, after a wrist fracture. Occasionally, it happens in association with other disease — such as rheumatoid arthritis.
* Terminal end of digit appears bent but cannot be straightened.

Splinting for six weeks may help cure cases caused by direct trauma.

In other situations, surgery may be needed.

■ RHEUMATOID ARTHRITIS
This disease affects the fingers and hands in a number of ways, including:
* Ulnar deviation of the fingers: the fingers appear to drift towards the side of the little finger, and the knuckle joints appear pronounced.
* Swan neck deformities; *see illustration.*
* Boutonnière's deformities; *see illustration.*
* Drop finger: the finger cannot be kept straight at the knuckle joint.
* Mallet thumb; *see above.*

■ DUPUYTREN'S CONTRACTURE
* A fibrous contracture of (commonly) the little and ring fingers, which cannot be completely straightened.
* Sometimes the fingers are so bent that cleaning of the hand is a problem.
* Thickening can be felt on the palm side of affected fingers and on the palm.

Often of unknown cause, but has been linked with excessive drinking, and with certain medications. It may also be hereditary.

■ GOUT
A generalized disease that may affect joints and skin. In the fingers and hands, the following may be seen:
* Tophi: lumps in the skin containing waxy, yellow material.
* Deformed joints of fingers and hand.
* Acute pain occurs with flare-ups.

RARE

■ ISCHEMIC CONTRACTURE
Direct or indirect injury to the blood supply of the forearm damages muscle, making it atrophy and shrink.
* Pale or bluish-looking skin on hand.
* Thin forearm.
* Hand is clawed — fingers flexed at both finger joints.
* Sensation diminished.
* Fingers can only be straightened when the hand is flexed at the wrist.
* Only able to grip when hand is flexed.

■ CONGENITAL DEFORMITIES
Present at birth.
* Failure of development — part or all of the fingers and hand may

be deformed or absent.
* Syndactyly or webbing: fusion of adjacent fingers.
* "Extra" digits: ranging from small lumps of flesh to entire digits (usually on the outer part of the limb).

■ CONGENITAL CONTRACTURE
* Present from birth.
* Fingers may be bent.
* Thickened tissue may be felt on the surface of the palm.
* May only affect one digit.

■ MALIGNANT TUMORS
See LUMPS IN THE SKIN, page 250.

■ BENIGN TUMORS
See LUMPS IN THE SKIN, page 250.

PAINFUL HIP

Likely to have different causes at different ages. Pain is often felt in the groin or the front of the hip, and may radiate down the thigh and to the knee. In children (who may not complain of pain) a limp may be the only evidence of pain. Accidental dislocation is excluded from this section because the cause – severe injury – is obvious.

PROBABLE
OSTEOARTHRITIS
FRACTURED NECK OF FEMUR
HIP STRAIN

POSSIBLE
IRRITABLE HIP
PERTHES' DISEASE
SLIPPED EPIPHYSIS
RHEUMATOID ARTHRITIS

RARE
CONGENITAL DISLOCATION OF THE HIP
SUBLUXATION OF THE HIP
INFECTIVE DISLOCATION OF THE HIP

PROBABLE

■ OSTEOARTHRITIS
From about 50 years of age. Osteoarthritis is a problem of growing old — of degeneration. All of us are affected to some degree by this form of arthritis, sometimes described as "wear and tear arthritis". Some pre-existing conditions predispose to an early appearance of osteoarthritis, including congenital dislocation of the hip, infective arthritis, Perthes' disease, and slipped epiphysis — the risk is increased if the diagnosis is missed or treatment delayed.
* Pain radiating from groin to knee.
* Pain after exercise, progressing to pain at rest or disturbing sleep.
* Progressive stiffness of leg.
* Difficulty in putting on shoes and socks.
* Progressive limp.
* Apparent shortening of leg.

Treatment is first aimed at relieving the pain (painkillers); then at improving function (exercises and physical therapy); eventually, severe cases may require joint replacement.

■ FRACTURED NECK OF FEMUR

See information on pathological fractures under BONES BREAKING EASILY, page 276.

■ HIP STRAIN

Pain following excessive use – climbing, running, jumping. Improves with painkillers and rest.

POSSIBLE

■ IRRITABLE HIP

In children or adults.
* Pain in groin or front of thigh, often to the knee.
* Limp.
* All movement of hip limited by pain.

This diagnosis tends to be made if all tests for other causes are normal. The hip settles with bed rest and, occasionally, traction. It is important, particularly in the young, to seek a specialist opinion to exclude more serious disease.

■ PERTHES' DISEASE

The blood supply to the femoral head is reduced, and it dies. Surprisingly, the symptoms can be quite slight.
* Patient aged five to ten years, occasionally older or younger.
* Ache in hip comes and goes.
* Limp comes and goes.
* Painful movements.

Slipped epiphysis

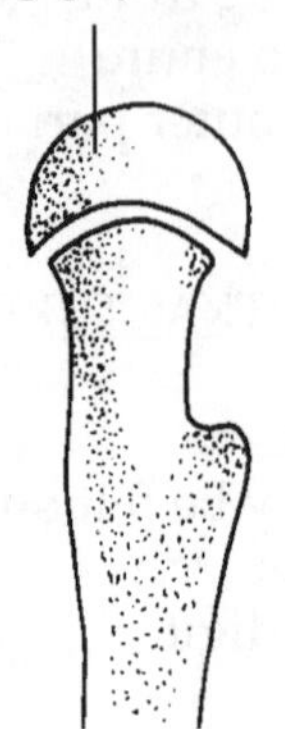

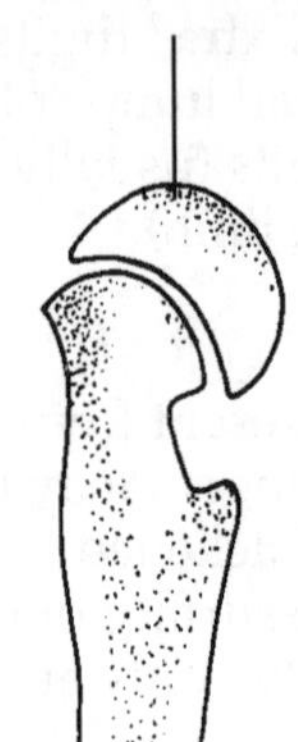

It is important to distinguish between this serious disease and irritable hip.

■ SLIPPED EPIPHYSIS

A disease of adolescents, usually between 11 and 13; commonest in boys. The top part of the femoral head slips off the lower part at the epiphysis. Hip injury may play some part in its development. People with this condition may be overweight and may have delayed sexual and physical development. The epiphysis may slip slowly, in which case the following symptoms develop:
* Slight pain in hip with reduced range of movement.
* The leg appears shortened.
* The foot appears to be twisted outwards.
* Hip rotation limited.
* Limp may be apparent.
* There may be muscle wasting on the affected side.
* The upper part of the femur — the greater trochanter — may appear higher on the affected side when felt through the skin.

Sudden slipping of the epiphysis gives the same symptoms as a fractured neck of the femur.

■ RHEUMATOID ARTHRITIS
Other generalized features of the disease will also be present. *See INFLAMMATORY ARTHROPATHIES, page 274.*
* Slow onset of groin pain.
* Limp which may be attributed to other joints.
* Muscle wasting can be severe.
* Both hips may be affected.
* Foot is turned outwards.
* Hip mobility is markedly reduced.

RARE

■ CONGENITAL DISLOCATION OF THE HIP
See DISLOCATED HIP, this page.

■ SUBLUXATION OF THE HIP
Early degeneration of the hip due to abnormal shape of the joint "cup". May well appear at about 20 years of age.
* Pain in groin.
* Worse on exercise.
* Progressive limp.

■ INFECTIVE DISLOCATION OF THE HIP
Most common in children and newborn babies. *See DISLOCATED HIP, below.*

DISLOCATED HIP

May be congenital (hereditary) or acquired, or caused by infection.

■ CONGENITAL DISLOCATION (CDH)
CDH tends to run in families and arises because of an abnormally-shaped hip joint socket, combined with weak joint ligaments. Breech birth (when the baby's feet, rather than the head, come out of the birth canal first) increases the likelihood. Babies are routinely checked for hip dislocation at regular check-ups. Symptoms before walking:
* Asymmetry of hip, seen at skin creases.
* Legs will not part fully.
* The baby may be late to start walking.

Symptoms after walking:
* Asymmetry of legs.
* Limp. Babies are checked for hip dislocation at regular checkings.

If both hips are dislocated, the waddling gait could pass as normal, in which case the dislocation will go undetected, causing damage. So the problem needs to be recognized at an early stage. Treatment is with different forms of splint.If untreated, the limp remains, and the hip joint is progressively distorted and damaged.

Ultimately, severe osteoarthritis develops and hip replacement may be needed as an adult.

CDH

This condition affects five times as many girls than boys. *Instability* of the hip — as opposed to outright dislocation — may be diagnosed in as many as 400 out of every 100,000 live births. However, this condition settles. True dislocation of the hip will not improve. Ultrasound can be used to check on the unborn baby, to avoid X-ray exposure.

■ ACQUIRED DISLOCATION

Acquired dislocation of the hip is caused either by injury or infection. Typically, an automobile or motorcycle accident, in which the individual is sitting with the knee bent, results in the femoral head being pushed backwards out of the socket. Extreme force is needed.

* Extreme pain.
* Deformity in extreme cases.
* Leg is shortened and twisted inwards.
* The knee is slightly bent.
* The leg cannot be moved.

The femoral head can be replaced in the socket, but recovery can be a lengthy process, often because there are other injuries.

Much less commonly, the hip may also dislocate forwards; also centrally, when the femoral head pushes through the socket into the pelvis.

■ INFECTIVE DISLOCATION OF THE HIP

Untreated infection (including tuberculosis) in any joint requires urgent orthopedic attention to remove pus and clear the infection, as the joint surface and surrounding structures can be rapidly destroyed.

Features include:

* Pain (of variable intensity).
* A limp.
* Eventually, loss of function.
* Feeling sick.
* Fever.

Neglected, or mistreated, episodes of infective dislocation may mean surgery at a later date to correct deformity.

BOW-LEGGEDNESS

This is, in most cases, an innocent variation of the normal, occurring in childhood. Most children grow out of it.

* Feet together.
* Knees splayed out.

May also, but much more rarely, be seen in rickets *(page 287)*, osteoarthritis *(page 285)*, and Paget's disease *(page 437)*.

LIMPING

Limping can be a symptom of many disorders and is caused by pain, or deformity or both. Look for a specific site of pain or deformity, and then refer to that section.

PAIN WHEN WALKING

Look at pages 316-21 first, then

consider alternatives in the following pages covering leg and knee; also the preceding pages covering hip.

WALKING WITH A WADDLING GAIT

See CONGENITAL DISLOCATION OF THE HIP, page 303; and MUSCULAR DYSTROPHY, page 270.

PAINFUL LEG OR THIGH

See the general bone and muscles symptoms pages 269-81; also back symptoms, pages 284-90.

PARALYSED LEG

See pages 404-6.

VEIN OR VEINS STANDING OUT IN LEG

See VARICOSE VEINS, page 310.

SWOLLEN LEG

See SWOLLEN ANKLE, page 310.

WEAK LEG

See WASTING AND LOSS OF POWER IN THE MUSCLES, page 269; also page 272.

LEG UNUSUALLY WHITE

This may indicate sudden blockage of an artery — a medical emergency — as a result of *PERIPHERAL VASCULAR DISEASE, page 318.*

KNEE PAIN AFTER INJURY

The precise cause of the pain will be governed by the force of the injury, and its site — so "probable", "possible" and "rare" are not relevant here.

The knee is made up from: bones — lower femur, upper tibia, patella; ligaments — medial and lateral collateral, anterior and posterior cruciate; the joint capsule; the menisci medial and lateral; and the surrounding soft tissues. All can be damaged.

The most significant injuries and their symptoms are listed below, and an indication of the type of injury that may cause them. All require immediate treatment.

Delaying treatment, especially if the injury is severe, will increase the risk of complications. All injuries to a joint increase the risk of early onset of osteoarthritis.

■ DISLOCATION OF THE KNEE

Enormous force is needed to disrupt the knee joint, including its capsules and ligaments.

* Severe pain.
* Marked deformity.
* Marked bruising.

Nerves and arteries to the leg may be damaged.

■ DISLOCATION OF THE PATELLA
See LOCKED OR LOCKING KNEE, this page.

■ FEMORAL CONDYLE FRACTURES
* May be sustained after a fall from a height.
* Severe pain in the knee, which cannot be moved.
* Immediate swelling and deformity.

■ LIGAMENTOUS TEAR
Can be complete or partial, and is often missed, the symptoms of swelling, pain and reduced function being put down to "sprain". If someone has a severe injury to the knee which still allows some movement, the knee should be assessed for stability by an expert when symptoms have settled and before any sporting activities are started again.

■ FRACTURED PATELLA
Probably caused by a falling on to knee, or by a direct blow.
* Immediate swelling over kneecap.
* The knee is bent.
* May be unable to straighten leg.

■ SUPRACONDYLAR FRACTURE OF THE FEMUR
Caused by severe, direct injury.
* Severe pain — knee cannot be moved.
* Immediate swelling and deformity.

■ FRACTURED TIBIAL PLATEAU
Caused by a direct blow or a fall from a height.
* Severe pain - knee cannot be moved.
* Immediate swelling and deformity.

■ UPPER TIBIAL EPIPHYSIS AND APOPHYSIS
Injury to the upper lower leg, below the knee cap (the shin just below the knee), can damage the point of attachment of the quadriceps tendon to the tibia.
* Knee swollen, particularly below the kneecap.
* Local tenderness at the upper tibia.
* Raising the leg when it is straightened is painful or impossible.

A similar condition in young adults, which develops spontaneously, or after sports like basketball, is known as Osgood Schlatter's Disease.

KNEE, SWOLLEN

See KNEE PAIN AFTER INJURY, page 305; KNEE, LOCKED OR LOCKING, below; INFLAMED OR ACHING JOINTS, page 278.

LOCKED OR LOCKING KNEE WHICH MAY COLLAPSE

The knee joint gets fixed at a particular angle. If it is completely locked it is not possible to

Ligamentous tear

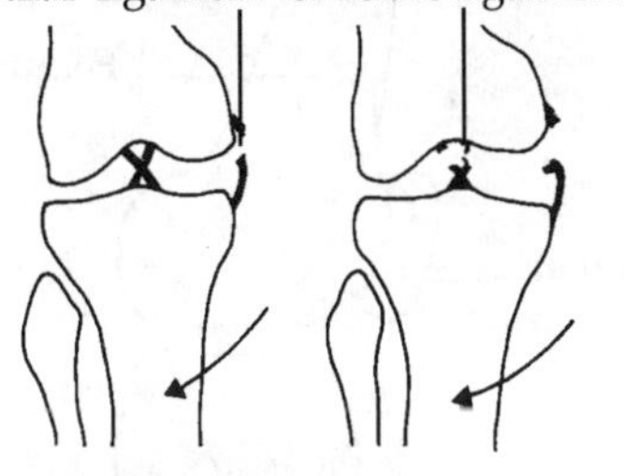

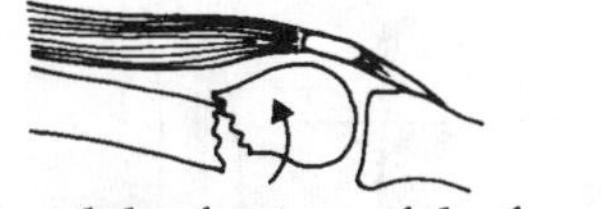

Supracondylar fracture of the femur

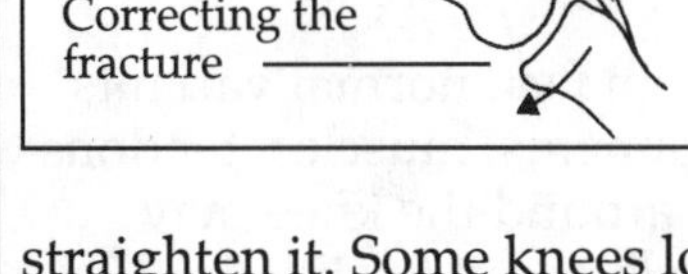

Fractured patella

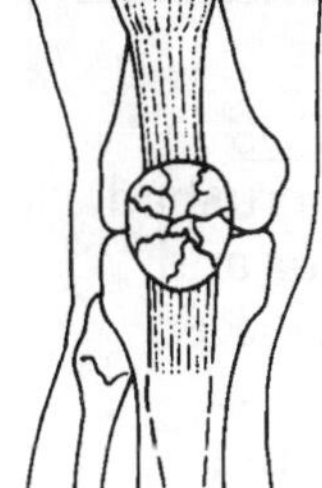

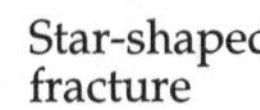

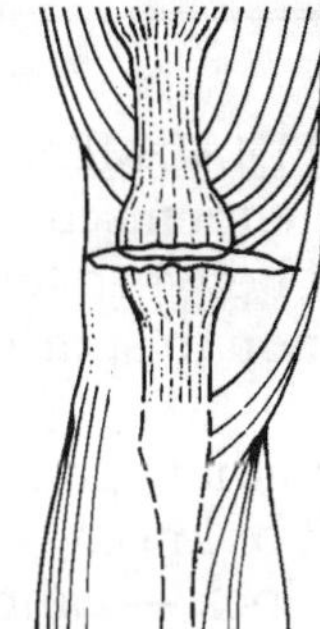

Knee injuries

straighten it. Some knees lock from time to time: they may appear to "catch", and then to straighten.

These symptoms suggest a problem within the knee itself, either a damaged cartilage (meniscus) or a loose body, which might be bone or cartilage. If injury to the knee predates the symptoms, it is important to remember exactly how it happened.

PROBABLE
LIGAMENT DAMAGE

POSSIBLE
TORN MEDIAL MENISCUS
LOOSE BODY
OSTEOARTHRITIS

RARE
RECURRENT DISLOCATION OF THE KNEECAP
TORN LATERAL MENISCUS
DISCOID LATERAL MENISCUS
CHONDROMALACIA PATELLA
OSTEOCHONDRITIS DISSECANS

PROBABLE

■ LIGAMENT DAMAGE
The most common reason for the knee to lock, collapse or give away is damage to one of the internal ligaments. Symptoms are often similar to those of damage to the cartilage; *see TORN MEDIAL MENISCUS, page 308.*

THE SKELETON

POSSIBLE

■ TORN MEDIAL MENISCUS
Typically, the meniscus is crushed and twisted between femur and tibia. Common in sports (soccer, basketball).
* Often immediate pain at the inner aspect of knee.
* Knee may lock — cannot be fully straightened.
* Swelling of the joint within a few hours.
After the first incident, symptoms may subside, only to recur with increasing frequency.

■ LOOSE BODY
Trapped between femur and tibia.
* Attacks of sudden pain on climbing or descending stairs.
* Inability to straighten leg.
* Swelling, due to fluid in the joint, may accompany each attack.
* Each attack resolves as the loose body moves from between the joints.
* The loose body may be felt in the joint, often above or at the side of the patella.

■ OSTEOARTHRITIS
Degenerative or osteoarthritic changes in the joint can cause formation of loose bodies; *see above*. Common in later middle age, and onwards.

RARE

■ RECURRENT DISLOCATION OF THE KNEECAP
Anatomical peculiarities, which

Knee joint

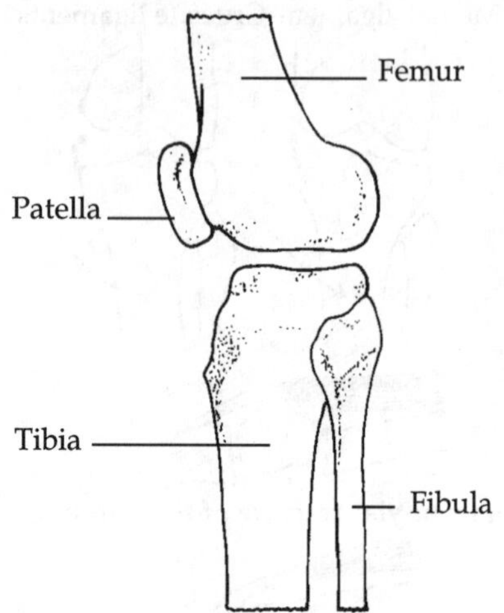

are often, in fact, normal variants of the ligaments, muscles, tendons or bones around the knee may allow the kneecap to slide sideways. Commonest in young females.
* Kneecap may appear very mobile from side to side.
* Knee gets stuck in a bent position (maybe only briefly), causing the individual to fall (collapsing knee).
* Kneecap can be felt to one side, and then moves.
* May occur in both knees.

■ TORN LATERAL MENISCUS
Less common than a torn medial meniscus; *this page*. Symptoms are the same, except pain is on the outer side of the knee.

■ DISCOID LATERAL MENISCUS
An abnormally-shaped lateral meniscus slips between the femur and tibia and the knee gives way. A "clunking" sensation is experienced. Eventually, surgery will be needed.

■ CHONDROMALACIA PATELLA
Degeneration of the cartilage at the back of the kneecap. Athletes, especially runners and joggers are affected.
* May have had recurrent patella dislocation *(page 308)* or a knee injury.
* Intermittent pain at the front of the knee, with swelling.
* Occasional locking of the knee.
* Knee occasionally gives away.

■ OSTEOCHONDRITIS DISSECANS
The lower part of the articular surface of the femur (the condyle) may be damaged after injury. Part of the articular cartilage flakes off, creating a loose body. The individual is often in his or her late teens.
* Intermittent ache.
* Intermittent swelling.
* Intermittent locking.
* Knee feels unstable, as though it will collapse.

"KNOCK" KNEES AND BOW LEGS

In the great majority of cases, knock knees are a normal feature of childhood. As the child grows, the knees gradually begin to look normal, usually by the time the child is seven.
* Feet appear splayed.
* Knees press against each other.

Physicians often watch the leg shape over a period of six months to see how the appearance changes. At three to four years, the gap between a child's inner ankle bones, when standing comfortably, should be less than 4 inches.

May also, but rarely, be seen in rickets *(page 287)*, osteomalacia *(page 287)*, Paget's disease *(page 437)* and Charcot's joints *(page 281)*.

BOW LEGS

Bow legs are common in infants. If the child is lying flat, with feet together, and there is a gap of more than 2 inches between the bottom of the femurs at the knee, an X-ray may be a useful precaution to exclude rare causes, such as rickets and problems of bone development.

Bowing on one side only should always be evaluated by a physician.

PAINFUL KNEE

See INFLAMED OR ACHING JOINTS, page 278; LOCKED OR LOCKING KNEE; page 306; PAINFUL HIP, page 301.

SWOLLEN ANKLE

Can be on one or both sides.

PROBABLE
ACUTE OR CHRONIC INJURY

POSSIBLE
VARICOSE VEINS
DEEP VENOUS THROMBOSIS
POST-PHLEBITIC LIMB
CELLULITIS
HEART FAILURE
GOUT

RARE
ANEMIA
LYMPHEDEMA
MISSED FRACTURE
NEPHRITIS

PROBABLE

■ ACUTE OR CHRONIC INJURY
See WEAK AND PAINFUL ANKLE, page 312.

POSSIBLE

■ VARICOSE VEINS
Enlarged leg veins caused by damage to valves in the veins. Blood fails to return to the heart at the proper rate and stays in the leg. This in turn can cause a swollen ankle and lower leg, often only on one side.
* Varicose veins visible.
* Increases during day or after exercise.
* Discomfort rather than pain.
* Disappears when leg is elevated, and at night.
* May be associated with ulcers, particularly inner-ankle swelling.
* Long-standing varicose veins cause brownish discoloration of the lower legs and feet. Sometimes described as varicose eczema.

■ DEEP VENOUS THROMBOSIS
Blockage of the veins by a thrombosis or blood clot deep inside the leg. May occur for no reason; or after an operation or prolonged bed rest. More likely in the elderly, the obese, smokers, and those on the contraceptive pill or with known malignant disease. If suspected, requires urgent medical attention.
* Sudden onset.
* Initially no pain, then mild discomfort.
* Calf and sometimes the thigh also swell.
* Pain may be caused by pressure on the back of the calf.
* Swelling is persistent and does not decrease.

If a piece of the clot moves from the legs to the lungs, there will be chest pain and shortness of breath. (*See also PULMONARY EMBOLUS, page 218.*) If the clot is large enough, death can follow in rare cases.

■ POST-PHLEBITIC LIMB
For months or years after a deep venous thrombosis (*above*) the limb may remain swollen and tender. Ulcers may develop at the ankle, plus discoloration of the skin. Best treated with support bandages.

■ CELLULITIS
A bacterial infection of the soft tissues. It may be localized in part of the foot, ankle or leg, or it may spread. Caused by a simple puncture wound, or by bacteria gaining access through broken skin on the foot or ankle (for example, via an ulcer or Athlete's foot).
* Redness; swelling.
* Can be very painful.
* Skin may be shiny, due to stretching.
* Sickness.
* Fever.

Rest and antibiotics are needed to treat this condition.

■ HEART FAILURE
If the heart fails to pump as well as it should, the body retains fluid. At worst this can cause congestion of the lungs, which makes breathing difficult. A mild case may cause ankle swelling.
* Swelling on both sides.
* Legs feel cool.
* May come and go.
* May be associated with shortness of breath.
* In bad (and untreated) heart failure, swelling may progress all the way up the leg.
* Associated symptoms can include distended neck veins and cyanosis.

The symptoms can be helped by diuretic tablets.

■ GOUT
See page 278.

RARE

■ ANEMIA
Ankle swelling may be the first symptoms noted by an anemic individual. This is because anemia may precipitate mild heart failure *(this page).*

■ LYMPHEDEMA
Obstruction to drainage of fluid via the lymphatic system. Rarely it may be primary (no underlying cause); the result of congenital abnormality; or it can arise from absence of the lymphatic system in that limb. Secondary lymphedema can be caused by operation on, or blockage of, the lymph glands in the groin (for example to control malignant disease), or by parasite infection — filariasis.
* Firm swelling.
* Does not vary in size.
* Infection or inflammation may develop; *see CELLULITIS, this page.*
* Skin becomes thickened.
* In severe cases the skin may acquire the texture of elephant hide — elephantiasis.

■ MISSED FRACTURE
Occasionally a small fracture of an ankle bone may go unrecognized at the time of injury, resulting in long-term swelling, pain and instability.

■ NEPHRITIS
Damage, acute or chronic, to the kidneys caused by disease, not injury, may also cause swelling of the ankles.

Other symptoms may include:

* Puffy face (particularly around the eyes).
* Protein and/or blood in urine.
* Sickness.
* Shortness of breath.
* Nausea and vomiting.

WEAK AND PAINFUL ANKLE

Almost always the result of injury, such as a twist (often caused by slipping on a step) or jumping from a height. The ankle joint is made up of three main bones: the tibia, fibula and calcaneum. Each may be damaged. The injury also damages the soft tissues (ligaments, tendons and muscles) surrounding the ankle. Pain originates from these structures. The ankle feels "weak" and likely to "give way". The symptoms only relate to the affected ankle.

Ankle injuries should be regarded seriously, since even untreated sprains can cause long-term disability. Pain killers, rest and physical therapy are often appropriate treatments if there is no fracture.

PROBABLE
ACUTE INJURY (SPRAIN)

POSSIBLE
CHRONIC INJURY
CELLULITIS

RARE
FRACTURE

Bones of the foot and ankle

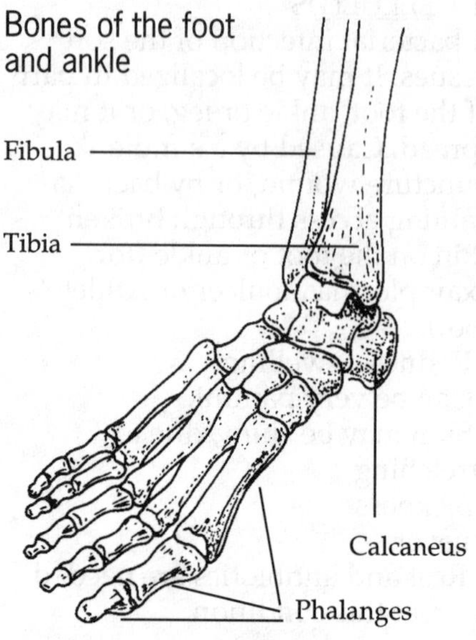

PROBABLE

■ <u>ACUTE INJURY (SPRAIN).</u>
* Clear story of injury.
* Painful to stand or bear weight.
* Swelling, local or general.
* Swelling appears after a few hours or the following day.
* Ankle feels as though it will "give way".

POSSIBLE

■ <u>CHRONIC INJURY</u>
* Injury some time in past — weeks, months or even years.
* Symptoms have persisted for some time.
* Constant feeling of "weakness" or "about to give way".
* Pain not so intense as with acute trauma.
* Swelling after exercise.

■ <u>CELLULITIS</u>
See page 311.

RARE

■ FRACTURE
In general, the symptoms are very obvious and confined to the affected bone.
* Pain severe.
* Unable to bear weight.
* Immediate swelling.
* Bruising within a few hours.

A break to the lower end of the tibia will cause symptoms on the inner aspect of the ankle; to the lower fibula on the outer aspect; to the calcaneus (heel bone) on both sides and at the back over the heel.

UNUSUALLY LARGE FEET

PROBABLE
NORMAL VARIANT

RARE
ACROMEGALY

PROBABLE

■ NORMAL VARIANT
Most individuals worried about their foot size have no physical abnormality or underlying disease. The size of their feet merely reflects the variation in size that would be expected in any population. And many people worry that their feet are too small.

RARE

■ ACROMEGALY
See page 275.

FLAT FEET

The term really means flattening of the arches. It can be a postural problem, in association with knock knees and a short Achilles tendon. It may occasionally be congenital, in association with spina bifida, but this is rare. It may also develop as a result of general lack of fitness, say after being bed-ridden. The muscles and tendons that support the arches become wasted and flat feet develop.
* Feet look flat — no arch on instep.
* Shoe soles wear badly.
* Pain is rare, but may develop later in the foot and leg muscles.

Treatment is rarely needed, although instep supports (orthotics) may be of some help.

Most commonly, no cause for flat feet is found, and unfortunately specialists can offer little in the way of help.

Flat feet often run in families.

PAINFUL ARCHES OF FEET

See FLAT FEET, previous page.

PAINFUL FEET

PROBABLE
PLANTAR WART

POSSIBLE
PLANTAR FASCIITIS
HALLUX VALGUS
HALLUX RIGIDUS

RARE
CLAW TOES
MORTON'S METATARSALGIA
PES CAVUS

PROBABLE

■ PLANTAR WART
Caused by a viral infection, hence outbreaks in schools and swimming pools.
* Local tenderness on sole of foot, where the wart is pushed into the surface.
* The plantar wart is visible and there may be several — normally on the weight-bearing areas.
* May vanish spontaneously. Can be treated with a product containing salicylic acid. Consult your pharmacist. Left alone, it will eventually disappear.

Hallux valgus or bunion
(normal position of toe shown with dotted line)

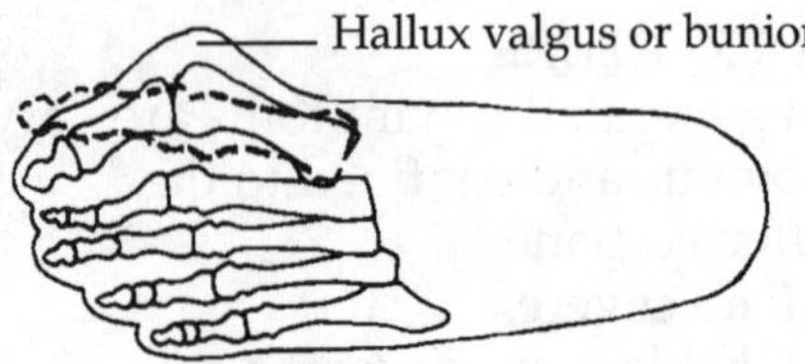

Morton's metatarsalgia

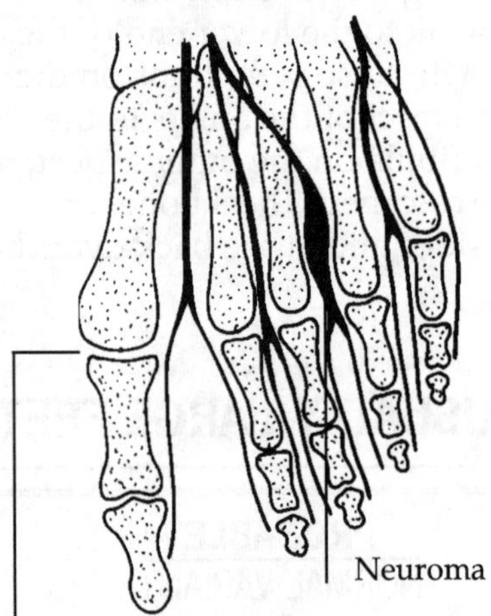

POSSIBLE

■ PLANTAR FASCIITIS
An inflammation of the layers of membrane, called fascia, which lie in the sole of the foot, just in front of the heel.
* Common after the age of 40.
* Local tenderness underneath the heel.
* Worse on walking/running.
* Commonest in occupations requiring individuals to be on their feet for long periods.

■ HALLUX VALGUS
The big toe becomes deformed. Commonest in women beyond middle age.
* Big toe tip points to outer side of foot.
* Base of big toe sticks out.
* The end of the metatarsal bone points to the inner side of the foot.
* A lump of bone is therefore felt under the skin.
* The overlying skin becomes thickened and painful (bunion) as does the bone on the sole of the foot. May eventually need surgery

■ HALLUX RIGIDUS
Caused by osteoarthritis of the first metatarsophalangeal joint.
* Pain on movement.
* Bony outgrowths may develop, appearing as lumps around the joint.
* Thickened skin may develop on the upper surface of the joint.
* Range of movement of the joint is eventually limited by stiffness and pain.

RARE

■ CLAW TOES
See PES CAVUS, this page.

■ MORTON'S METATARSALGIA
Affects the middle-aged.
* Enlargement of the nerve (neuroma) between the heads of metatarsal bones.
* Local pain, worse if foot is squeezed from side to side.
* Pain radiates to toes.
May require surgery.

■ PES CAVUS
The opposite of a flat foot: the arch of the foot is raised. Often associated with curling of the toes (claw toes). Thought to be caused by imbalance of the muscles that support the arches, and most likely to be seen in those with neurological disease of the lower limb, for instance poliomyelitis, spina bifida, cerebral palsy.
* Curled or clawed toes.
* High arch on instep.
* Calluses eventually develop on pressure points.
* Metatarsalgia (pain on the metatarsal heads) may develop.

SWOLLEN FEET

See SWOLLEN ANKLE, page 309.

ULCERATED OR INFECTED FEET

PROBABLE
INGROWN TOENAIL
ATHLETE'S FOOT
PLANTAR WART

POSSIBLE
DERMATITIS
DIABETIC COMPLICATION
VARICOSE VEINS
DEEP VENOUS THROMBOSIS
POST-PHLEBITIC LIMB
CELLULITIS
ATHEROSCLEROSIS

The Skeleton

RARE

ALCOHOLIC NEUROPATHY
MULTIPLE SCLEROSIS
RAYNAUD'S DISEASE
BUERGER'S DISEASE
FROSTBITE
SYPHILIS

PROBABLE

■ INGROWN TOENAIL
The big toe is the one almost always affected. The side of the nail cuts into the toe tissue causing local infection (paronychia). Caused by ill-fitting shoes and cutting the nail too short.
* Outer side of nail most commonly affected.
* Often on both feet.
* Recurrent pain.
* Recurrent infection — with redness, swelling and pus.

May ultimately need surgery to the nail bed.

■ ATHLETE'S FOOT
See ITCHING OR NUMBNESS OF THE FINGERS AND TOES, page 320.

■ PLANTAR WART
See page 314.

POSSIBLE

These diagnoses are discussed in detail on pages 321; under DIABETIC NEUROPATHY, page 317; on page 310; and under PERIPHERAL VASCULAR DISEASE on page 318.

RARE

These diagnoses are discussed in detail on pages *318, 488, 321 and 324,* respectively. Buerger's disease is painful ulceration caused by obliteration of blood vessels in the limbs; particularly in young male smokers of eastern European origin.

CORNS ON THE FEET

See page 255.

FINGERS AND TOES

Collected here is a group of symptoms which can particularly affect the fingers and toes (but also the arms and legs): parts of the body at the outer reaches of the blood's circulation. The nose and ears are similarly placed, and certain symptoms such as numbness, itching or discoloration can affect them just as they do the fingers and toes.

NUMB FINGERS AND TOES

The onset of numbness in any part of the body should be taken seriously. It is not a common symptom in isolation and may be an accompaniment to underlying

Pressure points of the feet

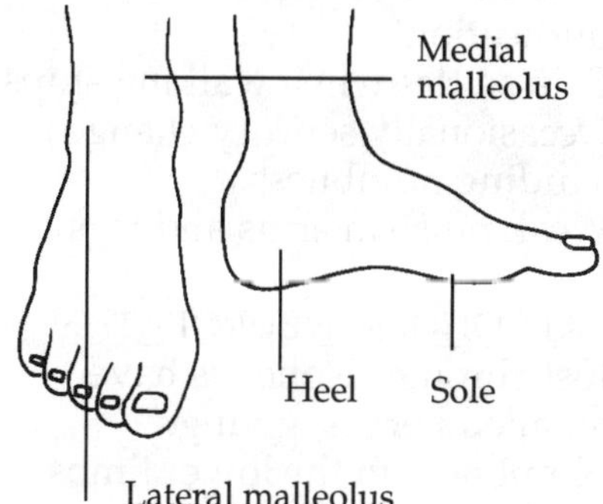

disease. Its main danger is that the "warning sign" of pain is not present: therefore skin damage, skin breakdown and ulcers may develop because the individual cannot feel the discomfort. This is particularly common over pressure points (eg heel, medial and lateral malleolus, sole of the foot).

Numbness of fingers and toes accompanied by back or neck pain is a serious symptom, and should be reported to your physician immediately. It can be a sign of direct pressure applied to a nerve by a disc or from a bone injury.

POSSIBLE

CERVICAL SPONDYLOSIS
DIABETIC NEUROPATHY
MULTIPLE SCLEROSIS
PERIPHERAL VASCULAR DISEASE
ALCOHOLIC NEUROPATHY

RARE

GUILLAIN-BARRE SYNDROME
FROSTBITE
LEPROSY

POSSIBLE

■ CERVICAL SPONDYLOSIS
See page 136.

■ DIABETIC NEUROPATHY
A long-standing complication of diabetes. Neuropathy means disease of the nerves. If you have diabetes, you may notice:
* Some tingling and pain (lower limbs).
* Stocking anesthesia (numbness over a leg to the upper thigh — the area covered by a stocking).
* Some muscle wasting and weakness.
* Painless ulceration over pressure points on feet.
* Cellulitis (*see above*) associated with ulcers.

Occasionally, only one nerve may be affected, causing numbness, muscle wasting and weakness in one limb.

Other neurological symptoms of diabetes may be:
* Radiculitis — localized scalding and painful sensory changes.
* Irregular shape to pupils.
* Impotence.
* Failure of orgasm.
* Night diarrhea.
* Feeling of dizziness on standing or changing position (postural hypotension).
* Loss of sweating in lower limbs.

THE SKELETON

■ MULTIPLE SCLEROSIS
Used to be known as disseminated sclerosis. Nervous tissue in the central nervous system is affected. Features may include:
* Numbness and tingling in hand(s) or feet (allowing ulcers to develop if pressure points are not treated carefully).
* Visual disturbance (poor vision, double vision).
* Weakness in limbs.
* Muscle wasting.
* Loss of balance.
* Dizziness.
* Bladder disturbance.
* Tremor.
* Speech disturbance.
* Swallowing difficulties.

May take several years to be diagnosed as it remits and relapses. The outlook is mixed: some unfortunate cases suffer, eventually, from paralysis and disability; in many, symptoms remain mild and can be helped with medication. But, as yet, no specific treatment exists.

■ PERIPHERAL VASCULAR DISEASE
As individuals age, the arteries become narrowed by fatty and calcified deposits, known as atherosclerosis. In certain individuals, particularly smokers and those with a genetic disposition, the arteries are affected more extensively and at a younger age. Progressive atherosclerosis will cause reduction of blood supply to the legs, with:
* Cold limbs (predominantly the legs).
* Legs may appear pale if lifted in the air.
* Cramp-like pain, particularly in the calf muscles, on walking any distance (intermittent claudication).
* Pain settles when walking stops.
* Occasionally sensory changes, including numbness.
* Weak pulse in arms and legs.

■ ALCOHOLIC NEUROPATHY
Most chronic alcoholics have damaged nerves, giving:
* Numbness in the lower limbs. Ulcers may develop.
* Tingling in the lower limbs.
* Burning in the lower limbs (especially in the feet).
* Weakness of the lower limbs.
* Wasting of the muscles of the lower limbs.

Walking will be affected. The problems can be reversed by giving up alcohol; proper diet; taking B vitamin supplements.

RARE

■ GUILLAIN-BARRE SYNDROME
Also known as acute inflammatory polyneuropathy.

An illness affecting the peripheral nervous system. It can occur at any age, often one to three weeks after an acute viral infection.
* Initially, tingling in the hands and feet.
* Weakness develops in the arms and legs and ultimately, in severe cases, the muscles controlling the lungs. Sometimes the individual needs artificial ventilation.
* Loss of sensation may be severe or minimal.
* Facial weakness is a possibility.

Gradual improvement takes place over weeks or months: complete recovery is normal.

■ FROSTBITE
See page 321.

■ LEPROSY
Essentially a disease of under developed countries acquired by close contact with an infected individual over a prolonged period. Under these circumstances, the diagnosis will probably be obvious. One of the early signs is numbness and tingling in the ends of the arms and legs. There are many other symptoms

COLD FINGERS AND TOES

See FEELING THE COLD, page 487.

ALTERED SENSATION IN THE FINGERS AND TOES

Any disease or injury of a nerve can cause altered sensation in the area of the skin supplied by that nerve. It can take many forms, from tingling, through pins and needles and burning, to complete absence of sensation if the nerve is destroyed.

PROBABLE
DISEASE OR INJURY OF A NERVE OR NERVES

POSSIBLE
DIABETIC NEUROPATHY
MULTIPLE SCLEROSIS
PERIPHERAL VASCULAR DISEASE
ALCOHOLIC NEUROPATHY
SUBACUTE COMBINED DEGENERATION OF (SPINAL) CORD

RARE
GUILLAIN-BARRÉ SYNDROME
FROSTBITE
LEPROSY

PROBABLE

■ DISEASE OR INJURY OF A NERVE OR NERVES
Perhaps the commonest form is pressure neuropathy — or nerve palsy. This can occur if you fall asleep in an awkward position. Nerves usually affected are the ulnar (at the elbow); the radial (at the upper arm); and the peroneal nerve by the knee.

Common to all these palsies are:
* Initial numbness on waking in the area served by the nerve.
* Initial loss of movement of the affected part.
* Within a few minutes, sensation returns.
* At first this is a mild tingling, but it progresses to painful pins and needles.
* After several more minutes, or longer, the sensations settle and full function returns.

Occasionally, if the local

pressure on the nerve has been unduly prolonged, full function may take weeks to return.

POSSIBLE

■ DIABETIC NEUROPATHY
■ MULTIPLE SCLEROSIS
■ PERIPHERAL VASCULAR DISEASE, *pages 317-8.*
■ ALCOHOLIC NEUROPATHY
See page 318.

■ SUBACUTE COMBINED DEGENERATION OF THE SPINAL CORD
This is a result of vitamin B12 deficiency, caused by a number of of factors, the most significant being pernicious anemia. Other causes include poor diet, extreme vegetarianism, poor absorption of food from the gut, certain medications and alcohol abuse. Damage is done to parts of the white nerve matter in the spinal cord, giving:
* Pins and needles (paresthesia) in the feet (hands and arms rarely affected).
* Inability to feel vibration and to sense position — affecting legs and body.
* Weakness in the legs; muscle wasting.
* Unsteady gait.

RARE

■ GUILLAIN-BARRE SYNDROME
■ FROSTBITE
■ LEPROSY
See pages 318, 321 and 319, respectively.

TINGLING FINGERS AND TOES

See ALTERED SENSATION IN THE FINGERS AND TOES, page 319.

ITCHING OR NUMBNESS OF THE FINGERS AND TOES

In an otherwise normal individual.

PROBABLE
ATHLETE'S FOOT
DERMATITIS

POSSIBLE
CHILBLAINS
ECZEMA

RARE
FROSTBITE

PROBABLE

■ ATHLETE'S FOOT
A fungal infection of the feet.
* Irritation between the toes.
* Burning and itching between the toes.
* Some redness, as a result of inflammation.
* Crusting and further infection can take place.
* Smelly feet.
* Cracking of skin, particularly between the toes.

Athlete's foot

To prevent fungal infection spreading keep the skin between the toes dry and treat with antifungal powder.

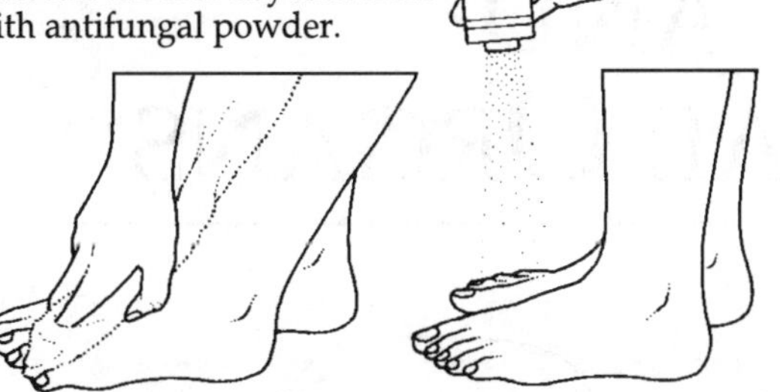

Keep the feet dry and well ventilated by wearing open toed sandals.

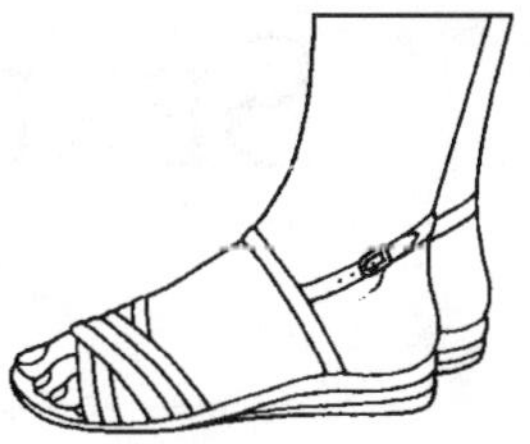

■ DERMATITIS

Acute dermatitis — inflammation of the skin — may be caused by an allergy to chemicals (for instance, deodorants or washing powders). So dermatitis can be caused by socks washed in a detergent to which an individual is allergic.

* Irritation.
* Burning.
* Inflammation, including weeping and crusting skin.
* Symptoms confined to areas which come in contact with the source of the allergy.

POSSIBLE

■ CHILBLAINS

Damage to blood vessels in the skin caused by exposure to cold. Treated best by slow rewarming.

* Local pain in fingers or toes.
* Itching and burning at first, followed by:
* Swelling .
* Local discoloration (reddish/ purple) at the site of pain.
* Blister formation.

■ ECZEMA

Chronic irritation of the skin, often associated with allergies.
See page 375.

RARE

■ FROSTBITE

In prolonged below-freezing temperatures, all extremities are at risk, including ears, nose, toes and fingers. People with poor circulation, typically the elderly, or those who lose heat fastest (for instance children) are most at risk.

* Initial pain and tingling in affected part.
* May become numb (pain-free) — a bad sign.
* Discoloration: may at first be reddish purple, but when the affected part becomes white, then the frostbite is serious.
* If untreated, the frostbitten areas will develop gangrene — death of tissue — because blood is no longer supplied. Ulcers develop and rapidly become infected.

Urgent medical help is needed to supervise the rewarming of the affected part, and to minimize the final damage.

THE REPRODUCTIVE AND SEXUAL ORGANS

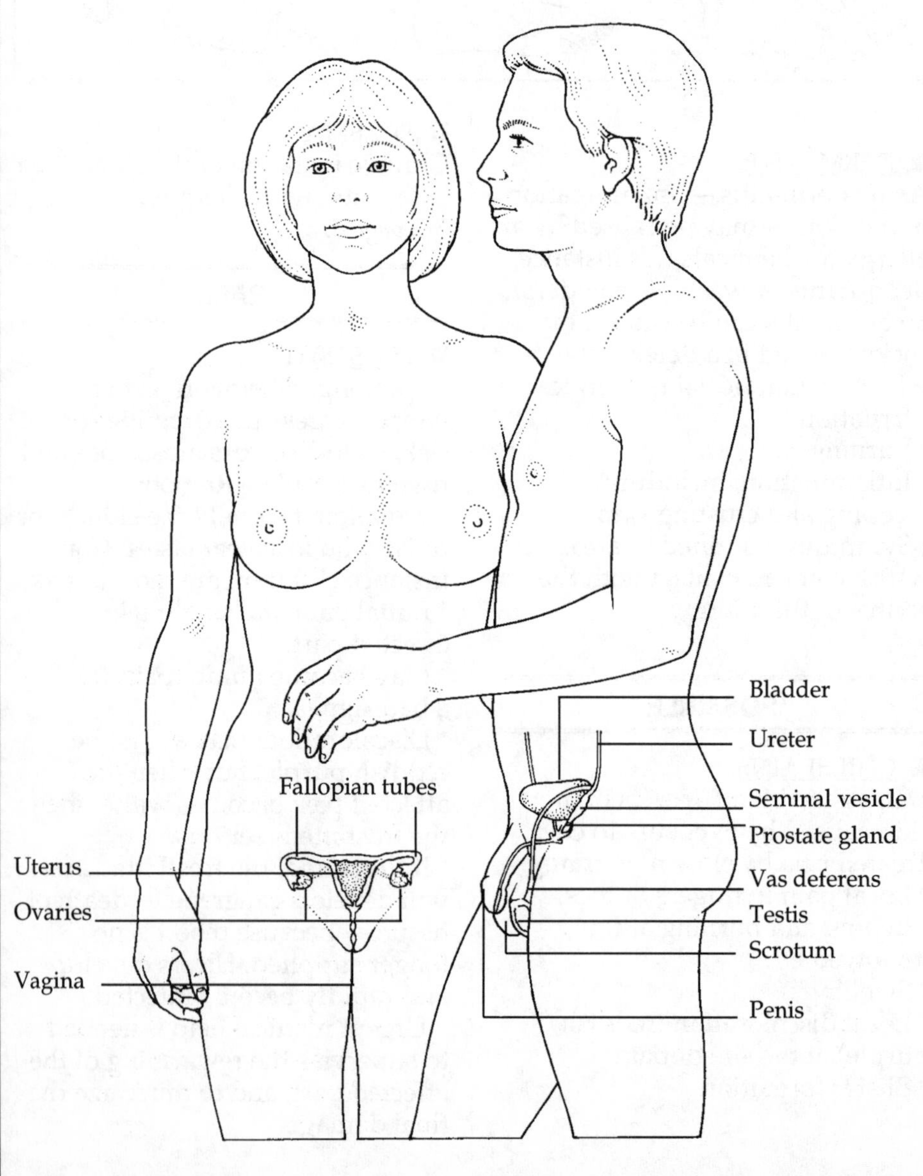

BLISTERS ON OR AROUND THE GENITALIA

PROBABLE
HERPES

POSSIBLE
MOLLUSCUM CONTAGIOSUM

PROBABLE

■ HERPES
The same virus that causes cold sores can cause these blisters on and around the genitalia. Commonest in women.
* A few blisters crop up from time to time.
* Intensely painful when they appear.

Anti-viral medications may be helpful. It is especially important, if you are pregnant, to report any previous or current attacks of herpes to your physician. Measures will be taken to reduce the risk of infecting the baby at birth, which can be dangerous.

POSSIBLE

■ MOLLUSCUM CONTAGIOSUM
Harmless, blister-like lumps, that occur in many parts of the body. Caused by a virus.
* Painless, unless they become infected.
* Dimple in the center.

These usually disappear on their own; simple treatment can speed the process.

GENITAL LUMPS, ULCERS AND SORES

Minor infections of the genitals are very common. Serious sexually transmitted diseases (STDs) are also increasingly common. It is important to be alert to early symptoms of STDs. You owe this not just to yourself but to your sexual partners, too.

PROBABLE
FURUNCLES
SCABIES OR CRAB LICE
WARTS

POSSIBLE
CYSTS
SYPHILIS

RARE
BEHCET'S DISEASE
TROPICAL STDs
CANCER

The Reproductive and Sexual Organs

PROBABLE

■ FURUNCLES
Tiny pimples on the skin, or at the base of pubic hairs.
* Sore, rapidly-appearing lumps.
* Come to a yellow head.
* Discharge pus and blood, then disappear.

Simple antiseptic creams help these go. Severe cases may require a course of antibiotics.

■ SCABIES OR CRAB LICE
Mites which bite the skin, causing:
* Itch, worse at night.
* Several small lumps appearing rapidly around the genitals.
* Scabies commonly bite also between the fingers, and on the wrist.

Treatment is with shampoos and skin applications, plus careful decontamination of bedding and clothing.

■ WARTS
Fleshy growths a few millimeters in length are fairly common, and as harmless on the genitals as elsewhere. Quite different are masses of spreading warts:
* Appear like tiny, branching corals.
* Often also found around the anus.

As these may also be associated with syphilis it is important to seek medical care.

POSSIBLE

■ CYSTS
Women can often develop a cyst, known as Bartholin cyst or abscess.
* Painless swelling in one lip of the vagina.
* May cause no other problem.
* If infected, becomes very swollen and tender; fever.

Surgical drainage or antibiotics are needed.

■ SYPHILIS
The symptoms of infection with syphilis appear two to four weeks after contact. Either partner may be infected.
* Painless ulcer on the genitals, turning into a firm lump. The ulcer, known as a chancer, may appear around or in the vagina, in the mouth, or around the anus, depending on the nature of the sexual activity.
* Lymph nodes enlarge in the groin.
* Heals after several weeks.
* After a few months, secondary features appear, such as rashes on the palms and soles, joint pains, swollen lymph nodes, genital warts.Years later, syphilis can rampage through the body, affecting just about every organ and causing dementia. Early disease is cured by penicillin. Sexual partners must be treated.

RARE

■ BEHCET'S DISEASE
A combination of:
* Painful, single ulcers on genitals and in the mouth.
* Red eyes, either conjunctivitis or iritis.
* Symptoms tend to come and go.

■ TROPICAL STDs
By rare, we mean rare in Europe and the U.S.A; sexually promiscuous travellers to the tropics are at risk. These diseases are chancroid, *lymphogranuloma venereum* and *granuloma inguinale*. They all produce:
* Genital ulcer, within a few days of infection.
* May remain small, or become very large.
* Usually painful.
* Swollen local lymph glands.

The diagnosis is made on appearance, and results of taking a specimen for culture; treatment with antibiotics usually leads to a cure.

■ CANCER
Skin cancer may be the reason for a persistent, ulcerated area on the penis or vagina: see a physician immediately.

Delay reduces the chance of a complete cure.

LUMPS IN THE GROIN

The groin is the region at the top of the thighs, by the side of the genitals in front of the hip joints. Lumps on the genitals themselves are considered under specific headings. Lumps in the groin are very common and are noticed early, being such a visible part of the body. They are not usually serious.

There are several different structures in the groin. Lumps in that region may have many causes. In practice, it is usually possible to make a confident diagnosis based only on the appearance of the lump and an examination.

PROBABLE
INGUINAL HERNIA
ENLARGED LYMPH NODES

POSSIBLE
VARICOSE VEINS
FEMORAL HERNIA
LIPOMA
UNDESCENDED TESTICLE

RARE
ANEURYSM OF BLOOD VESSEL
TUMORS AND ABSCESSES

PROBABLE

■ INGUINAL HERNIA
An extremely common type of hernia, caused by weakness in the muscle wall of the abdomen, which bulges forward as a soft lump. Although typically a problem of adulthood, and made worse by lifting and straining, it may also be seen in very young babies.
* Bulges on straining.
* Often completely disappears when relaxed, lying flat.
* Slight aching is common.
* If it becomes painful and firm, bowel may be trapped within it.

THE REPRODUCTIVE AND SEXUAL ORGANS

Seek medical help immediately. Hernias in children should always be treated. Inguinal hernias in adults who are engaged in physical activity or lifting of heavy materials can be extremely troublesome. In an elderly person who is not particularly active, repair may not be necessary.

■ ENLARGED LYMPH NODES
Just like the neck, the groin has groups of lymph glands, whose job is to protect against infection. It is normal to feel a few small glands in the groin; they are about half a centimeter in size, painless and mobile under your finger. Minor scratches on the legs, or a virus infection, or pimples around the groin, will cause these glands to enlarge for a few days, and it is best to check on these until they shrink again. Glands which remain swollen for longer, which are painful or unusually large, need to be carefully checked. There are so many possibilities that enlarged glands are treated as a separate topic in *SWOLLEN LYMPH NODES, page 488.*

Enlarged glands with any of the following symptoms should be taken seriously.
* Enlarged glands elsewhere, such as neck, armpits.
* Sores on the genitals.
* Bleeding from the rectum.
* Fever, feeling sick.
* Anemia.
* Bruising.
* Vaginal or penile discharge.
* Vaginal bleeding.
* Low belly pain.
* Growth on the leg.

POSSIBLE

■ VARICOSE VEINS
Enlarged veins are often seen and felt in the groin.
* Swelling is very soft, easily squeezed by finger pressure.
* A bluish tinge may be noticeable.
* Usually, also varicose veins further down the leg.
* Slight aching after standing.

■ FEMORAL HERNIA
A femoral hernia arises from a weakness at the very top of the thigh, and is different from an inguinal hernia. It carries a higher chance of blockage, and also requires surgical treatment.
* Commonest in older women.
* Often appears rapidly as a small tender lump..
* Blockage causes a painful, hard lump, vomiting, intestinal obstruction.

■ LIPOMA
A soft mass, present for many weeks and growing slowly, if at all, is probably a lipoma — a fat lump.
* Painless.
* Often others elsewhere.

There is no need to the remove the lump unless there is some doubt about the diagnosis.

■ UNDESCENDED TESTICLE
In males, the testicle may lodge just above the groin.
* Noticeable in babies and children, when it may be seen soon after birth. The scrotum is usually checked during the first

year to make sure both testicles are present.
* No testicle felt in that side of the scrotum.
The testicle should be surgically brought down into the scrotum, as soon as possible. Failure to do so increases the risk of infertility and the development of cancer in the affected testicle.

RARE

■ ANEURYSM OF BLOOD VESSEL
The large femoral artery, which carries blood to the leg, passes near to the surface in the groin. Its wall can weaken and it expands like a balloon, producing:
* A lump, pulsating in time with your heart beat, but delayed by a fraction of a second.
* Often tender.
Can be repaired surgically.

■ TUMORS AND ABSCESSES
As with lumps anywhere on the body, the possibility of a tumor or an abscess has to kept in mind. In such cases the lump may:
* Be tender.
* Feel as if it is attached to surrounding tissues.
* You may be generally unwell.

LOSS OF PUBIC HAIR

Although this is not a common problem, it is alarming to the individual when it happens. Thinning of the hair is a normal feature of aging, and it occurs as an expected side effect of chemotherapy for cancer. Otherwise, it is probably caused by hormone disturbances.

PROBABLE
ALOPECIA

POSSIBLE
ADRENAL INSUFFICIENCY
CIRRHOSIS OF LIVER

RARE
UNDERACTIVE PITUITARY GLAND

PROBABLE

■ ALOPECIA
A general term for hair loss of unknown cause. In the most common form, it causes thinning of hair, perhaps with some actual hairless patches. Only in severe cases is there complete, generalized hair loss.
* Baldness in men or women.
* Loss of eyebrows, armpit hair.
Usually cures itself. *See also LOSS OF HAIR OR BALDNESS, page 263.*

POSSIBLE

■ ADRENAL INSUFFICIENCY
A consequence of underactive adrenal glands, causing:
* Profound weakness.
* Dark patches in the mouth, on the gums or on old scars.
* Weight loss.
* Nausea, stomach cramps.

Treatment is by hormone replacement, once the underlying cause has been established.

■ CIRRHOSIS OF THE LIVER
Usually due to alcoholism.
* Hair thins rather than disappears.
* Small, dilated veins appear on face, chest.
* Red palms.
* Impotence.
* Swollen ankles.
* Nausea, indigestion.
* Easy bruising.
* Possibly blood in vomit, or in bowel movement.
* Variable degree of confusion.
Treatment, of course, requires complete abstention from alcohol.

RARE

■ PITUITARY GLAND DISEASE
Failure of this gland in the brain, which is involved in so many functions of the body, causes: extremely pale skin.
* Hairlessness.
* Great tiredness, weakness.
* In women, menstrual periods.
Lifelong hormone replacement allows a return to health.

HOT FLASHES

Sudden waves of heat passing over the whole body, occurring at any time. Often worse at night, and in social gatherings.

PROBABLE
MENOPAUSE

POSSIBLE
OVER-ACTIVE THYROID GLAND

RARE
CAUSES OF FEVERS OR SWEATS

PROBABLE

■ MENOPAUSE
Known also as "the Change", or "the change of life", and linked to the drop in the level of female hormones present in the blood.

Menopause is said to have begun if a woman has not menstruated for one year. However, hot flashes can begin before menstruation stops — blood tests are a useful check. On average, the menopause begins at about 50 years. But, it is entirely normal to enter menopause earlier or later in life. The best guide is the age at which your mother began her menopause. Other symptoms are:
* Irregular menstruation.
* Skin texture coarsens.
* The skin of the vagina becomes drier.
* Aches and pains are common.
Some features are more a reflection of personal adjustment to this major event in a woman's life:
* Loss of sexual desire.
* Headaches.
* Depression.

* Irritability.

Hot flashes often continue for two to three years; a few unlucky women continue to have them for 10 years or more.

Hormone replacement therapy (HRT) can control hot flashes, vaginal dryness and reduce the aches and pains. A decision about HRT needs detailed discussion with your physician about the pros and cons. The treatment is particularly advisable if you go into a very early menopause. Many studies now show that HRT (also called ERT, estrogen replacement therapy) reduces the bone loss of osteoporosis and also reduces the risk of heart attack in post-menopausal women.

POSSIBLE

■ OVER-ACTIVE THYROID GLAND

* Occurs at any age.
* Sweating, increased appetite, weight loss.
* Intolerance to heat.
* Tremor of hands.
* Consistently rapid pulse, possibly palpitations.
* Protruding eyes (in some cases).

Treatment reduces the excessive output of thyroid hormone from the thyroid gland.

RARE

■ PERSISTENT FEVER OR SWEATS

It is worth considering whether any of the many causes of fevers or sweats might be responsible. The subject is covered in detail on

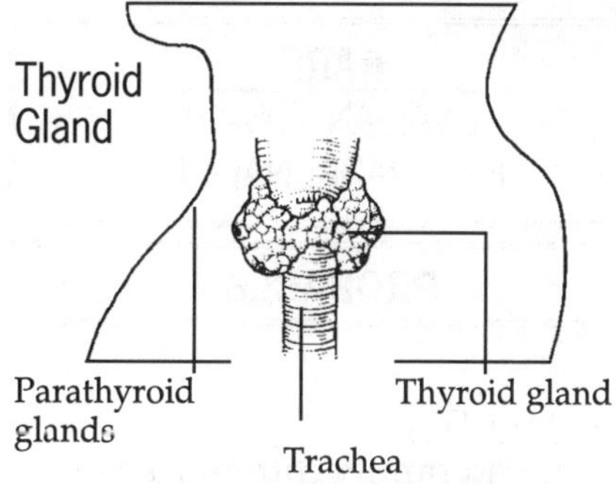

pages 440-51 and 455-459. Suspicious symptoms include:
* Hot flashes beginning abruptly.
* Menstruation regular.
* Drenching sweats at night.
* Feeling sick; weight loss.
* Exposure to unusual infections through travel, occupation.
* Enlarged lymph glands.

MASCULINE CHANGES

Masculine changes in a woman may be due to an upset in the balance between male and female hormones. If periods are normal, there is probably no serious hormonal problem. Typical masculine changes are:
* Growth of hair on the face, chest, abdomen.
* Balding.
* Deepening voice.
* Disruption of periods.

PROBABLE

HEREDITY

POSSIBLE

HYPOTHYROIDISM
POLYCYSTIC OVARIES
MEDICATIONS

THE REPRODUCTIVE AND SEXUAL ORGANS

RARE
OVARIAN TUMOR
HYPERADRENALISM

PROBABLE

■ HEREDITY
Racial and family differences in hairiness are well known; for example, both men and women from Mediterranean races tend to be hairier than Nordic peoples. This is in the normal range and there is no effect on fertility.

POSSIBLE

■ HYPOTHYROIDISM
An underactive thyroid gland may often be the reason for masculinization, as it causes:
* Gruff voice, coarse skin.
* Menstrual changes.

Additional features of an underactive thyroid gland are:
* Weight gain.
* Slow thinking.
* Slow pulse.
* Weakness.

The diagnosis is made by blood tests.

■ POLYCYSTIC OVARIES
A disease in which the ovaries have many cysts, and produce male hormones. It is *not* a form of cancer. It affects women in their teens or early 20s, and its symptoms are:
* Hairiness.
* Absent menstruation.
* Severe acne.
* Obesity.

The severity varies. Ultrasound examination of the ovaries, together with measurement of hormones in the blood, have made this disease easy to diagnose. Treatment can improve fertility, as well as improving other symptoms.

■ MEDICATIONS
Hairiness is a side effect of several widely used medications. The most common is phenytoin, used to control epilepsy; steroids, used to treat a range of arthritic diseases, may also be a cause.

RARE

■ OVARIAN TUMOR
Suspected in a previously healthy woman who develops signs of masculinization. There are no other symptoms of an early tumor, which must be detected by examination and ultrasound investigation.

■ HYPERADRENALISM
There are many causes of this syndrome, which involves the production of excessive amounts of natural male hormones and steroids by the body's glands. Synthetic hormones (anabolic steroids), used by athletes to build muscle, will cause excess hair. Among its symptoms are:
* Obese body, but thin limbs.
* Masculine features.
* Easy bruising.
* Excessive production of urine.
* Purple stripes across the hips, and other fat-bearing areas.

PAIN IN THE PELVIS

Pains in the lower belly are common in women, and are frequently difficult to diagnose. Apart from gynecological causes, there are plenty of other organs to consider: the intestines, the bladder and kidneys; pain from irritation of nerves in the back; diseases of the major arteries which run through the lower abdomen. The belly is also a sensitive index of emotional distress, at all ages and in both sexes. It is important to consider emotional factors which may be contributing to the complaint or aches and pains.

Pains associated with the following symptoms suggest a gynecological cause:
* Painful menstruation.
* Unusual vaginal discharge.
* Abnormal vaginal bleeding.
* Pain on intercourse.
* Infertility.
* Swelling of the belly, which comes and goes monthly.

For further details *see pages 343-61, 335 and 332.*

Symptoms pointing to a non-gynecological cause are:
* Diarrhea or constipation.
* Frequent desire to urinate; stinging or burning when you do.
* Pain varies on moving your back.
* Throbbing in your abdomen, pain in legs on walking.
* Rectal bleeding.
* Depression, marital problems.

Your overall condition may point to one of the many non-gynecological diseases which can cause recurrent abdominal pains. Your physician will use the pattern of symptoms, and the results of tests, before making a diagnosis.

INFERTILITY

Fifteen percent of couples who have regular sexual intercourse will not have conceived after one year. About 10 percent of all couples remain sterile. Before anything else, it is essential to establish that normal intercourse is taking place. Also, a sperm count should be taken early on, to avoid fruitless and unpleasant tests for the woman. About 55 percent of cases are due to problems in the woman's reproductive system.

PROBABLE
FAILURE OF EGG PRODUCTION
BLOCKED FALLOPIAN TUBES
LOW SPERM COUNT
CAUSE UNKNOWN

POSSIBLE
ENDOMETRIOSIS
GENERAL DISEASE

RARE
WOMB ABNORMALITIES

The Reproductive and Sexual Organs

PROBABLE

■ FAILURE OF EGG PRODUCTION
This involves hormone imbalance, and would be suspected if there are:
* Irregular or absent menstruation.
* Delay in beginning periods.
See specific headings on pages 343-353.

■ BLOCKED FALLOPIAN TUBES
These are the tubes through which eggs travel to the womb. Blocked tubes usually follow repeated pelvic infections, suspected from:
* Recurrent pelvic pain.
* Recurrent, infected vaginal discharges.
* Deep pain on intercourse.
See also PAINFUL PERIODS, page 351 and PAIN IN THE PELVIS, page 331.

■ LOW SPERM COUNT
Occurs in 25 percent of cases of infertility. Sometimes it is the result of diseases of the testicle, blockage of the tubes from the testicles, but mostly unknown. Treatment of varicose veins in the testicle may improve fertility.

■ CAUSE UNKNOWN
Despite thorough investigation, many cases remain unexplained.

POSSIBLE

■ ENDOMETRIOSIS
See page 349.
* Deep pain on intercourse.

■ GENERAL DISEASE
Any serious, general disease can reduce fertility, but should already be obvious.

RARE

■ WOMB ABNORMALITIES
Investigations sometimes show a range of unsuspected abnormalities, such as a malformed womb, which prevents implantation of the egg.

LACK OF INTEREST IN SEX

Most enduring relationships eventually balance the partners' sexual desires so that neither partner is left feeling frustrated or guilty. The road to that adjustment can be a difficult one. Sexual problems are never the fault of one party alone: recognizing that there is a problem is the first step to resolving it.

Natural variations in a woman's sexual desire occur during the monthly cycle, reaching a peak in mid-cycle (before ovulation) for some women. Major illness and stress can affect desire in both sexes. Childbirth and breast feeding often decrease sexual desire.

PROBABLE
PSYCHOLOGICAL FACTORS

POSSIBLE
BAD SEXUAL EXPERIENCES
DEPRESSION

PROBABLE

■ PSYCHOLOGICAL FACTORS
Psychological factors are most likely if you feel:
* Sex is dirty or bad.
* Dislike of being touched sexually by your partner.
* That things in the relationship should be better than they are.
* Guilty about your lack of enjoyment of sex.

Family counselors and other therapists can be very helpful.

POSSIBLE

■ BAD SEXUAL EXPERIENCES
Problems include painful intercourse, misunderstanding about sexual anatomy and sexual response, fear of pregnancy and, most importantly, the memory of early sexual experiences, particularly if either partner was abused. The techniques for dealing with such problems involve explanation, honesty and patience. Gradually exploring your anatomy and sexual response with your partner, without progressing to sexual intercourse, may be helpful.

■ DEPRESSION
A decreasing interest in sex in either a man or a woman may signal depression. Some other features of depression are:
* Feelings of sadness.
* Loss of self-worth.
* Disturbed sleep.
* Easy crying.
* Thoughts of suicide.
* Slowing of thought.

ORGASMIC FAILURE

A popular view places orgasm during intercourse right up there alongside other major goals of Western society. However, orgasm is not essential to a satisfactory sexual relationship.

Men may be unable to achieve orgasm for much the same reasons as women.

Some facts about female orgasm:
* It is a real physical and psychological event.
* Stimulation of the clitoris is usually important.
* It is not necessary for enjoyable sex each time.
* It may take longer to achieve for a woman than for a man.
* Women are capable of multiple orgasms; they do not need a resting period like most men.

Failure to achieve orgasm may be due to difficulty within the partnership, or because of the techniques used during intercourse. Some women are unable to experience orgasm until they start to masturbate. It is helpful to share and explore with your partner what forms of stimulation lead to orgasm so that they can be enjoyed together.

PROBABLE
PSYCHOLOGICAL
POOR TECHNIQUE

POSSIBLE
PARTNER'S PROBLEM

PROBABLE

■ PSYCHOLOGICAL
This refers to the array of experiences that make a relationship: affection, trust, previous positive experiences. It is common knowledge that uncertainty in these, and other, aspects will lead to problems with sex and orgasm.

■ POOR TECHNIQUE
It is necessary to take the female anatomy into account. Female orgasm requires:
* Adequate foreplay.
* Clitoral stimulation.
* Avoidance of pain.
* Proper lubrication.
* For some, affectionate warm communication.

This is a matter of trial and error.

POSSIBLE

■ PARTNER'S PROBLEM
Failure to achieve orgasm can be a result of a partner's:
* Premature ejaculation;
* Impotence.

See pages 365, 366 and 363.

PAINFUL SEXUAL INTERCOURSE

PROBABLE
VAGINAL INFECTION
VAGINAL SPASM (VAGINISMUS)

POSSIBLE
VAGINAL DRYNESS
ENDOMETRIOSIS
CHRONIC PELVIC INFECTION

RARE
PHYSICAL BARRIER TO INTERCOURSE

PROBABLE

■ VAGINAL INFECTION
Perhaps a raw area in or near the vagina.
* Pain is superficial, not deep inside.
* Probably discharge.
* Probably an itch.

Possible causes are thrush and herpes. *See page 357.*

■ VAGINAL SPASM
Vaginismus. A term for a contraction of the muscles around the vagina which will prevent intercourse. This important symptom is nearly always the result of a psychological fear of penetration. Occasionally, it follows an unpleasant injury to the vagina, such as a painful tear or cut (episiotomy) after childbirth.
* Other aspects of sexual behavior may be normal.
* Gynecological examination may be difficult or impossible; this frequently gives the first clue to the problem.

Treatment encourages familiarity with one's own genitals, building up gradually to sexual intercourse.

POSSIBLE

■ VAGINAL DRYNESS
See also BLEEDING AFTER THE MENOPAUSE, page 352. Mainly a post-menopausal problem. Can also occur because of inadequate foreplay.
* Vagina feels generally sore.
* Watery discharge, possibly bloodstained.

This can be greatly helped by the use of locally applied estrogen creams or hormone replacement therapy (HRT). *See page 329.*

■ ENDOMETRIOSIS
* Intercourse causes pain deep inside.
* Heavy menstruation.
* Infertility.

See page 349.

■ CHRONIC PELVIC INFECTION
Also causes:
* Deep pain on intercourse.
* Heavy periods.

See PELVIC INFLAMMATORY DISEASE, page 349.

RARE

■ PHYSICAL BARRIER TO INTERCOURSE
The hymen, the membrane across the entrance to the vagina that is normally broken at first sexual intercourse, can be too thick to break. Rarely the entrance to the vagina is unusually narrow. Surgical help is needed here.
* You may see or feel an obstruction.
* Pain on attempting intercourse.
* Pain around entrance to vagina.

BREAST DISORDERS INTRODUCTION

It is wise for women to check their breasts from time to time, to familiarize themselves with how they feel normally so that changes can be picked-up early. Remember that the tissues of the breast extend into the armpit, so checks should include that area. X-ray mammography is an effective way to screen for breast lumps and cancer. It may detect changes in the breasts before *you* notice a problem. Such screening is not 100 percent reliable, and it may turn up apparent abnormalities which, on further testing, prove harmless. Screening is very useful for women over 50, when it should be done every year. Between 40 and 49 the test is not so accurate but many experts believe it is still important to get a mammogram, especially if there is a family history of breast cancer.

Many women believe that the only breast disease is breast cancer, and that any change whatsoever in their breast must be a symptom of this disease. But it is not usually the most likely cause.

Fear of a breast cancer diagnosis makes some women avoid reporting symptoms. However, more often than not, skilled examination alone will produce a reassuring diagnosis, while tests, will show that all is well. Also, when cancer is confirmed, any delay in reporting symptoms will delay treatment and treatment is now very effective.

LUMP IN THE BREAST

At some time in their lives, most women will feel a lump in one of their breasts. Breasts are frequently lumpy, and some of these lumps are easily felt. In nine out of ten cases it will be entirely harmless (a benign cyst). That leaves a one in ten chance of a lump being cancerous.

Breast cancer is one of the most closely studied forms of cancer, but physicians will admit that there is still much they do not know about it. Fundamental questions remain unanswered, such as why the cancer starts, how quickly it grows and how best to treat it. Expert opinion about therapy is constantly changing, following the results of treatment trials which are being carried out worldwide.

In this situation, some women with cancer are tempted to search for miracle cures. Be very careful. There is a big difference between unconventional approaches that give support, hope, and self-reliance, and those which are just a means of peddling treatment which does not, and will not, stand up to the simplest scientific assessment.

There is a myth that physicians wash their hands of women who do not wish to follow conventional treatment. It is very rarely true. Begin by seeing your physician as soon as you feel an abnormality in your breast. Your physician will often be able to reassure you on the basis of examination alone.

PROBABLE
FIBROADENOMA
FIBROCYSTIC DISEASE
DUCT PAPILLOMA

POSSIBLE
BREAST CANCER
FAT NECROSIS

RARE
OTHER TUMORS

PROBABLE

■ FIBROADENOMA
Commonest in women between 20 and 40 years old.
* Firm, painless lump.
* Freely mobile: which is why this lump has been described as a "breast mouse".

Some women have several of these over many years, but each one should be surgically removed. They are not thought to lead to cancer.

■ FIBROCYSTIC DISEASE
This is a misleading technical term for something that is not really a disease at all. The breasts are generally lumpy, and within that lumpiness there may be more definite, large lumps which are usually fluid-filled cysts.
* Commonest in women 30 to 50 years of age.
* Lumpiness varies during the menstrual cycle.
* Often pain before menstruation.
* Often areas of the breast are tender.

Mammograms (X-rays of the breast) are useful in differentiating these lumps from cancer. Many physicians will drain obvious cysts, using a needle and syringe, and send the contents for detailed analysis. No other treatment is necessarily needed.

■ DUCT PAPILLOMA
A lump felt just behind the nipple, and associated with a bloody discharge from the nipple. This should always be reported to your physician.
See page 341.

POSSIBLE

■ BREAST CANCER
You feel a lump; it may be tiny but you are sure it has appeared recently. Some of the features that would suggest that a lump is likely to be cancerous are:
* A firm, irregular lump.
* Not freely mobile, seems stuck in one place.
* Skin over it is dimpled and puckered.
* A newly indrawn nipple, or any nipple changes occurring at the same time.
* Swollen glands felt in armpit.
* Pain in the region of the lump.
* Bleeding from the nipple.

It may be possible to take a biopsy from the lump, allowing a definite diagnosis before any surgery is planned. Mammograms also help with diagnosis. In other cases, the diagnosis may not be

THE REPRODUCTIVE AND SEXUAL ORGANS

made until the lump has been removed and analyzed.

Treatment for pre-menopausal women is a combination of surgery, radiotherapy and chemotherapy in varying proportions. In post-menopausal women, surgery is commonly combined with radiotherapy and anti-estrogen medications, such as tamoxifen.

■ FAT NECROSIS
A hard knock to the breast can damage fat cells, leading to a lump that feels indistinguishable from a cancer.
* A firm lump.
* Does not move freely.
* Skin over it may be dimpled.

The only safe way to deal with this is a biopsy.

RARE

■ OTHER TUMORS
It is possible for cancers elsewhere to spread into the breast. The diagnosis will probably only be made on biopsy.

PAIN IN THE BREASTS

If pain is felt over the whole breast, it is usually caused by a variation in hormone levels. It may be confined to one area, when you should feel for a localized abnormality, such as a lump or dimpled skin. Breast pain may be no more than a nuisance, but for some women it is a great problem, which has only attracted recent attention. Mammography makes it possible to be confident that there is no underlying disease. Treatments currently under study include hormones, Vitamin B6, and evening primrose oil.

PROBABLE
BREAST ABSCESS
FIBROCYSTIC DISEASE
BREAST FEEDING

POSSIBLE
BREAST CANCER
PAIN FROM THE RIBS
PREGNANCY

PROBABLE

■ BREAST ABSCESS
See DISCHARGE FROM NIPPLE, page 340.
* Pain.
* Redness of one breast.
* Fever.

■ FIBROCYSTIC DISEASE
See page 337.

A frequent cause for a general ache in one or both breasts, with localized areas being especially tender.

■ BREAST FEEDING
Breasts that get overful with milk, when a woman is nursing, can become lumpy and sore.

POSSIBLE

■ BREAST CANCER

See page 338. Pain is unusual as an early symptom of breast cancer; though it can be present at an advanced stage.

■ PAIN FROM THE RIBS

Inflammation of the muscles between ribs, or where the rib and the breast bone meet.
* One breast affected.
* Pain is sharp, and highly localized.
* Pain reproduced by pressing between the ribs, or by pressing on the breast bone.

A harmless symptom that settles over a few weeks.

■ PREGNANCY

Aching in the breasts due to pregnancy often occurs even before a period has been missed. Other early symptoms of pregnancy are:
* Frequent urination.
* A vague tiredness.

BREAST SIZE

The popular Western attitude to breast size equates large size with femininity. This attitude is largely shaped by male opinion and the media, but many women are dissatisfied with the size of their breasts, considering them either too small or too large. Breast size does not affect the ability to breast feed a child. It is normal for the two breasts to be slightly different in size and shape.

PROBABLE
HEREDITY

POSSIBLE
HORMONAL

RARE
LYMPHATIC OBSTRUCTION

PROBABLE

■ HEREDITY

Breast size is mainly determined by in-built factors, with influence from grandparents on both the mother's and the father's side. Race also plays a part, with Asiatic women generally having smaller breasts. Reasons for breast surgery might include:
* Psychological distress.
* Neck and back pains from very heavy breasts.

POSSIBLE

■ HORMONAL

The contraceptive pill and hormone replacement therapy often cause a slight increase in breast size. Pregnancy, of course, makes the breasts enlarge, also under the influence of hormones. Many women notice a slight variation in size during their menstrual cycle. Breast size bears no relationship to a woman's ability to have children.

THE REPRODUCTIVE AND SEXUAL ORGANS

RARE

■ LYMPHATIC OBSTRUCTION
Interference with normal drainage of tissue fluid from the breast via the armpit will lead to one swollen breast.
* Often after radiotherapy to the chest wall, when the arm on that side is also very swollen.
* You may feel glands in the armpit; if so, report immediately.
* Breast becomes generally firm.
Unfortunately, little can usually be done to cure this problem.

DISCHARGE FROM THE NIPPLE

During pregnancy it is normal for a milky fluid to ooze from the breasts. Mothers who nurse their babies will find that even the sound of the baby crying will trigger this entirely normal response. Abnormal discharges are milk in the absence of pregnancy, clear fluid, blood or yellow/green pus. Discharges are commonly due to disease of the duct system, that is, one of the 20 or so channels through which milk flows to the nipple from the milk-producing glands deeper within the breast.

PROBABLE
BREAST ABSCESS
HORMONE DISTURBANCE

POSSIBLE
DUCT PAPILLOMA
CANCER OF DUCTS
DUCT ECTASIA

RARE
BREAST CANCER
PAGET'S DISEASE OF THE NIPPLE

PROBABLE

■ BREAST ABSCESS
A frequent problem in the first few weeks of breast feeding, and thought to be caused simply by infection entering the breast via the constantly damp and sometimes cracked nipple.
* Symptoms build up over a few hours.
* Aching in one part of the breast.
* Often you see a firm red area of the breast.
* Bloody discharge, mixed with milk, may be present.
* Frequently chills, high fevers, sweats.
* Pain can be severe.
Antibiotics nearly always settle this disorder. Occasionally there is a chronic abscess, caused by persistent infection deep within the breast.

■ HORMONE DISTURBANCE
Milk production is controlled by a hormone, prolactin, from the pituitary gland within the brain. An excess of prolactin causes:
* Discharge of milk from both breasts for months on end.
* Scanty menstruation.

Blood tests will show abnormal levels of prolactin. The usual reason is a tiny growth in the pituitary gland; this can be controlled with appropriate medications. A few medically prescribed medications can cause this problem, particularly powerful sedatives and methyldopa, widely used to treat high blood pressure.

POSSIBLE

The three following possibilities give similar symptoms, and in all cases will require further testing, since examination alone is not enough to decide definitely between them.

■ <u>DUCT PAPILLOMA</u>
A wart-like, benign growth within one of the ducts leading to the nipple.
* A bloody discharge, perhaps just a spot of blood on the bra.
* Sometimes just a clear, yellowish discharge.
* A lump may be felt near the nipple.

■ <u>CANCER OF DUCTS</u>
* Bloody discharge.
* Possibly a prickling sensation behind the nipple.

■ <u>DUCT ECTASIA</u>
In this condition, enlarged ducts allow the build-up of normal secretions, which then appear as:
* A brown or green discharge.
* Discharge is firm, cheese-like.

The breast

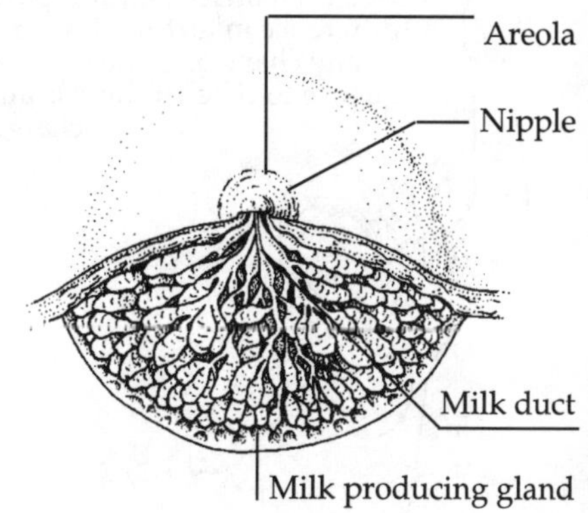

RARE

■ <u>BREAST CANCER</u>
See page 338. Occasionally a breast cancer some distance from the nipple causes bleeding.
* A breast lump is likely.
* Some discomfort is likely.

■ <u>PAGET'S DISEASE OF THE NIPPLE</u>
A distinctive condition, most common in older women:
* Cracked dry, red skin around one nipple.
* Oozes blood.
* The nipple becomes distorted.

This disease is nearly always due to breast cancer.

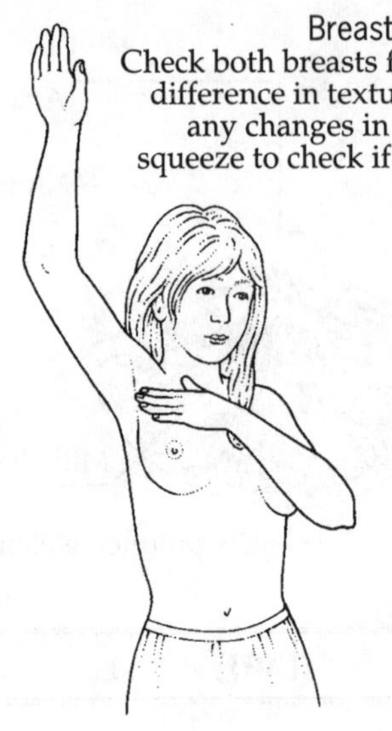

Breast examination
Check both breasts for lumps or difference in texture. Look for any changes in the nipples, squeeze to check if there is any discharge.

RETRACTION OF THE NIPPLE

Both nipples normally project a little, becoming flatter when warm or relaxed, and more protuberant if cold, or sometimes if sexually aroused. Retracted nipples appear sunken into the breast.

PROBABLE
CONGENITAL

POSSIBLE
BREAST CANCER

PROBABLE

■ CONGENITAL
Commonly seen in baby girls who grow up with one or both nipples retracted. It is not a sign of disease, but might affect the ability to breast feed.

There are many "cures" for retracted nipples, but there is little evidence that they work.

POSSIBLE

■ BREAST CANCER
The retraction of a previously normal nipple must be taken as a symptom of breast cancer until proven otherwise. You should search for:
* Lump in the breast.
* Discharge from the nipple.

Always inform your physician of any changes to your nipples. Don't delay.

MENSTRUATION INTRODUCTION

During the monthly cycle, the lining of the womb (uterus) thickens and prepares to accept a fertilized egg. If conception does not take place, the lining breaks down and is shed — this is the menstrual discharge. This complex process involves hormones from the brain, the ovaries and the egg, all directed towards a common goal: a successful pregnancy. Problem-free menstruation depends on a healthy balance between mind and body: it is more likely to be upset by psychological factors than most other bodily functions.

The length, frequency and heaviness of menstruation vary greatly, from person to person and from month to month, and this is not necessarily a symptom of any abnormality. Sudden changes are a different matter and should be a warning to seek medical advice.

ABSENT OR INFREQUENT MENSTRUAL PERIODS

This section concerns women who have previously had normal menstrual periods. If menstruation has never started, *see DELAY IN BEGINNING MENSTRUATION, page 347.* In young women, stress is so often the reason for irregular periods that further testing is usually unnecessary, except for reassurance, or to exclude pregnancy. Irregularities in women in their late 30s or early 40s are likely to have a physical or hormonal cause. In particular, women with infrequent periods should be examined to make quite sure that normal but infrequent periods are just that, and are not in fact occasional, abnormal episodes of bleeding from the womb or cervix. Bleeding out of the blue, without your usual pre-menstrual symptoms, should definitely be evaluated.

PROBABLE

PREGNANCY
STRESS
BREAST FEEDING

POSSIBLE

MENOPAUSE
RAISED PROLACTIN
MAJOR WEIGHT CHANGE
POLYCYSTIC OVARIES
POST-PILL ABSENT PERIODS
SERIOUS GENERAL DISEASE

THE REPRODUCTIVE AND SEXUAL ORGANS

RARE

THYROID DISEASE

ADRENAL DISEASE

PROBABLE

■ PREGNANCY

It is a useful and proven medical rule of thumb that, if in doubt, any woman of child-bearing age with absent menstrual periods should have a pregnancy test if intercourse has taken place. After any missed period, you should be on the lookout for other symptoms of pregnancy, such as:

* Morning sickness.
* Tender breasts.
* Feeling tired, weight gain.
* Passing urine more frequently than usual.
* Appetite changes.

Have a pregnancy test if you are uncertain.

■ STRESS

An extremely common reason, especially in young women. Stress is caused not just by obvious emotional turmoil but major changes in lifestyle, such as changes of job, travel, illness. Even what appears to be "everyday" stress, such as preparing for exams, can be sufficient to stop menstruation.

* In conditions of obvious tension, the absence of periods for two or three months should not be a concern, as long as pregnancy is excluded.

Tests are rarely needed, unless symptoms persist for more than six months.

■ BREAST FEEDING

Menstruation often does not return during breast feeding, since hormones stop the normal menstrual cycle. It is, however, possible to become pregnant while breast feeding, for egg release may still occur.

POSSIBLE

■ MENOPAUSE

To be considered in women from 30 years of age onwards, especially given a family history of early menopause. Any woman whose ovaries have been removed, for example, in the treatment of breast cancer or at a hysterectomy, will experience rapid onset of menopausal symptoms.

■ RAISED PROLACTIN

See HORMONE DISTURBANCE, page 340. Absent menstruation, plus a milky discharge from the breasts, suggest an excess of prolactin, one of the hormones that normally contribute to the production of breast milk.

Rarely, the condition can be caused by a tumor in the brain. Blood tests and simple X-rays can sometimes detect this.

■ MAJOR WEIGHT CHANGE

Both excessive weight gain and loss will disrupt periods, because they affect some brain centers. Very athletic young women with little body fat will stop menstruating, as will those who diet excessively. The most extreme form is due to *anorexia nervosa*:

* Skeletal thinness.
* Obsession with weight.
* Fine hair grows on body.

■ POLYCYSTIC OVARIES.
In a young woman, a diagnosis suggested by:
* Absent periods.
* Hairiness.
* Acne.
* Above-average weight.
See page 330.

■ POST-PILL ABSENT MENSTRUAL PERIODS
Commonest in women whose periods were irregular before they began to take oral contraception.
* Otherwise sound health.
* Periods return after three to six months.

If you have not had a period for more than six months after you stop taking the pill, seek professional advice.

■ SERIOUS GENERAL DISEASE
Remember that tension can stop your menstrual cycle (*see above*). The strain of another illness on your body may also be a cause. Other symptoms might be:
* Weight loss.
* Tiredness.
* Chronic cough.
* Fever, diarrhea.

Menstruation should return after recovery.

RARE

■ THYROID DISEASE
Over-excitability or tiredness, combined with changes in your menstrual pattern may suggest an over or under-active thyroid gland. *See page 350.*

■ ADRENAL DISEASE
A possibility if absent menstruation is associated with:
* Hairiness.
* Weight gain.
* Weakness.

See also MASCULINE CHANGES, pages 329-31.

BLEEDING BETWEEN PERIODS OR AFTER INTERCOURSE

The older the woman, the greater the chance that there is a serious cause. It is important to get medical advice about this problem. Check that the cause is not blood in your partner's semen.

PROBABLE
BREAKTHROUGH BLEEDING ON THE PILL
EROSION OF THE CERVIX
HORMONE IMBALANCE

POSSIBLE
POLYP OF THE CERVIX
CANCER OF CERVIX
CANCER OF THE WOMB
INFLAMMATION OF THE VAGINA

RARE
URETHRAL CARUNCLE

The Reproductive and Sexual Organs

PROBABLE

■ BREAKTHROUGH BLEEDING ON THE CONTRACEPTIVE PILL
In a young woman:
* Otherwise normal cycle.
* Scanty show of blood for a day or two.
* Occurs at about the same time each month.

If this occurs for more than a few months, a change of pill may be advised. This bleeding does not, however, mean that the pill is not working. Don't stop taking the pill because you see bleeding. Finish the packet as you would normally.

■ EROSION OF THE CERVIX
A harmless raw area on the cervix, which may cause:
* Heavy, clear vaginal discharge.
* Bleeding after intercourse.
* Brief, irregular blood-spotting between periods. Blood appears on underclothing and toilet tissue.

■ HORMONE IMBALANCE
Caused by changes in natural estrogen levels during the cycle.
* A possibility in young women.
* Regular, scanty, intermenstrual bleeding.
* Periods are otherwise normal.

The diagnosis is made only after the other possibilities have been ruled out.

POSSIBLE

■ POLYP OF THE CERVIX
A small fleshy outgrowth, which causes no other symptoms, and which may be visible on pelvic examination. Polyps should always be removed and biopsied, though it is rare for one to be malignant.

■ CANCER OF THE CERVIX
It is hoped that widespread cervical (Pap smear) screening will reduce the frequency of this disease. Publicity may give the impression that it is a disease of young women; in fact, it is most common in women in their 40s and 50s. It is known that early sexual activity and having many partners increase the risks significantly. Though early cancer of the cervix has no symptoms, the disease later causes:
* Irregular bleeding.
* Unusual vaginal discharge.
* Pain, though this is unusual unless the cancer has spread inside the pelvis.

Treatment, at an early stage, is an outpatient procedure. The diseased part of the cervix is treated with cryotherapy (freezing) or surgical removal, and this usually cures the problem. Advanced disease requires extensive surgery and radiotherapy. All sexually active women should have regular smears — at least every three years. Annual smears are recommended for women who have had a previously abnormal smear, or who have the wart virus (human papilloma virus — HPV), or herpes virus, present on the cervix, or who have greater risk factors: many partners, sexually transmitted disease, smokers.

■ CANCER OF THE WOMB
Many older women with irregular bleeding are offered a "D&C", meaning dilatation and curettage. This simple operation, sometimes called a scrape, involves removal of part of the womb's lining: the object is to relieve symptoms and to provide cell material for analysis. The analysis may detect cancer cells as a cause of the bleeding. For details *see page 353.*

■ INFLAMMATION OF THE VAGINA
Through infection or, in post-menopausal women, when vaginal skin becomes thin and raw.
* Dry vagina.
* Itch.
* Thin, watery, blood-stained discharge.

Treatment aims to eradicate the infection, and put female hormones back into the walls of the vagina, with estrogen cream or hormone replacement therapy (HRT).

RARE

■ URETHRAL CARUNCLE
An outgrowth at the outlet from the bladder, causing pain and bleeding. *See page 353.*

DELAY IN BEGINNING MENSTRUATION

By the age of 16, most Western girls are menstruating, and it is reasonable to be concerned about those who are not.

PROBABLE
NORMAL BUT DELAYED

POSSIBLE
HORMONE DISORDERS
ANOREXIA NERVOSA

RARE
OBSTRUCTION TO MENSTRUAL FLOW
GENETIC DISORDERS OR CONGENITAL MALFORMATION

PROBABLE

■ NORMAL BUT DELAYED
This is likely if there is:
* Normal development of breasts, pubic and underarm hair.
* Normal growth.
* Family history of menstruation starting late.

In addition, hormone blood tests would be normal. In these circumstances, it is a matter of "wait and see", sometimes using hormone treatment to "jump-start" the system.

POSSIBLE

■ HORMONE DISORDERS
Suggested if the girl has the following symptoms:
* Short stature.
* Poor development of breasts.
* Either an absence or an excess of body hair.
* Obesity.

* Very severe acne.

Investigation of the girl's hormones, and treatment with hormones, may be needed.

■ ANOREXIA NERVOSA
See page 423.

RARE

■ OBSTRUCTION TO MENSTRUAL FLOW
A membrane across the vagina can block the discharge of normal menstrual blood.
* Normal sexual development.
* Recurrent, lower abdominal pain.
* A bulge may protrude from the vagina, containing menstrual blood.

Treatment is simply the removal of the membrane.

■ GENETIC DISORDERS OR CONGENITAL MALFORMATION
There is a wide range of disorders which can lead to malformation of the womb, ovaries and vagina, or even a complete absence of these organs. There are no characteristic symptoms; it is a matter of specialist assessment after other causes have been excluded.

HEAVY MENSTRUAL PERIODS

Just what constitutes a heavy menstrual period is a highly individual matter, but a reasonable definition would be periods which:
* Involve flooding.
* Last for more than seven days each month.
* Produce clots of blood.
* Cause anemia, with weakness, tiredness, pallor.

Blood loss which is significantly heavier than you would expect is worth discussing with your physician.

PROBABLE
DYSFUNCTIONAL BLEEDING

POSSIBLE
ENDOMETRIOSIS
FIBROIDS
PELVIC INFECTION
MISCARRIAGE

RARE
THYROID DISEASE
ABNORMAL BLOOD CLOTTING
TUMORS OF THE CERVIX AND WOMB

PROBABLE

■ DYSFUNCTIONAL BLEEDING
A medical way of saying "we don't think there is anything very wrong; this is a time when, for one reason or another, your bleeding pattern is disturbed." This diagnosis should only be made when serious causes and other possibilities have been

investigated and no abnormality found. It is the commonest diagnosis in young women, less so in older women, where other causes are more likely. Treatment is with various combinations of hormones, and it can be expected to settle with time. Emotional upset may play a part for some women.

POSSIBLE

■ ENDOMETRIOSIS
A puzzling disease, in which tissue that is an entirely normal part of the womb grows outside the womb. Frequently-affected sites are the ovaries and the lining of the belly. The cause is unknown, though there are many theories. Whatever the cause, it is a disease that brings much misery and heartache.
* Commonest in women who are in their 20s to 40s.
* Menstruation may be heavy, painful, or irregular.
* Difficulty in conceiving.
* Deep pain on intercourse.
* Sometimes abdominal pain and bladder symptoms.

Treatment involves hormones, destruction of localized deposits of endometriosis, or — as a last resort — hysterectomy.

■ FIBROIDS
The womb has walls of powerful muscle; fibroids are overgrowths of muscle fibres, which form swellings in the wall of the womb. They can be tiny or large (five pounds); they are not cancerous.
* Commonest between 30 to 55 years of age, especially in women who have not borne children.
* Heavy, sometimes irregular, menstruation.
* Swelling of lower abdomen, if the fibroids are very large.
* Occasionally, sudden pain (if a fibroid becomes inflamed).

Fibroids are easy to diagnose and can then be safely watched by the physician unless causing problems. Single fibroids can sometimes be cut out, but usually the only effective treatment if fibroids are very troublesome is a hysterectomy.

■ PELVIC INFECTION
A wide range of infections can smoulder within the womb and Fallopian tubes. Risk factors are:
* Having intercourse with many partners.
* Previous, acute pelvic infections, with pain, fever and vaginal discharge.
* Deep pain on intercourse.
* Irregular menstruation.
* Infertility.
* Presence of an intra-uterine contraceptive device (IUCD).

Prolonged, intensive antibiotic therapy is often necessary.

■ MISCARRIAGE
It is thought that as many as one in eight pregnancies miscarries. Heavy bleeding or a "late period" may be a miscarriage.

Sudden, severe bleeding in any woman of childbearing years raises the possibility of pregnancy and its complications — regardless of contraception, moral rectitude or denial, as every physician knows to their dismay. A negative

pregnancy test does not exclude the diagnosis.
* A period may or may not have been missed.
* Other symptoms of pregnancy, such as nausea, tender breasts.
* Lower abdominal pain.
* Heavy bleeding.
* Passage of jelly-like material.

A reliable diagnosis can usually be obtained by having an ultrasound scan of the womb and Fallopian tubes.

RARE

■ THYROID DISEASE
Both overactive and underactive glands are associated with heavy periods. *See also HOT FLASHES, page 328, and MASCULINE CHANGES, page 329.*

■ ABNORMAL BLOOD CLOTTING
Heavy menstrual flow may result from any condition which makes the blood clot less well than it should. Also look for:
* Easy bruising.
* Gums which bleed easily.
* Look pale.
* Enlarged lymph glands.
* Blood in urine, vomit or from bowels.

■ TUMORS OF THE CERVIX AND WOMB
Though heavy periods are a possible symptom, these diseases are more likely to cause:
* Irregular bleeding.
* Unusual discharges.
* Post-menopausal bleeding, especially cancer of the womb.

Routine evaluation of heavy menstruation will discover these tumors. *See also page 353.*

IRREGULAR MENSTRUAL PERIODS

Common at the beginning and end of a woman's reproductive life. This must be distinguished from intermenstrual bleeding which is more serious. *See ABSENT OR INFREQUENT MENSTRUAL PERIODS, page 343.*

PROBABLE
DYSFUNCTIONAL BLEEDING

POSSIBLE
PRE-MENOPAUSE
POST-MENOPAUSE

PROBABLE

■ DYSFUNCTIONAL BLEEDING
See page 348.

Irregularity in the mechanism of menstrual control is particularly common in teenage girls. Most women experience at least one episode of dysfunctional bleeding at some time in their life. It needs investigation if symptoms are at all troublesome or severe. Again, it is very important to distinguish between irregular periods and either heavy periods *(see page 348)* or bleeding between periods or

after intercourse *(see page 345)*.
See also DELAY IN BEGINNING MENSTRUATION, page 347.

POSSIBLE

■ PRE-MENOPAUSE
While irregular menstrual periods are common, medical advice is needed if you notice:
* Bleeding between periods.
* Bleeding after intercourse.
* Heavy, painful menstruation.

As there is often doubt about the health of the womb, an endometrial biopsy is often done.

■ POST-MENOPAUSE
All bleeding after the menopause, or after one year without menstruation, must be investigated. Never ignore bleeding after the menopause. Always check with your physician since this can be due to serious, but treatable, disease. Early treatment is important. Don't delay.

See also BLEEDING AFTER THE MENOPAUSE, page 352.

PAINFUL MENSTRUAL PERIODS

Fortunate is the woman who has never experienced pain with her menstrual periods. However, levels of pain vary widely, as does the amount which different women will tolerate. Pain can certainly be regarded as a problem when time is regularly lost from work, or when menstruation is accompanied by debilitating cramps, faintness and vomiting. In older women, these symptoms should be investigated, particularly if previously acceptable periods become intolerable, and are accompanied by pain on intercourse or heavy bleeding.

However, it is often the case that no disease is found.

PROBABLE
UNKNOWN CAUSE

POSSIBLE
ENDOMETRIOSIS
FIBROIDS
PELVIC INFLAMMATORY DISEASE

RARE
ABNORMAL SHEDDING OF THE WOMB LINING

THE REPRODUCTIVE AND SEXUAL ORGANS

PROBABLE

■ UNKNOWN CAUSE
Painful menstrual periods are common in young women for the first few years of menstruation. They are thought to be caused by painful contractions of the womb during menstruation.
* Pain begins 12-24 hours before menstruation.
* Continues for first one to two days of period.
* Pain frequently felt in upper legs and back.

Medications related to aspirin are extremely helpful in relieving symptoms. One particular drug called mefenamic acid is increasingly used and can be very effective. The contraceptive pill can be useful for cases resistant to these drugs. The problem is sometimes relieved after a first pregnancy.

POSSIBLE

■ ENDOMETRIOSIS
Suggested by a combination of:
* Pain for several days before menstruation.
* Heavy menstruation.
* Deep pain on intercourse.
* Infertility.

This is a fairly common condition. *See also page 349.*

■ FIBROIDS
Benign muscular growths in the wall of the womb, also responsible for heavy menstruation.
See page 349.

■ PELVIC INFLAMMATORY DISEASE (PID)
Painful periods are one part of a picture which may include:
* Recurrent lower abdominal pain.
* Heavy menstruation.
* Deep pain on intercourse.
* Symptoms of infection.

It is especially important to catch this condition early, and treat it quickly. Otherwise, it may lead to infertility. *See the section on PELVIC INFECTION, page 349.*

RARE

■ ABNORMAL SHEDDING OF THE WOMB LINING
During menstruation, the lining of the womb is shed in many small pieces. But in this condition, called membranous dysmenorrhea, the whole lining is lost in a few large pieces.
* Very severe abdominal pain.
* Passage of fleshy material.

This can happen once, or on a regular basis, in which case hormonal treatment is given.

BLEEDING AFTER THE MENOPAUSE

Bleeding more than a year after menstrual periods have apparently finished. This is a very important symptom, which should not be ignored, even if it happens only once, or if the blood looks pink rather than the usual full red.

There can easily be confusion with bleeding in urine, or from the rectum, so be prepared for your physician to examine those regions, too.

PROBABLE
THIN VAGINAL SKIN
POLYP

POSSIBLE
CANCER OF THE WOMB
CANCER OF THE CERVIX

RARE
URETHRAL CARUNCLE

PROBABLE

■ THIN VAGINAL SKIN
An effect of low estrogen levels.
* Vagina feels dry.
* A pink discharge is more common than outright blood.
* Skin feels sore.

Treatment is with estrogen cream or medication.

■ POLYP
A fleshy outgrowth from the cervix, which oozes blood.
* Intermittent, fresh blood.
* Possibly a heavy or offensive discharge.

A polyp can be seen on examination, but always needs to be biopsied to ensure that it is benign.

POSSIBLE

■ CANCER OF THE WOMB
There is no escaping the fact that this disease is a possibility. Unless the tumor is advanced, when pain arises, there will be no symptoms other than bleeding.

Diagnosis is made by sampling the lining of the womb, and treatment is hysterectomy plus radiotherapy of the pelvis. If it is caught early, the outlook is positive, but advanced cancer has a poor outlook, underlining the need to report post-menopausal bleeding as soon as possible.

■ CANCER OF THE CERVIX
* Possibly bleeding after intercourse, as well as at other times.
* Possibly an offensive discharge.

Diagnosed by examination plus cervical smear. Treatment depends on the size of the tumor, varying from a local removal, to removal of the womb and all surrounding tissues.

RARE

■ URETHRAL CARUNCLE
An oddity in which the outlet from the bladder, the urethra lying just in front of the vagina, becomes swollen and inflamed.
* Painful to touch.
* Pain on intercourse.
* Pain when passing urine.

The inflamed area is easily removed.

PRE-MENSTRUAL TENSION

Feelings of tension and stress are are just two from a group of physical and emotional changes, which appear up to two weeks before menstruation and which go soon after bleeding begins. Among the many possible symptoms, the commonest are:

* Feeling bloated.
* Irritability.
* Tiredness.
* Headache.
* Tender breasts.
* Depression.

No one reason satisfactorily explains the symptoms, nor is there any agreed treatment. However, women report benefit from many different remedies. The most promising are:

Vitamin B6: taken pre-menstrually, this undoubtedly helps some women.

Diuretics ("water pills"): increase the output of urine and so relieve bloating.

Herbal and alternative remedies: many different substances are for sale. Price is no indication of their likely efficacy. Physicians are sceptical of their benefits. It is usually worth trying conventional treatments first.

Hormonal preparations: physicians may advise a trial, either of progesterone (a female hormone), to be taken pre-menstrually, or the contraceptive pill. Both may possibly decrease pre-menstrual symptoms.

Beta-blockers: these drugs, originally introduced for control of blood pressure, can sometimes help to decrease physical symptoms of tension and irritability.

Some women find that simply knowing that they have a real condition, albeit one which medicine is relatively ignorant about, enables them and their families to adjust to their swings of mood.

FEMALE REPRODUCTIVE SYSTEM: THE VAGINA

BLEEDING FROM THE VAGINA

This topic refers to bleeding which is unexpected. Menstrual problems are dealt with under specific headings.

PROBABLE
MISCARRIAGE
ECTOPIC PREGNANCY

POSSIBLE
COMPLICATIONS LATE IN PREGNANCY
DISEASE OF THE CERVIX
DISEASE OF THE WOMB
ATROPHIC VAGINITIS

RARE
DISORDERS OF BLOOD CLOTTING

PROBABLE

■ MISCARRIAGE
It cannot be repeated too often that pregnancy is a possibility for any woman of childbearing years who experiences unusual vaginal bleeding. The chances are increased in the presence of:
* A missed period.
* Tender breasts, morning sickness.
* Lower abdominal pain.

There is often great difficulty in deciding between a miscarriage and an ectopic pregnancy (*see below*). Miscarriages up to the twelfth week after conception happen in as many as one in eight pregnancies, and possibly more often.

■ ECTOPIC PREGNANCY
Occurs if a fertilized egg implants not within the womb, but somewhere else, usually inside a Fallopian tube. The egg can only grow a little before its size starts to swell the tube, causing:
* Severe, one-sided lower abdominal pain (not always present).
* Bleeding.
* Faintness, if internal bleeding is severe.
* These may occur in women using an IUCD.

This is a life-threatening emergency. Urgent removal of the egg and tube is needed. Later fertility can be affected.

POSSIBLE

■ COMPLICATIONS LATE IN PREGNANCY
In an established pregnancy, bleeding suggests a possible abnormality of the placenta. Painless bleeding happens if the placenta is lying too low in the womb (termed *placenta previa*). Painful bleeding, especially after 26 weeks, may mean that part of the placenta has detached from the womb (abruption). In either case, a full and urgent obstetric assessment is essential.

■ DISEASE OF THE CERVIX
A possibility if the symptoms include any of the following, each of which is dealt with under specific headings:
* Heavy vaginal discharge.
* Irregular bleeding.
* Bleeding after intercourse.

See page 345.

■ DISEASE OF THE WOMB
This is the likeliest cause of vaginal bleeding after menopause, an extremely important symptom.
See page 353.

■ ATROPHIC VAGINITIS
A thin, watery, bloody discharge.
See THIN VAGINAL SKIN, page 353.

RARE

■ DISORDERS OF BLOOD CLOTTING
As well as bleeding from the vagina, there will probably be:

* Easy bruising.
* Blood from bowels, in urine.

See also pages 426-7.

DISCHARGE FROM THE VAGINA

Normal discharge from the vagina is clear, or slightly yellow. It varies in volume and consistency during the monthly cycle, reaching a peak at the time of ovulation, which is roughly mid-cycle. If you have an IUCD fitted, the amount of discharge may increase. Any change in the amount, consistency or smell of the discharge from what you would normally expect can be considered abnormal.

PROBABLE
THRUSH/YEAST
CERVICAL EROSION

POSSIBLE
ATROPHIC VAGINITIS
CERVICAL POLYP
VAGINAL INFECTION
PELVIC INFECTION
FOREIGN BODY

RARE
GONORRHEA
TUMOR
SEXUAL ABUSE

PROBABLE

■ THRUSH/YEAST
The commonest cause of discharge is a yeast infection. It is not something you "catch" from your partner: it occurs as the normal balance of the various vaginal constituents is disturbed, allowing the yeast to grow until it gives rise to symptoms. It is possible for your partner to develop some symptoms on his penis as a result of contact with the yeast. Both partners should be treated at the same time.
* Itchy, white discharge.
* Curd-like deposits, visible on the walls of the vagina.

The risk increases after a course of antibiotics. There is a wide range of treatments, including creams, vaginal tablets and medication by mouth. For some women, thrush can be a regular problem. Any woman with frequent attacks should have a urine test for diabetes, a disease which predisposes to yeast infection.

■ CERVICAL EROSION
A cause of persistent, heavy, usually clear discharge. *See page 346.*

POSSIBLE

■ ATROPHIC VAGINITIS
Mainly a post-menopausal condition.
* Watery, possibly blood-tinged discharge.

See THIN VAGINAL SKIN, page 353.

■ CERVICAL POLYP
These fleshy outgrowths may also cause a persistent, heavy sometimes bloody discharge. *See POLYP, page 353.*

■ VAGINAL INFECTION
Apart from thrush, three other infections are commonly caused by these organisms:
Trichomonas: a greenish, frothy discharge.
Gardenerella: a grey discharge, with a fishy smell.
Chlamydia: a recurrent discharge. Your partner may have had a penile discharge, termed non-specific urethritis.
There are specific antibiotic treatments for each of these.
Chlamydia, in particular, can lead to pelvic infection and infertility, making it especially important to diagnose. It requires special tests to make a diagnosis for chlamydia.
For all these infections, both partners should be treated.

■ PELVIC INFECTION
See page 349.
An acute pelvic infection causes:
* Heavy, yellow or green vaginal discharge.
* Severe pelvic pain.
* Fever, sickness.
Aggressive treatment aims to reduce any internal damage which might lead to infertility.

■ FOREIGN BODY
Probably the commonest is a tampon lodged deep inside the vagina. Young children sometimes push small toys inside themselves.
* Yellow or green discharge, increasingly heavy.
* Bad smelling.
* Possibly fever.
Tampons and the like are easily removed; children may need a specialist's help.

RARE

■ GONORRHEA
Unfortunately, this venereal disease causes only slight symptoms in women, so that cases are often detected by tracing the contacts of men who have had this diagnosis confirmed.
* A slight increase in discharge.
* Possibly persistent burning on passing urine.
* Possibly a yellow discharge.
Gonorrhea can progress to pelvic infection with pain, profuse discharge and fever. It can cause infertility.

■ TUMOR
Growths in and around the vagina may be a rare cause of a persistent discharge, but should be visible on pelvic examination.

■ SEXUAL ABUSE
This upsetting possibility needs to be considered for girls who have recurrent or unusual vaginal discharges. Signs of sexual interference might include:
* Tears, bruising around vagina or anus.
* Disturbed behaviour.
The possibility of abuse needs the utmost care, both to avoid false conclusions and yet to uncover hidden misery. If suspected, the case should be evaluated by

professionals who are trained to assess this problem.

VAGINAL PROTRUSION

Often called a prolapse of the womb, caused by weakening of the muscles around the vagina. Part of the womb "drops" down into the vagina.

PROBABLE
PROLAPSE OF THE WOMB

POSSIBLE
PROLAPSE OF THE BLADDER OR RECTUM

RARE
TUMOR

PROBABLE

■ PROLAPSE OF THE WOMB
* A firm lump, felt to be central in the vagina.
* Worse on coughing, straining.
* Improves on lying flat or relaxing.
Surgical repair is possible.

POSSIBLE

■ PROLAPSE OF THE BLADDER OR RECTUM
* Bladder prolapse is felt in the front of the vagina.
* Usually causes leakage of urine on coughing, laughing.
* Rectal prolapse is felt at the back of the vagina.
Surgical repair is possible.

RARE

■ TUMOR
The growth could arise from the womb, or the walls of the vagina; pelvic examination will pinpoint this.

VAGINAL ODOR

PROBABLE
NORMAL

POSSIBLE
INFECTION
RETAINED FOREIGN BODY
PSYCHOLOGICAL

RARE
CANCER

PROBABLE

■ NORMAL
* Some vaginal odor is normal.

POSSIBLE

■ INFECTION
See page 357. Suggested by odors which are:
* Very bad smelling or fishy.

* Accompanied by itch and discharge.

■ RETAINED FOREIGN BODY
It is not unusual for a forgotten tampon to cause a foul-smelling discharge.
* Brown discharge.
* Unpleasant odor.
* No pain or symptoms of illness.

Other possible causes are contraceptive sponges or condoms which have been left in the vagina in error. Physicians or nurses can remove these easily if you have difficulty.

■ PSYCHOLOGICAL
* An odor, but your partner or physician smell nothing unusual.
* A worry that the odor is obvious to others.

A sympathetic ear may allow concerns and fears to be expressed, typically about cancer of the womb.

RARE

■ CANCER
Cancer of the cervix, womb, or even of the bowel, may cause:
* A persistent, foul-smelling vaginal discharge.
* Bleeding.
* Pain.

Things should not reach this stage unless warning symptoms have been neglected, such as unusual vaginal bleeding, discharges and changes of bowel habit.

VAGINAL PAIN

The causes overlap with those symptoms described under *PAINFUL SEXUAL INTERCOURSE, page 334.*

PROBABLE
INFECTIONS
ATROPHY OF VAGINAL SKIN

POSSIBLE
VAGINISMUS

RARE
CANCER

PROBABLE

■ INFECTIONS
Any vaginal infection will cause soreness, plus:
* Itch.
* Discharge.
* Vaginal odour.

Sometimes herpes will cause vaginal pain.

See page 357.

■ ATROPHY
In post-menopausal women, discomfort is due to thinning of the skin of the vagina, which becomes sore. This is easily remedied by estrogen creams or hormone replacement therapy (HRT).

See THIN VAGINAL SKIN, page 353.

POSSIBLE

■ <u>VAGINISMUS</u>
Spasm of the muscles around the vagina. The effect is pain, which prevents intercourse. It has a psychological cause: *see VAGINAL SPASM, page 335.*

RARE

■ <u>CANCER</u>
Cancer growing within the vagina can cause pain, but it is highly unlikely to be an early or only symptom. Previously there is likely to have been:
* Bleeding after intercourse.
* Discharge.

See also pages 345 and under CANCER OF THE CERVIX, page 353.

VULVAL ITCH

PROBABLE
INFECTION

POSSIBLE
ALLERGY
PINWORMS/CRAB LICE
ECZEMA OR PSORIASIS

RARE
LEUKOPLAKIA
CANCER
GENERAL DISEASE

PROBABLE

■ <u>INFECTION</u>
* Rapid onset of intense itch.
* White or colored discharge.

The appearance of the associated discharge is usually diagnostic, for example, yeast, trichomonas (*see VAGINAL DISCHARGE, page 356*). If yeast infection is recurrent, diabetes may be a possibility and should be tested for.

POSSIBLE

■ <u>ALLERGY</u>
The sensitive skin in and around the vagina may itch because of allergy to over-vigorous douching, bubble baths, vaginal deodorants or condoms. Diagnosis is arrived at by eliminating all possible irritants, and then testing each one individually. Special low-allergy condoms are available.

■ <u>PINWORMS/CRAB LICE</u>
Pinworms are extremely common, particularly in childhood.
* Intense itch.
* Especially at night.
* Itching around the anus.

Worms or lice will be visible on careful inspection. Treatment will clear the problem.

■ <u>ECZEMA/PSORIASIS</u>
Common skin disorders, causing:
* Dry flaking areas.
* Psoriasis spreads around anus.
* Usually skin elsewhere is affected.

RARE

■ LEUKOPLAKIA
* Whitish, cracked skin.
* Spreads around anal area.
* Commonest in the elderly.
As this may progress to skin cancer, biopsy and medical follow-up is usual.

■ CANCER
Skin cancer may present the following symptoms:
* An itchy sore.
* Grows slowly.
* Bleeds.
Treatment is usually curative, but the earlier the diagnosis the better.

■ GENERAL DISEASE
Several disorders may cause generalized itch. Specific features might include:
* Swollen lymph glands.
* Jaundice.
* Changes in volume of urine produced.
* Widespread skin involvement.
* Joint pains.
See also ITCHING — WITHOUT A RASH, page 259.

FEMINIZATION

Adult men who start to develop female features need a full hormonal assessment. Female features include loss of body hair, development of breasts, loss of sexual drive, and shrinking testicles.

THE REPRODUCTIVE AND SEXUAL ORGANS

PROBABLE
MEDICATION EFFECTS

POSSIBLE
GENETIC PROBLEMS
ALCOHOLISM

RARE
TUMORS

PROBABLE

■ MEDICATION EFFECTS
Common offenders are cimetidine, used for treating peptic ulcers; estrogens for treating cancer of the prostate; spironolactone and digoxin in heart disease.

POSSIBLE

■ GENETIC PROBLEMS
* Unusually tall individuals.
* Infertile.

■ ALCOHOLISM
* Impotence.
* Breast development.
* Decreased fertility due to diminished sperm count.

RARE

■ TUMORS
If the above causes are excluded, it is essential to search for cancers in

the testicles, lungs or elsewhere, which may be secreting female hormones. Possible symptoms include:
* Lump in or on a testicle.
* Coughing blood, chest pains, weight loss.

PAIN IN THE CROTCH

PROBABLE
INJURY

POSSIBLE
PROSTATITIS

RARE
CANCER OF PROSTATE

PROBABLE

■ INJURY
Injury to the genital area and lower pelvis may irritate the prostate gland, causing:
* A dull ache in the groin, crotch or rectal area.
* Slight discomfort on passing urine.
* Blood in urine, if there has been a severe injury, such as falling astride a bicycle crossbar.

POSSIBLE

■ PROSTATITIS
Infection of the prostate gland causes:
* Pain.
* Fever, chills.
* Burning sensation when passing urine.
* Urine may appear cloudy.

This can be a difficult problem to eradicate, often needing long courses of antibiotics.

RARE

■ CANCER OF PROSTATE
An advanced cancer may produce the following:
* Ache or pain in the lower pelvis.
* Pain in back or pelvis because of spread to bones..

More usually, cancer of the prostate is painless, and is found on investigation after:
* Difficulty passing urine, caused by enlargement of the prostate, which obstructs the passage of urine.

Other symptoms of an enlarging prostate, not normally cancerous, include:
* Difficulty in starting to pass urine.
* Dribbling at the end of passing urine.
* Frequency of passing urine increases: typically, you starthaving to get up in the night.

BLOOD IN SEMEN

A fairly common symptom, which looks alarming but one which hardly ever has an underlying cause. In fact, the reason remains unknown for most cases.
* Commonest in elderly men.
* Blood may obviously be in the semen.
* May be mistaken for bleeding from the vagina after intercourse.

It is sensible to have your genitals examined, plus a urine check, to ensure that the blood does come from the bladder. Otherwise, nothing else needs to be done unless the symptom recurs, when an internal check of the bladder and prostate gland may be advisable.

IMPOTENCE

Impotence means difficulty in achieving, or maintaining, a firm erection or premature ejaculation. It is a common disorder, that is not easy for many men to discuss. Brief episodes of impotence accompany tiredness, and any serious, general ill-health. After ejaculation, there is loss of erection which takes longer and longer to recover with age, perhaps several hours by old age. Psychological factors are still the most likely reasons for impotence, but it is increasingly clear that medical causes are more common than once thought, especially problems with blood flow to the penis.

There is, accordingly, a great range of physical treatments now available at specialized centers, such as medications injected into the penis, and pump devices.

See also PREMATURE EJACULATION, page 366.

PROBABLE
PSYCHOLOGICAL

POSSIBLE
DIABETES MELLITUS
BLOOD FLOW PROBLEMS
MEDICATIONS
ALCOHOL
POST-OPERATIVE

RARE
NEUROLOGICAL DISEASE
HORMONE DISORDERS

PROBABLE

■ PSYCHOLOGICAL
Factors here include depression, problems between partners and, most especially, the vicious cycle of past impotence causing impotence again. Symptoms strongly suggestive of a psychological cause are:
* Normal erections during sleep or on waking.
* Ejaculation during sleep.
* Impotence with one particular partner.
* Sudden onset of impotence.

Therapy will include

explanation, exploration of psychological problems, and gradual return to sexual intercourse.

POSSIBLE

■ DIABETES MELLITUS
Diabetes affects the nerves and blood supply involved in erection. Undiagnosed diabetes may cause:
* Excessive passage of urine at night and during the day.
* Thirst.

■ BLOOD FLOW PROBLEMS
An erection is caused by engorgement of the penis's spongy tissues with blood. If the veins carrying this blood supply are leaking, inadequate erection may follow. Arterial disease can also affect the blood supply, both to the penis and to the nerves controlling erection.

Sophisticated tests of blood flow are available.

■ MEDICATIONS
Many medications used to treat high blood pressure may cause impotence, as do tranquillizers and some other medications.

■ ALCOHOL
Chronic alcoholism actually leads to hormonal and neurological changes that make permanent impotence a risk.

■ POST-OPERATIVE
Surgery to the bowel, and to the prostate gland, runs the risk of damaging the nerves involved in an erection.

RARE

■ NEUROLOGICAL DISEASE
Of these, the commonest is multiple sclerosis, giving rise to:
* Numbness in various parts ofthe body.
* Unsteady gait.
* Visual disturbances, transient blindness in one eye.
* Difficulty in controlling passage of urine.

Anything else damaging the lower spine may cause impotence.

■ HORMONE DISORDERS
A wide range of possibilities. A possible cause if the individual has:
* Absent or small testicles.
* Lack of body hair.
* Breasts.
* Unusually short or tall stature.
* Extreme obesity.

Hormone treatment may help such cases.

See also HORMONAL, page 480.

MALE INFERTILITY

Male problems account for about 25 percent of infertility cases where couples have been trying to conceive for a year or more without success (the conventional definition of infertility). An early sperm count is always advisable, looking for low numbers of sperm, or increased numbers of abnormal sperm. Obviously, normal sexual intercourse should be taking place at regular intervals. Temporary infertility can follow a severe illness, after which it takes a few months for sperm production to recover.

See also INFERTILITY (female), page 331.

PROBABLE
DAMAGE TO TESTICLES

POSSIBLE
MEDICATIONS
VARICOCELE
ALCOHOLISM
HORMONE DISORDERS

RARE
CHROMOSOME DISORDERS

PROBABLE

■ DAMAGE TO TESTICLES
The testicles may:
* Feel small.
* Be soft.

A number of different testicular problems may account for damage or impaired function. One example is undescended testicles, when the testicles may not be in the scrotum at birth and surgery is required to draw them down from the groin into the scrotal sac. Failure to do this at an early age, ideally before three years of age, can lead to impaired fertility later in life.

Torsion of the testicles, mumps, radiation and chemotherapy for cancer may all lead to a diminished sperm count.

Cigarette smoking, drinking, and high temperatures in the area of the scrotum can also decrease sperm production.

See also PAIN IN TESTICLES, page 372.

POSSIBLE

■ MEDICATIONS
Several medications reduce sperm production. The medications used to treat cancer in children may damage the testicles.

■ VARICOCELE
See page 373.

These soft masses in the scrotum, which are enlarged veins, may cause reduced sperm production.

THE REPRODUCTIVE AND SEXUAL ORGANS

■ ALCOHOLISM
See also IMPOTENCE, page 363.
Chronic drinking reduces sperm production.

■ HORMONE DISORDERS
See page 364.
A possibility if there is:
* Absent body hair.
* Development of breasts.

RARE

■ CHROMOSOME DISORDERS
* Unusual height.
* Enlarged breasts.
* Small or absent testicles.
* Absent body hair.
* Abnormally-formed penis.

PRECOCIOUS PUBERTY

Sexual development before the age of nine years is abnormal; that includes the appearance of body hair, enlarged penis, deepening voice. All cases are rare; all require urgent evaluation.

RARE
PITUITARY DISEASE
TESTICULAR TUMORS
ADRENAL DISEASE

RARE

■ PITUITARY DISEASE
This gland in the brain controls many hormones. A disorder is likeliest if:
* The boy was normal at birth, and during early childhood.
* Later, shows abnormal growth, either too short or too tall.

■ TESTICULAR TUMORS
* A lump may be felt.
* There may be a change or swelling in one testicle.

Blood tests may detect abnormally high levels of hormones in the blood.

■ ADRENAL DISEASE
Adrenal glands function abnormally, producing excess hormones. The glands, which lie over the kidneys, when affected, usually make a baby very ill within days of birth.

PREMATURE EJACULATION

This means ejaculation before the penis enters the vagina, or very soon after entry. While this is not a disease, it can be very troublesome for many men. Considerable time and patience are needed, as well as courage to explore the problem.

PROBABLE

■ PSYCHOLOGICAL FACTORS
Premature ejaculation is fairly common in young men, perhaps because of sexual inexperience. Psychological approaches encourage concentration on aspects of sexual behavior other than intercourse, for example stroking and massaging.

An aid to this is the "squeeze technique", when the partner, told that ejaculation is near, squeezes around the base of the penis for some seconds. This usually delays progress to orgasm without destroying the erection. Further information should be sought from professionals who specialize in sexual counseling.

CURVED PENIS

Known medically as chordee. Extreme curvature may prevent sexual intercourse.

PROBABLE
CONGENITAL

POSSIBLE
PEYRONIE'S DISEASE

RARE
INJURY

PROBABLE

■ CONGENITAL(BIRTH DEFECT)
* Noticed at birth.
* The opening for urine (external meatus) is underneath the penis, not at the end — medical term, hypospadias.

Delicate surgery to correct these abnormalities makes use of the foreskin, which should therefore not be circumcised.

POSSIBLE

■ PEYRONIE'S DISEASE
A band of firm tissue forms on part of the shaft of the penis. In the middle-aged, or older male.
* Pain and curvature on erection.
* A firm area felt on the shaft.

Treatment is difficult. Sometimes disappears spontaneously.

RARE

■ INJURY
Vigorous sexual intercourse or other injury may damage the erect penis. Needs early treatment.
* Sudden pain; bruising.

DISCHARGE FROM PENIS

Whether clear or colored, is highly suggestive of sexually transmitted disease, with non-specific urethritis and GONORRHEA, *both page 357*, the likeliest. Partner also likely to be infected. Requires urgent treatment.

DISEASED FORESKIN

The foreskin is subject to infection, resulting in cracking and scar tissue formation. It may cause pain, interfere with passing urine and make sexual intercourse difficult.

PROBABLE
BALANITIS
PHIMOSIS

POSSIBLE
PARAPHIMOSIS

RARE
CANCER OF THE PENIS

PROBABLE

■ BALANITIS
An infection of the foreskin and adjacent penis.
* Mild pain.
* Discharge around the foreskin, not from the opening of the penis itself.
* Itch.

Antibiotics and local cleaning are the treatment. Diabetes may be the cause of repeated attacks.

■ PHIMOSIS
In uncircumcised boys, inability to retract the foreskin over the tip of the penis. (In boys it is normal to be unable to retract the foreskin until the child is five years old and it is wrong to attempt to do so.) It may be abnormal if there is:
* Recurrent balanitis.
* Ballooning of the foreskin on passing urine.

Circumcision or stretching of the foreskin is then advisable.

POSSIBLE

■ PARAPHIMOSIS
* The foreskin becomes stuck, like a collar, rolled behind the tip of the penis.
* Pain.
* Swelling of tip of penis prevents unrolling of foreskin back over the tip of the penis.

This calls for rapid treatment to reduce swelling; sometimes the only remedy is surgical.

RARE

■ CANCER OF THE PENIS
It is unusual among circumcised men, the exact reason being unclear.
* Begins as a red area on tip of penis, or hidden within the foreskin.
* Grows, ulcerates.
* Discharge, pain, bleeding.

Treatment is radiotherapy and surgery.

PAINFUL PENIS

PROBABLE
INFECTION
DISEASE OF FORESKIN

POSSIBLE
STONE

RARE
PEYRONIE'S DISEASE

PROBABLE

■ INFECTION
* Pain, burning on passing urine.
* Need to urinate frequently.
* Possibly blood in urine.
* Urine cloudy.
* A discharge suggests sexually transmitted disease.

Infection, whether in a boy or adult, should always be investigated. There is usually an important cause.

■ DISEASE OF FORESKIN
* Tender, swollen foreskin.

See page 368.

POSSIBLE

■ STONE

See KIDNEY STONES, page 184.

* Pain radiating to tip of penis from groin, or from kidney region.
* Blood in urine.
* Nausea, sweating.

Stones can stick anywhere in the urinary tract, from the kidney to the tip of the penis. Strong painkillers make it possible to tolerate the severe pain, and some may even help get rid of the stone.

RARE

■ PEYRONIE'S DISEASE

See page 367.

* Pain and curvature of penis when erect.

PROLONGED ERECTION

Also known as priapism.
A very painful, prolonged erection in the absence of sexual desire. The tip of the penis remains soft. Whatever the cause, it needs urgent treatment to avoid long-term damage to the penis.

PROBABLE
CAUSE UNKNOWN

POSSIBLE
BLOOD DISORDERS

RARE
ALL OTHER CAUSES

PROBABLE

■ CAUSE UNKNOWN
Accounting for about three out of five cases: it may follow prolonged sexual activity.
* Otherwise sound health.

POSSIBLE

■ BLOOD DISORDERS
Blood tests to check for leukemia or sickle cell disease.
* Easy bruising, sickness, enlarged glands suggest leukemia.
* Recurrent joint, abdominal pains or lung problems suggest sickle cell disease.
See pages 419 and 487.

RARE

■ ALL OTHER CAUSES
A routine search is always made for growths in the pelvis, medications affecting erection, or damage to the spinal cord.

SMALL PENIS

An objective assessment of size is difficult because of variations at different temperatures, and degrees of erection. Worry about a small penis may be justified in the presence of some of the following features:
* Absent or small testicles.
* Absence of body hair.
* Excessive height.
* Breast development.
* Obesity.
* Previous injury, twisting of testicles.

In boys, a normal penis may appear very small if it is sunk in fat in the groin.

Investigations such as chromosome analysis, hormone profiles and brain scans may be needed. As treatment is possible for boys, cases of true micro-penis are worth reporting to a physician, sooner rather than later.

ABSENT TESTICLE

Absence may be discovered at routine child health checks.
* A testicle which is not brought down into the scrotum is at risk of decreased fertility and also at greater risk of cancer in later life.

PROBABLE
UNDESCENDED TESTICLE

POSSIBLE
RETRACTILE TESTICLE

RARE
ECTOPIC TESTICLE

PROBABLE

■ UNDESCENDED TESTICLE
* Normal general development.
* Testicle often felt as a lump in the groin.

Three to four percent of male babies have undescended testicles at birth. By the age of one, only 0.8 percent will still have the condition: the testicles tend to descend into the scrotum of their own accord.

Undescended testicles should be surgically brought down into the scrotum, ideally around the age of two and, if possible, before three years old. This helps to reduce the risk of future subfertility.

POSSIBLE

■ RETRACTILE TESTICLE
An exaggeration of a normal reflex, which pulls the testicles up into the groin.
* Testicle is present at certain times.
* Cold, and emotion, can cause retraction.

Usually no treatment is needed for this condition.

RARE

■ ECTOPIC TESTICLE
The testicle may lodge itself somewhere in the lower abdomen. It may be felt in the groin, at the base of the penis, or even the upper thigh. Surgical correction is recommended to preserve fertility.

LUMPS IN THE TESTICLE OR SCROTUM

A firm structure felt at the back of the testicles is the epididymis. Small lumps within the skin of the scrotum are common, being minor infections or yellow fat-filled cysts.

See also PAIN IN TESTICLES, page 372.

PROBABLE
VARICOCELE
EPIDIDYMAL CYST

POSSIBLE
CANCER OF TESTICLE

RARE
SYPHILIS
TUBERCULOSIS

PROBABLE

■ VARICOCELE
A harmless swelling caused by enlarged veins, "like a bag of worms", felt behind the testicle.
See also page 373.

■ EPIDIDYMAL CYST
Another harmless swelling, arising from the epididymis.
* Commonest in elderly men.
* Often, cysts on both sides of the scrotum.
* The swelling feels separate from the testicle.

Once confirmed, nothing need be done about a cyst unless it is causing discomfort.

POSSIBLE

■ CANCER OF THE TESTICLE
This is a rare cancer, but is the most common one to affect men between 15 and 40 years of age. Twice as many now develop it each year, compared with 25 years ago.

Just as women examine their breasts for lumps, men should check their testicles every month for any signs of changes.
* A lump in a testicle is cancer until proven otherwise.
* Feels hard.
* A feeling of heaviness.
* Often also a swollen scrotum.
* Pain is unusual.

The treatment depends on the precise kind of tumor, but carries a very positive outlook, particularly if any changes are found early.

Don't delay — report any changes in your testicles to your physician immediately.

RARE

■ SYPHILIS
* A slowly growing lump.
* Previous features of syphilis; *see page 324.*

■ TUBERCULOSIS
Increasingly common:
* A painless lump.
* May discharge like an abscess, but without throbbing.
* Other features of tuberculosis, such as cough, sickness, sweats, weight loss.

PAIN IN TESTICLES

In boys and young men, pain equals torsion (*see below*) until proved otherwise. In adults there is a wider range of possible diagnoses.

PROBABLE
EPIDIDYMITIS
TORSION
INJURY

POSSIBLE
VARICOCELE
STONE
HERNIA

RARE
MUMPS ORCHITIS
PANCREATITIS

PROBABLE

■ EPIDIDYMITIS
The epididymis is a structure involved in the transport of sperm from the testicles, and can normally be felt at the back of the testicle. Inflammation usually occurs for no obvious reason, but if there is also a discharge from the penis, a physician must test for sexually transmitted disease and non-specific urethritis (NSU).

Epididymitis is unlikely in a boy before puberty. Torsion is far more likely.
* Pain, initially behind testicle, builds up over a few hours.
* Swelling of testicle and scrotum which are very sore.
* Fever, nausea.

Antibiotic treatment is needed, plus rest, for a couple of weeks.

■ TORSION
The testicles hang on a cord which can twist. Other structures near the testicles can also twist, giving a similar condition. Deciding which has happened can only be done during surgery.
* Sudden, severe pain in one testicle.
* Nausea, vomiting.
* Affected testicle swells and is tender.

An urgent operation is nearly always needed to untwist the testicle, and to anchor it into place to prevent recurrence. It is usual to operate on the other testicle also: if one has twisted, the other is likely to do so in the future. Neglected torsion will inevitably lead to death of the affected testicle, with future effects on fertility.

■ INJURY
* A definite history of injury to the scrotum, such as a kick in the crotch.
* Often bruising or swelling.
* Modest pain and tenderness.
* Normal urinary stream and no blood.

Support, painkillers and time to heal are the only treatment.

POSSIBLE

■ VARICOCELE
Rather like a varicose vein, this is a sheath of enlarged veins, felt at the back of the testicle.
* Increasingly common with age.
* You notice an ache, not pain.
* Aching slowly increases over months.

No treatment is needed unless the varicocele is affecting fertility, or the pain is too uncomfortable.

■ STONE
A stone in the urinary system gives rise to:
* Pain of rapid onset, lasting an hour or so.
* Pains recur over days and weeks.
* Appears to radiate from the low back (kidney region) to the testicles, or to the tip of the penis.
* Nausea, vomiting.
* Blood in urine.

Often a stone will pass; if it sticks, surgical removal is needed.

■ HERNIA
See INGUINAL HERNIA, page 325.
This frequently gives an ache, felt generally around the scrotum or testicles.

RARE

■ MUMPS ORCHITIS
Mumps is an increasingly rare disease which in a very few cases gives rise to inflammation of the testicles, called orchitis.
* Mumps causes swellings, like chipmunk cheeks, just in front of the jaw joint.

* After three to four days, one or both testicles may swell.
* Fever, pain.

The risk of orchitis is much less than once thought. Although sterility may follow, it appears that this, too, is much less of a risk than was once feared.

■ PANCREATITIS

See page 149.

SMALL TESTICLE

Testicles vary slightly in size and the left testicle usually hangs lower than the right one. Alcoholism, and medications used in treating cancer of the prostate, may cause previously normal testicles to decrease in size.

PROBABLE
PREVIOUS INJURY OR INFECTION

POSSIBLE
HORMONE DISORDERS

RARE
GENETIC DISORDERS

PROBABLE

■ PREVIOUS INJURY OR INFECTION

Likely if:
* Only one testicle is small.
* Previous pain.
* Previous swelling.

Possible causes include twisted testicle and orchitis. *See PAIN IN TESTICLES, pages 372-4.*

POSSIBLE

■ HORMONE DISORDERS
* Both testicles are small.
* Individual is often very tall.
* Absent or decreased body hair.
* Breast development.
* Infertility.

Hormone blood tests are needed to diagnose the exact cause.

RARE

■ GENETIC DISORDERS

Often there is uncertain sexual development.
* Testicles and penis may be abnormally formed.
* Man is likely to be abnormally tall or short.
* Infertility.

SWOLLEN TESTICLE OR SCROTUM

This means swelling without any obvious lump. For lumps in the testicle or scrotum, see the appropriate section. Swellings may be due to an underlying cancer, and should always be medically examined.

Don't delay in reporting to your physician any changes you notice in your testicles — early treatment has a very significant effect on getting a full cure.

PROBABLE
HYDROCELE
ORCHITIS

POSSIBLE
HERNIA
ECZEMA

RARE
FILARIASIS

PROBABLE

■ HYDROCELE
An accumulation of fluid around the testicle.
* Tense, swollen testicle.
* Pain may or may not be present.
* If chronic, can be very large.
* In children, often accompanies a hernia.
* Not uncommon at or soon after birth.

Specialist opinion should be sought, since there may be an underlying cause such as infection or cancer of the testicle. May need surgery.

■ ORCHITIS
A general term for a swollen, inflamed testicle.
* Pain builds up over a few hours.
* Scrotum usually also swells with fluid.

Underlying causes include injury, infection and mumps. *See MUMPS ORCHITIS, page 373.*

An acutely painful testicle may be twisted, with a risk of future sterility. Medical attention is essential, especially for children.

POSSIBLE

■ HERNIA
When the bowel bulges through a weakness in the wall of the abdomen.
* Usually just a lump in the groin.
* In children, commonly extends into the scrotum, which appears to be swollen.
* Less common in adults.
* Swelling may disappear after lying flat.

See page 325.

■ ECZEMA
Chronic skin irritation often with secondary infection will give a swollen, leathery-looking testicle. May also be associated with yeast infection. Needs medical attention.

RARE

■ FILARIASIS
A parasite which blocks the drainage of tissue fluids, leading to swelling of the affected region.
* A disease of the Far East.
* Repeated inflammation of the testicles, epididymis.
* After several infections, the scrotum remains permanently swollen.

Advanced disease needs surgical treatment.

The Brain and Nervous System

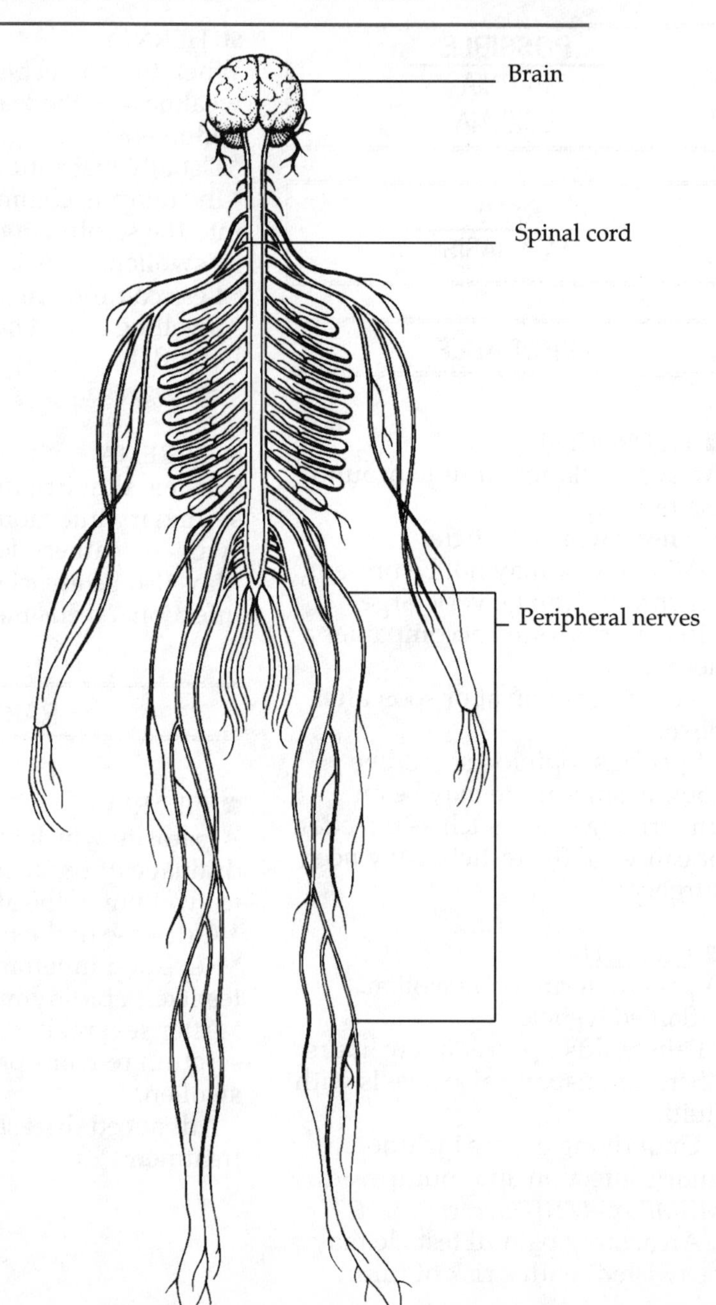

The Brain and Nervous System

Symptoms in this section are arranged alphabetically.

ANXIETY

Anxiety can be defined as a state of concern and fear. Mild degrees of anxiety are normal and increase the individual's readiness to deal with problems of life.

Anxiety becomes abnormal when it is out of proportion to the situation or when one problem or event becomes the focus of severe concern and starts to interfere with daily life *(see OBSESSIONS AND PHOBIAS)*. The symptoms are multiple and include:

* A feeling of tension mingled with apprehension.
* Headache.
* Sweating: hands, armpits and forehead are particularly affected.
* Palpitations.
* Dry mouth.
* Tremor.

But many other symptoms occur, too, such as overbreathing, impotence, diarrhea, dizziness, restlessness.

PROBABLE
ANXIETY STATE

POSSIBLE
OTHER PSYCHOLOGICAL DISEASE
OVER-ACTIVE THYROID GLAND
DRUG AND ALCOHOL EFFECTS

RARE
LOW BLOOD SUGAR
PHEOCHROMOCYTOMA

PROBABLE

■ ANXIETY STATE
Worry comes naturally to human beings, more naturally to some than to others; heredity plays a part. Every society has its own anxieties: the problem of choosing perfectly matched table decorations does not, on the face of it, compare with the fear of being mugged. But who are we to judge? Childhood experiences, repressed sexual urges, the stresses of modern society: all are theoretically reasonable explanations for anxiety.

Diagnosing anxiety is usually straightforward, based on the symptoms given above; sympathetic discussion will usually reveal an underlying cause of stress. Physical symptoms as alarming as breathlessness may need a medical check-up before a person can accept that the symptom is psychological in origin. Treatment includes medications, counseling and psychotherapy.

POSSIBLE

■ OTHER PSYCHOLOGICAL DISEASE
Possible when anxiety:
* Appears in a previously stable personality.

THE BRAIN AND NERVOUS SYSTEM

* No obvious source of stress.
* Other disturbance of mood, thought, or concentration.

Possibilities which are dealt with separately, and should be followed up, include *DEPRESSION, DEMENTIA* and *SCHIZOPHRENIA* *(the latter on page 386)*.

■ OVER-ACTIVE THYROID GLAND
Gives all the symptoms of anxiety, but there are suggestive additional features:
* Fine trembling of hands.
* Weight loss.
* Increased appetite.
* Intolerance of heat.
* Rapid pulse.
* Bulging eyes.
* Swelling in neck.

Where there is doubt, a blood test will help to confirm diagnosis.

■ DRUG AND ALCOHOL EFFECTS
Withdrawal of many abused drugs and of alcohol may cause:
* Shaking.
* Anxiety.
* Sweating.

There may be other features of drug abuse such as:
* Neglected appearance.
* Hallucinations.
* Needle marks on limbs.

Specialized clinics are available to help with these problems.

RARE

■ LOW BLOOD SUGAR
Commonest in diabetics on treatment with pills or insulin.
* The symptoms appear rapidly.
* Light-headedness.
* Sweating.
* Irritability.
* Hunger.
* Drowsiness.

All diabetics should recognize the warning symptoms, keeping some glucose at hand in an easily absorbed form (for example, hard candy, sugar tablets or orange juice).

■ PHEOCHROMOCYTOMA
A tumor which produces a hormone that causes high blood pressure. The level of hormone can rapidly increase, causing:
* Sudden anxiety, sweating, palpitations.
* Pallor.

When an attack is in progress, blood pressure will be very high.

COMA

A precise medical term meaning a state of unrousability and unresponsiveness to voice, touch or pain. At its most severe there is:
* No response to pain.
* No movement.
* No speech.

Stupor is less severe: the individual can be roused by painful stimuli. The causes are the same. There are many stages in between the two, such as sleepiness and confusion and there may be some delirium, too.

Cases of coma require urgent hospital admission in order to search for the many possible causes. You will be providing extremely useful information to the hospital if you can report on:
* A history of diabetes; any

drowsiness and confusion in the preceding hours.
* Drug or alcohol abuse; evidence such as bottles, syringes.
* Epilepsy, with details of previous seizures and of medication.
* A head injury in the previous few weeks.
* Previous strokes; treatment for high blood pressure.
* Depression and suicidal intent: empty pill containers.

PROBABLE
STROKE
HEART ATTACK
DRUGS OR ALCOHOL
MEDICATION OVERDOSE

POSSIBLE
EPILEPSY
INFECTION
METABOLIC DISEASE
INJURY

RARE
HYPOTHERMIA
OTHER CAUSES

PROBABLE

■ STROKE
Usually in the elderly.
* Sudden collapse.
* One-sided paralysis *(see PARALYSIS, RAPID ONSET).*

■ HEART ATTACK
See page 229.
Coma following:
* Chest pain.
* Breathlessness.
* Sweating and blue lips.

■ DRUGS OR ALCOHOL
Diagnosis tends to depend on a knowledge of the person's habits and other pointers, such as the smell of alcohol. Drug abuse is a strong possibility if there are:
* Deep, shallow breathing.
* Pinpoint-sized pupils.
* Signs of intravenous injections (red marks on the arms or thickened hard veins).

■ MEDICATION OVERDOSE
Overdosing with various medications such as anti-depressants, pain killers and sedatives can produce coma.

POSSIBLE

■ EPILEPSY
After a severe convulsion someone suffering from epilepsy may be comatose for a few minutes. *See page 384.*

■ INFECTION
Although any severe infection may cause coma through shock *(see page 471)*, meningitis is the most likely, especially in babies. It should be suspected in any infant showing otherwise unexplained:
* Irritability, drowsiness.
* Increasing drowsiness.
* Purple rash on body.
* In a baby, a bulging soft spot on the skull.

In adults there may also be:
* Neck stiffness.
* Sensitivity to bright lights.

An emergency. Take the individual to hospital without delay.

■ METABOLIC DISEASE
Most probably kidney or liver disease or diabetes, usually already known.
* Diabetics may have developed another illness or missed injections.
* Urine output either greater or much less than usual.
* Deep, heavy breathing.
* Possibly jaundice.
The coma can often be reversed, especially with diabetics.

■ INJURY
A head injury is the commonest injury causing coma, usually following an accident. The diagnosis will be obvious. Stupor or coma occurring a few weeks after a serious head injury may be due to a blood clot on the brain resulting from that injury. Surgical removal of this blood clot usually allows full recovery.

RARE

■ HYPOTHERMIA
A profound drop in body temperature, most common in the elderly, in winter, following a fall or a stroke. *See page 451.*

■ OTHER CAUSES
A book could be written about the other causes of coma, since it can be the final scenario of any serious upset to the body's working.

LACK OF CONCENTRATION

Peoples' attention span is very variable and depends on factors such as mood, conditions of work, age and stress. There is rarely any serious reason for this symptom. Children have a much shorter attention span than adults.

PROBABLE
TIREDNESS
HYPERACTIVITY
POOR HEARING

POSSIBLE
ANXIETY

RARE
MINIMAL BRAIN DISORDER

PROBABLE

■ TIREDNESS
May affect adults and children.
* Normally sound health and adequate concentration.
* Obvious lack of rest or overwork.
* Concentration returns after rest.

■ HYPERACTIVITY
Some physicians disagree as to whether such a specific condition exists in children and, less commonly, in adults. It is true, however, that some children exhibit:
* Inability to settle down to a task.

* Rapid loss of interest in one activity.
* Frequent movement and restlessness.

Social circumstances and food ingredients such as colorants have both been blamed for this condition. It is likely that a number of factors are responsible. There may be an overlap with minimal brain disorder *(see below)*.

■ POOR HEARING
Children who have had chronic ear infections may have reduced hearing. The hearing loss may not be very obvious but it leads to lack of concentration and learning problems. Needs medical evaluation.

POSSIBLE

■ ANXIETY
See page 377.
* Tension.
* Sweating.
* Palpitations.

RARE

■ MINIMAL BRAIN DISORDER
A somewhat controversial childhood diagnosis.
* Child shows abrupt changes in behavior.
* Poor learning ability.
* Disruptive behavior.

Treatment is very difficult, and such children often need special schooling.

CONFUSION

A combination of disorientation and emotional upset. Gradual confusion is most likely to occur in the elderly (*see also DEMENTIA*). Sudden confusion at any age may have an acute underlying cause and will probably need investigation.

PROBABLE
SENILE CONFUSION

POSSIBLE
DIABETIC COMPLICATIONS
DRUGS OR ALCOHOL
HEART FAILURE
INFECTIONS
MINOR STROKE
RESPIRATORY FAILURE
HYPOTHERMIA

RARE
UNDERACTIVE THYROID GLAND
METABOLIC FAILURE
SUBDURAL HEMATOMA

PROBABLE

■ SENILE CONFUSION
There is a breakdown of memory for recent events. Confusion follows as the individual forgets why they are where they are and what for. At its worst, it develops into *DEMENTIA,* but for many

THE BRAIN AND NERVOUS SYSTEM

elderly people confusion is just a nuisance.
* General health normal for age.
* No confusion or problem with familiar tasks and journeys.
* Can cope by using notes, lists.
* Deterioration occurs only gradually, but major changes in lifestyle, for example, a vacation, may bring it on.

POSSIBLE

■ DIABETIC COMPLICATIONS
Confusion can be caused by either too little or too much sugar.
* Onset over hours or minutes and may progress to *COMA* *(see page 471).*
* Irritability, drowsiness.
* Deep, sighing breathing, thirst.
* Hunger, light-headedness.

Diabetics should be aware of the early signs and take appropriate action — increasing their dose of insulin, or taking glucose.

■ DRUGS OR ALCOHOL
This diagnosis tends to rely on knowledge of a previous history of drug abuse or alcoholism. In alcoholics, an acute state of confusion needs urgent medical attention.

■ HEART FAILURE
Confusion as a symptom of heart failure is most likely to affect the elderly.
* Breathlessness, swollen ankles.
* Inability to lie flat.
* Recent chest pain or tiredness could signal a heart attack.

■ INFECTIONS
In the elderly, any acute infection may worsen a tendency to confusion. There may or may not be a fever.
* Cough.
* Need to pass urine frequently suggests a bladder infection.

In a younger person, the combination of:
* Confusion,
* Headache,
* Sensitivity to light, suggests meningitis, needing emergency hospital care.

■ MINOR STROKE
* Sudden confusion.
* Sudden slurring of speech or difficulty finding words.
* Face may droop on one side.
* Possibly loss of function of an arm or leg.

Recovery from such minor strokes is often rapid. Such an episode should be reported to your physician.

■ RESPIRATORY FAILURE
Most likely in someone with chronic bronchitis or emphysema *(see page 222).*
* A chest infection may be the trigger.
* Blue lips and tongue.
* Warm hands.
* Breathlessness.

Needs hospital treatment.

■ HYPOTHERMIA
Confusion is a common early symptom of low body temperature. Usually affects the elderly.

RARE

■ UNDERACTIVE THYROID GLAND
* Weight gain; sluggishness; intolerance of cold; yellowish, puffy appearance.
* Slow pulse.

■ METABOLIC FAILURE
This includes liver and kidney disease.
* Liver disease suggested by previous history of alcoholism; jaundice; easy bruising; red palms; swollen ankles.
* Kidney disease suggested by either very high or very low urine output; anemia; feeling sick, yellow tinge to skin.

■ SUBDURAL HEMATOMA
A collection of blood, which has built up following an injury to the skull and which puts pressure on the brain.
* Symptoms emerge over several weeks.
* History of head injury.
* A fluctuating degree of confusion and abnormality of behaviour.
* One-sided weakness of arm and leg may develop.

Though uncommon, a subdural hematoma is a treatable form of confusion, now relatively easy to diagnose, thanks to brain scans.

CONVULSIONS

The features of a convulsion, also known as a seizure or epileptic attack, are:
* Possibly a warning of an impending attack, called an aura; it may be a feeling, a visual disturbance, a smell, a headache.
* The individual may cry out, then collapse unconscious.
* Remains stiff; may turn blue around the lips for about 30 seconds.
* Arms and legs then begin to jerk in a coordinated manner.
* Possibly incontinence of urine, frothing at mouth.
* Afterwards, drowsiness, confusion, before return to normal.

Not all convulsions are as dramatic. One form of convulsion is no more than a brief absence of consciousness, which may be misinterpreted as a blank look.

A convulsion is different from a simple faint, where there is no aura, no incontinence, no shaking of limbs. Tests are needed if there is any doubt.

PROBABLE
EPILEPSY
FEBRILE SEIZURE

POSSIBLE
ECLAMPSIA OF PREGNANCY
ALCOHOL RELATED
MENINGITIS

RARE
METABOLIC DISORDER

THE BRAIN AND NERVOUS SYSTEM

PROBABLE

■ EPILEPSY
Epilepsy is caused by abnormal electrical discharges in the brain. Most cases are of unknown origin, but it can result from previous brain injury, for instance a stroke, a head injury or cerebral palsy. Anyone having a seizure for the first time needs careful assessment since occasionally it may be a symptom of brain disease, such as a tumor or abnormal blood vessels.

Most epileptics can lead a full life, taking care to avoid situations which would be dangerous if they had a seizure, such as climbing ladders, driving or using hazardous machinery.

■ FEBRILE SEIZURE
A convulsion in a child who is feverish. Anyone with a high enough temperature may go into convulsions: but children's brains are more sensitive to relatively minor fevers. It is to reduce the chances of a seizure that children with fevers should be given paracetamol and kept cool.

Febrile seizures are common, occurring in some 10 percent of all children, and do not mean that the child will grow up epileptic. A child having a febrile seizure for the first time needs immediate medical attention: often admission to hospital will be advised to test for meningitis. Children who have recurrent febrile seizures can be managed at home, as long as the parents know how to give an anti-convulsant if the seizure becomes prolonged. They are uncommon after the age of five.

* Child is feverish, typically with a cold or ear infection
* Sudden stiffness, rolling of eyes, breathing stops.
* Then, co-ordinated jerking, of limbs and possibly incontinence.
* May last five to ten minutes.
* Child becomes responsive, but remains drowsy for a few hours.
* The seizure usually occurs early on in the fever, as the temperature rises. In children below six months or older than five years, it is not safe to make a diagnosis of febrile seizures and other causes must be considered by a professional.

POSSIBLE

■ ECLAMPSIA OF PREGNANCY
A risk of later pregnancy: the blood pressure suddenly rises too high and the mother starts to have a convulsion. The situation should be avoided by routine pre-natal care. Warning symptoms are:
* Fingers and feet swell rapidly.
* Headache, flashing lights.

Tests will also detect protein in the urine (besides the high blood pressure). This is an emergency, calling for urgent reduction in blood pressure to reduce risks to mother and baby.

■ ALCOHOL-RELATED
Both excess alcohol and sudden abstention from it can bring on seizures, the diagnosis usually being obvious from previous knowledge of the individual. Alcoholics are as likely as anyone else to develop true epilepsy, so the usual full assessment should be made.

■ MENINGITIS
An infection around the brain possible at all ages but an especial worry in childhood. *See also Drowsiness.*

RARE

■ METABOLIC DISORDER
This usually means breakdown in the function of the kidneys or liver and should be detected on routine investigation of epilepsy.

DELIRIUM

Meaning the rapid appearance of:
* Confusion.
* Restlessness.
* Hallucinations.
* Incoherent speech and thought.
* Often worst at night.

Often, the confusion fluctuates, with severe symptoms interspersed with relatively normal phases.

The causes are those given under *CONFUSION*, but with an added urgency because of the greater risk of serious underlying illness, and with a higher chance of an infection being the cause.

Older people are more likely to become delirious during an otherwise moderately serious illness. In children, delirium frequently accompanies a harmless feverish illness and should be treated by bringing the temperature down. If there is any suspicion of:
* Headache,
* Sensitivity to light,
* Neck stiffness: meningitis must be checked for – immediate medical attention is needed.

DELUSIONS

There is no reliable definition of a delusion: conventionally, it is a belief which appears not to be founded in reality — reality as judged by a reasonable group of people sharing the same cultural background — which gives scope for gross abuse of the term. It has, indeed, been a convenient way of labelling as mentally ill those who have held such shocking beliefs as liberty, democracy and freedom.

Nevertheless, there are individuals who hold beliefs so bizarre that they are taken as prime signs of mental illness: the unshakeable conviction, for instance, that you are Napoleon Bonaparte or that if your left knee itches your wife is being unfaithful. The deluded person may then act on that belief, so that what appears to be a motiveless crime proves to have been the logical outcome of delusions. With appropriate caveats, psychiatrists therefore take delusions seriously.

PROBABLE
SCHIZOPHRENIA

POSSIBLE
EARLY DEMENTIA
DEPRESSION

THE BRAIN AND NERVOUS SYSTEM

PROBABLE

■ SCHIZOPHRENIA
A common mental illness in which the sufferer experiences a breakdown of reality and a disintegration of personality. About one percent of the population is schizophrenic or goes through an episode of schizophrenia. A "schizoid state" is a less serious condition and describes individuals who have an abnormal set of emotional responses and relationships with others and are frequently loners.

Schizophrenia is not the "split personality" of popular myth, although it is true that a schizophrenic may appear unremarkable until you happen to touch upon his or her particular delusion. Most specialists believe that schizophrenia is the result of disorders of the chemistry of the brain. Treatment based on this view is quite successful, allowing many schizophrenics to lead quiet, undemanding, but self-sufficient lives.

* Delusions ranging from single ideas to whole networks of belief about the nature of reality.
* Hallucinations.
* Mood is often flat and emotionless.
* Apathy, self-neglect.
* Onset may be slow or rapid.

Treatment is with medication, usually for years.

Schizophrenics often need long-term support and supervision: the toll on their families, forced to witness the disintegration of a personality, can be appalling.

POSSIBLE

■ EARLY DEMENTIA
See DEMENTIA, below. In the early stages, memory loss may result in giving delusional explanations for events, whose cause the individual has forgotten: for example, believing that a mislaid handbag has actually been stolen.

■ DEPRESSION
Those with severe depression may come to hold delusions about their own health or that of their families — for example, they may think that a loved one has an incurable disease. People in deep depression have tragically murdered their own children in the delusional belief that they were giving relief from a terrible illness.

DEMENTIA

General breakdown of the mind, with the basic defect being loss of memory. Dementia becomes more common with age. About 20 percent of those over 80 suffer from it.

* Memory loss an early feature.
* Personality change.
* Forgetfulness about who you are, where you are and "when you are".
* Self-neglect.
* Depression and anxiety accompany early awareness of deterioration.
* Memory for childhood events is preserved.

* Gradually increasing confusion.

Despite this picture, the individual appears fully conscious, with no drowsiness. Although most cases are incurable, there are a few treatable causes which blood tests and brain scans can detect, and of which everyone should be aware.

PROBABLE
ALZHEIMER'S DISEASE

POSSIBLE
MEDICATION EFFECTS
ALCOHOLISM
MULTIPLE STROKES

RARE
HUNTINGTON'S CHOREA
HYPOTHYROIDISM
HYDROCEPHALUS
LIVER OR KIDNEY DISEASE
MENINGIOMA
BRAIN HEMATOMA
B12 DEFICIENCY
SYPHILIS
AIDS

PROBABLE

■ ALZHEIMER'S DISEASE

This term is replacing the old ones of senile and pre-senile dementia, especially as more is learned about the changes in the brain that cause dementia. However, there is at present no treatment and the outlook is progressive decline to a state needing nursing care.

* The symptoms are those of dementia, as above.

* Deterioration occurs steadily.

POSSIBLE

■ MEDICATION EFFECTS

Might be suspected if:

* Dementia appears rapidly and fluctuates.

* The individual is on multiple treatments, especially common with tranquillizers and medications to treat Parkinson's disease.

The test is to stop treatment and to see what happens.

■ ALCOHOLISM

Gives rise to a distinct form of dementia, due to lack of B vitamins.

* Profound loss of memory for recent events.

* A tendency to make up excuses to cover up for memory loss.

* Disorders of eye movements, for instance, jerking.

* Unsteady gait.

This condition is treatable.

■ MULTIPLE STROKES

Dementia follows when a series of small strokes destroys more and more of the brain.

* Dementia worsening as a series of small, abrupt steps.

* Often specific weakness of an arm or leg.

* Mood swings rapidly from tears to laughter.

Occasionally, investigation detects a treatable source of the strokes.

THE BRAIN AND NERVOUS SYSTEM

RARE

■ HUNTINGTON'S CHOREA
* Family history.
* Dementia with trembling of limbs begins in the 30s or 40s.
* Physical and mental deterioration is progressive and inevitable.

■ HYPOTHYROIDISM
A severely under-active thyroid gland.
* Apathy, sluggishness; weight gain.
* Slow thought, intolerance of cold, slow pulse.
* Rarely, a yellowish tinge to skin.
Treatment with thyroid hormone will reverse this condition.

■ HYDROCEPHALUS
An uncommon condition of increased pressure within the brain, but found much more often now that brain scans are widely available. Treatable.
* The degree of confusion fluctuates.
* Urinary incontinence.
* Unsteady gait.
* Clumsiness.

■ LIVER AND KIDNEY DISEASE
Should be detected on routine screening. *See under METABOLIC FAILURE, page 383.*

■ MENINGIOMA
A very slowly growing brain tumor. Apart from dementia, dependent on its position, it may cause:
* Epilepsy.
* Weakness of an arm or leg.
* Progressive headache.
* Loss of sense of smell.
Diagnosis will be confirmed by a brain scan.

■ BRAIN HEMATOMA
A blood clot on the brain, following a head injury. A possible cause of dementia of rapid onset. *See SUBDURAL HEMATOMA, page 383.*

■ VITAMIN B12 DEFICIENCY
Pernicious anemia.
* Pallor from anemia.
* Tingling in hands and feet.
Another rare but treatable cause of dementia.

■ SYPHILIS
In its final stages, many years after first infection, syphilis can cause dementia, plus:
* Unsteady gait.
* Drooping eyelids.
* Delusions, often of grandeur.
* Small, irregular pupils.
Blood tests will confirm the diagnosis and antibiotic treatment can then halt, though not reverse, the condition.

■ AIDS
A diagnosis to be considered in a younger person developing dementia. Other pointers include: being in a high-risk group (homosexuals, bisexuals, prostitutes, intravenous drug-abusers); unusual chest infections; weight loss; persistently enlarged glands.

DEPRESSION

When is it an illness? And when is it just a natural response to life's problems? Depression as a result of bereavement used to be considered something different from severe depression arising by itself. Now it seems that there is not a clear-cut distinction. All forms of depression may benefit from treatment with anti-depressants, although these medications need to be used with caution.

Everyone has a duty to be aware of depression as a severe illness in its own right. Growing out of unhappiness, or perhaps from long-term stresses and crises, clinical depression goes beyond unhappiness and carries the real risk of suicide.

Mood, appearance and speech are usually enough to make a firm diagnosis of significant depression. The symptoms are:
* Loss of enjoyment.
* Lack of energy, concentration and difficulty making decisions.
* Loss of sexual desire, or impotence.
* Sadness.
* Tearfulness.
* Frequently, headaches, like a band around the head.
* Breathlessness.

Severe depression gives rise to:
* Loss of appetite.
* Palpitations – fluttering of the heart.
* Constipation.
* Early-morning waking from sleep.
* Self-disgust.
* Thoughts that you have other serious diseases.
* Suicidal thoughts.

Telling people to pull themselves together is as useless as telling someone with appendicitis to snap out of it. The elderly deserve particular attention, as does anyone who has attempted suicide; also women experiencing severe depression after childbirth. Treatments range from counseling to anti-depressants to hospital admission.

Other causes of depression to be considered are:

POSSIBLE
POST-VIRAL SYNDROME
EARLY DEMENTIA
EARLY SCHIZOPHRENIA

RARE
HYPOTHYROIDISM
PARKINSON'S DISEASE
HORMONE DISORDERS

POSSIBLE

■ POST-VIRAL SYNDROME
* Follows a vague illness with fever, aches, pains.
* Mild depression and easy tiring.
* Most cases clear up within a few weeks.
* Occasionally becomes prolonged, with profound weakness and tiredness.

The cause of post-viral syndrome is controversial.

THE BRAIN AND NERVOUS SYSTEM

There are no tests to monitor the condition. The basic treatment is rest, but sometimes a low dose of an anti-depressant helps. Improved treatments may be available in due course.

A variant of this is called Chronic Fatigue Syndrome and can last for months causing great disability.

■ EARLY DEMENTIA
See DEMENTIA. In the late middle-aged or elderly.
* Memory loss is marked.

Depression is probably the result of the individual's awareness that his or her mind is going. Some idea of how this must feel can be found in the film 2001, where, in a scene of great poignancy, the circuits which give the super-computer HAL its "mind" are stripped away, one by one.

■ EARLY SCHIZOPHRENIA
See page 386.
* A possibility in a young person with depression.
* Possibly delusions and hallucinations.

RARE

■ HYPOTHYROIDISM
A severely under-active thyroid gland may give a state simulating depression. *See page 383.*

■ PARKINSON'S DISEASE
In the elderly.
* Shaking of hands.
* Stiff, shuffling gait.
* Impassive appearance.

This can be helped by medications.

■ HORMONE DISORDERS
Might be considered in someone with rapid onset of depression who appears otherwise unwell, especially with:
* Rapid weight gain or weight loss.

DIZZINESS

A common symptom, but rather difficult to define since it can mean different things. For some, it appears to be an inability to concentrate, with feelings of lightheadedness; for others, things really seem to spin, either inside the head or outside it. You will find that your physician will try hard to pin down just what you mean by dizziness.

DIZZINESS WITH VERTIGO

There is dizziness, unsteadiness, a feeling of falling and the room spins when you turn your head.

PROBABLE
VESTIBULITIS

POSSIBLE
MÉNIERE'S SYNDROME

RARE
DISEASE OF BRAIN OR SPINAL CORD

PROBABLE

■ VESTIBULITIS
A harmless viral infection of the inner ear giving rise to:
* Abrupt onset of dizziness.
* Worse when turning head.
* No pain or ringing in ear.
* Lying flat, you feel fine.

Though alarming, the symptoms fade over a few days with the help of anti-nausea medications.

POSSIBLE

■ MENIERE'S SYNDROME
A gradual process of degeneration in the ear.
* Ringing (tinnitus) is an early feature.
* Gradually worsening deafness.
* Sudden attacks of vertigo, in which the above symptoms worsen for a few minutes.

RARE

■ DISEASE OF BRAIN OR SPINAL CORD
Although highly unlikely as a cause of a few episodes of sudden dizziness, there are several diseases such as multiple sclerosis which can cause dizziness in combination with:
* Unsteady gait.
* Tingling or numbness of hands or feet.
* Visual disturbances such as double vision.
* Weakness of an arm or leg.

It is essential to get medical advice.

DIZZINESS WITHOUT VERTIGO

Feeling light-headed, unsteady, but no spinning feeling. The crucial clues are: in what circumstance the dizziness occurs; at what time of day; for how long; how often; and how you feel before and afterwards.

PROBABLE
CAUSE UNKNOWN
EMOTIONAL FACTORS

POSSIBLE
ANEMIA
LOW BLOOD PRESSURE
LOW BLOOD SUGAR

RARE
HEART AND CIRCULATION PROBLEMS
POLYCYTHEMIA
TEMPORAL LOBE EPILEPSY

PROBABLE

■ CAUSE UNKNOWN
Accounts for the great majority of cases. A safe conclusion as long as:
* You are otherwise well.
* Attacks of dizziness are not prolonged or recurrent.

Dizziness can occur in situations such as excess alcohol intake, over breathing, over exertion in the heat, lack of food.

A medical check-up may be reassuring.

THE BRAIN AND NERVOUS SYSTEM

■ EMOTIONAL FACTORS
Here dizziness is used to mean:
* Inability to concentrate.
* A fuzziness in the head.
* Muddled thinking.
* Difficulty in making decisions.

Try to review what in your life is giving rise to unusual degrees of stress and concern.

POSSIBLE

■ ANEMIA
* Pale.
* Tiredness.
* Breathlessness.
* A lightheaded feeling when you stand up.

Unless the cause of the anemia is obvious, for instance, very heavy menstruation, your physician will probably recommend some tests.

■ LOW BLOOD PRESSURE
* Dizziness when you stand up.
* Passes off after a few seconds.

This is common in older people, whose circulation is less efficient at making the rather complex adjustment for standing up.

Occasionally, it is because treatment for high blood pressure has been over-effective and sometimes medication must be changed. It is also common in pregnancy. Can occur if there has been significant blood loss internally, for example, a bleeding stomach ulcer.

■ LOW BLOOD SUGAR
As experienced by anyone missing a meal, and especially a risk for people with diabetes.
* Rapid onset.
* Difficulty concentrating.
* Irritability.
* Sweating.

Symptoms are quickly relieved by eating, or taking glucose (orange juice, candy).

RARE

■ HEART AND CIRCULATORY PROBLEMS
These can really only be confirmed by medical examination. They become commoner with age, and pointers include:
* Palpitations.
* A pulse rate that feels unusually fast, unusually slow, or irregular.
* Breathlessness.
* Chest pains.
* Dizziness when looking up.
* Symptoms of a minor stroke, with temporary limb weakness, disturbed speech or vision.

The underlying problem may be abnormal heart rhythms or narrowed valves of the heart, conditions which can be treated. Most likely, arteries to the brain have become narrowed.

Medications or even surgery may help.

■ POLYCYTHEMIA
The opposite of anemia, in which there is an over-concentration of blood. Commonest in those with chronic lung problems such as bronchitis and emphysema; *see page 222.*
* A red complexion.
* Headaches.
* Itchiness of skin.

Treatment depends on the underlying cause.

■ TEMPORAL LOBE EPILEPSY
Difficult to diagnose if dizziness is the only symptom. Other symptoms may include:
* A warning sensation (an aura) preceding the dizziness.
* Awareness of unusual smells, tastes or visual disturbances just before the dizziness.
* Associated drowsiness.

SLEEPINESS

Sleepiness caused simply by lack of sleep or by excess alcohol is not covered here.

Sleepiness in someone otherwise expected to be alert is an important symptom, and in children this is a warning symptom which always needs medical assessment.

PROBABLE
MEDICATION EFFECTS
NON-SPECIFIC INFECTION

POSSIBLE
HEAD INJURY
ENCEPHALITIS

RARE
BRAIN TUMOUR
NARCOLEPSY
SLEEP APNEA SYNDROME

PROBABLE

■ MEDICATION EFFECTS
* Most likely in the elderly.
* Common in the morning for people who take sleeping tablets or anti-depressants.
* Drowsiness clears during the day.

The dose may need adjustment, or a shorter-acting medication may be appropriate.

■ NON-SPECIFIC INFECTION
Drowsiness commonly accompanies the early stages of many illnesses, especially viral ones. There may also be:
* Muscle aches and pains.
* Fever.
* Aching eyes.

The infection soon shows itself, typically, as a cough or sore throat.

POSSIBLE

■ ENCEPHALITIS
A non-specific irritation of the brain, commonly caused by mild viral infections, but which may accompany meningitis.
* Severe, persistent sleepiness.
* Confusion.
* Headache.
* Bright lights hurt the eyes.
* As it worsens, seizures, coma, paralysis of limbs.

If you suspect encephalitis in a child, get medical advice; adults should also see a doctor unless the above combination of symptoms is very mild.

THE BRAIN AND NERVOUS SYSTEM

■ HEAD INJURY
Sleepiness occurring after a blow to the head may signify bleeding within the skull. Other warning signs are:
* Confusion.
* Nausea and vomiting.
* Loss of use of a limb.
* Double vision.
* Slow pulse.

Requires immediate medical evaluation in the Emergency Room.

RARE

■ BRAIN TUMOR
Brain tumors really are rare and when they occur have usually spread to the brain from a tumor elsewhere, typically the lung or breast. The features of a brain tumor are:
* Progressively worsening headache, more painful at night.
* Change of personality.
* Double vision.
* Later, loss of use of one side of the body.

Treatment depends on the type of tumor.

■ NARCOLEPSY
* Sudden sleepiness, totally out of the blue.
* For a while, the individual cannot be roused.

This unusual illness tends to run in families. Medication can help.

■ SLEEP APNEA SYNDROME
A condition now recognized more widely than before. During sleep, breathing becomes very shallow and stops altogether for brief periods. The resulting disturbed sleep causes marked daytime sleepiness.
* In the grossly overweight.
* Usually, in those with chronic bronchitis or emphysema.

EMOTIONAL INSTABILITY

If this happens to a previously stable person, emotional instability may be significant if there are also:
* Changes in personality.
* Irritability.
* Mood swings.

In some highly-strung people, apparent emotional instability is merely an exaggeration of the normal. They have abrupt swings of mood, often intensified by alcohol. They are not "ill" as long as:
* Emotional states do not interfere with work, social and domestic life.
* The person understands his or her own personality.
* General health and thought processes appear normal – for instance, no delusions.

However difficult such people may be to cope with or to live with, they are often useful and creative.

That leaves relatively few underlying causes of emotional instability:

PROBABLE
ANXIETY

POSSIBLE
MENTAL ILLNESS
EARLY DEMENTIA
DRUG ABUSE
HYPOGLYCEMIA

RARE
BRAIN TUMOR
BRAIN DISEASE

PROBABLE

■ ANXIETY
Anyone, whatever their previous personality, can become emotional under conditions of stress and tension.
* Difficulty concentrating.
* Tension headaches.
* Abrupt outbursts.
They will be aware of the changes and can discuss their distress.

POSSIBLE

■ MENTAL ILLNESS
When emotional instability really does appear to exceed the normal, psychiatrists will look for:
* Delusions.
* Hallucinations.
* Lack of understanding about own behavior.
* Severe depression.
* Manic, irresponsible behavior.
Diagnoses include manic depression, severe depression and schizophrenia.

■ EARLY DEMENTIA
See page 386. With breakdown of mental function, there is a loss of emotional control.

■ DRUG ABUSE
Various street drugs can produce irrational mood swings. Some prescribed medications can do this also, such as long-term steroids, anti-depressants.

■ HYPOGLYCEMIA
Low blood sugar in diabetes can produce mood swings.

RARE

■ BRAIN TUMOR
See page 394.
Highly unusual:
* Widespread changes in personality.
* Possibly feels sick.
* Headache.

■ BRAIN DISEASE
Numerous conditions can affect emotional control and are covered under *DEMENTIA.*
Suspected if there is:
* Memory loss.
* Disturbances of speech, walking, use of limbs.

FAINTING

A very short block in the flow of blood to the brain will cause lightheadedness; any longer pause is very likely to become a faint. Serious causes are unusual, unless fainting is regular or abrupt.

THE BRAIN AND NERVOUS SYSTEM

PROBABLE
HARMLESS CAUSES

POSSIBLE
LOW BLOOD PRESSURE

RARE
HEART PROBLEMS
BLEEDING
EPILEPSY
MINOR STROKE

PROBABLE

■ HARMLESS CAUSES
The great majority of causes are trivial: standing too long in the heat, missing a meal, over-tiredness. Fainting is common in pregnancy, after emotional shock and in reaction to severe pain.
* Recovery occurs within moments.
* No seizures or incontinence.

POSSIBLE

■ LOW BLOOD PRESSURE
See page 392.
* Frequent lightheadedness on standing.
* Most likely if you are diabetic, if you take medications which affect your blood pressure, or if your body is short of fluid.

RARE

■ HEART PROBLEMS
Worth considering if there is:
* Faintness on exercise.
* Palpitations.
* Slow, rapid or irregular pulse rates.

Most of the heart problems that will lead to fainting are treatable.
See also pages 193-203.

■ BLEEDING
Faintness, in combination with injury or pain, may be a symptom of serious blood loss.
* Sweating.
* Pale skin.
* Thirst.

Careful examination will reveal the source of the bleeding. If you suspect internal bleeding, for example, after a car accident, seek medical help immediately.
See also page 426.

■ EPILEPSY
Look for:
* Seizures.
* A warning aura.
* Urinary incontinence.

See page 384.

■ MINOR STROKE
* Possibly short-term loss of speech, or of the use of a limb.

See page 404.

HALLUCINATIONS

An experience without any basis in reality: a vision, a sound, a sensation. Dreams are "normal" hallucinations. Hallucinations occurring in clear consciousness are symptoms of major mental disease.

PROBABLE
DELIRIUM
CONFUSIONAL STATES

POSSIBLE
DRUG OR ALCOHOL ABUSE
SCHIZOPHRENIA
DEPRESSION

RARE
TEMPORAL LOBE EPILEPSY

PROBABLE

■ DELIRIUM
The hallucination occurs during a period of restless confusion.

■ CONFUSIONAL STATES
In this context, hallucinations are part of a general breakdown of personality. *See DEMENTIA.*

POSSIBLE

■ DRUG OR ALCOHOL ABUSE
* Bizarre behavior.
* Unresponsive.
* Trembling hands suggest alcoholism.

■ SCHIZOPHRENIA
Hallucinations, wound into a web of delusion, are prime symptoms of schizophrenia. *See DELUSIONS.*

■ DEPRESSION
Very severe depression may give rise to hallucinations. *See page 386.*

RARE

■ TEMPORAL LOBE EPILEPSY
* Hallucinations of smell and taste are commonest.
See page 393

HYPERACTIVITY

Typically a childhood problem (in adults, *see MANIA)* combining:
* Restlessness.
* Inability to settle down to an activity.
* Destructive, aggressive behavior.
* Poor concentration.

It is unclear whether this is a result of disease or an exaggeration of normal personality traits.

PROBABLE
CHILDHOOD HYPERACTIVITY
PSYCHOLOGICAL CONFLICT

POSSIBLE
NORMAL CHILD

RARE
FOOD ALLERGY
MINIMAL BRAIN DAMAGE

THE BRAIN AND NERVOUS SYSTEM

PROBABLE

■ CHILDHOOD HYPERACTIVITY
Doctors disagree as to whether such a specific condition exists in children. It is true, however, that some children exhibit:
* Inability to settle to one task.
* Rapid loss of interest in the current activity.
* Frequent movement and restlessness.

Social circumstances and food additives such as artificial colorings have both been blamed for this condition. It is likely to be due to many factors acting together, and it may overlap with minimal brain damage (*see below*).

■ PSYCHOLOGICAL CONFLICT
A possible diagnosis where the close family displays:
* Emotional conflict.
* Alcoholism.
* Mental illness.

POSSIBLE

■ NORMAL CHILD
Some parents have a low tolerance for usual childhood behavior, which is normally active or noisy.

RARE

■ FOOD ALLERGY
A highly controversial diagnosis, which can only be proved after careful dietary experiment.

■ MINIMAL BRAIN DAMAGE
Most likely if there is also:
* Clumsiness, difficulty in completing simple manual tasks.
* Severe learning difficulties.

Such children often need special schooling. This syndrome is new and not fully defined. Not all doctors agree on its cause or how best to manage affected individuals.

HYSTERIA

The popular definition of hysteria is wild, reckless, exaggerated behavior. The (more precise) medical definition is:
* Symptoms that have no physical basis, which appear to arise without conscious desire to deceive.

It can be difficult, if not impossible, to prove that the behavior is not motivated by a need to deceive.

Hysterical symptoms include blindness, paralysis of a limb, loss of speech.

PROBABLE
PSYCHOLOGICAL FACTORS

POSSIBLE
UNDETECTED PHYSICAL DISEASE

RARE
BRAIN DISEASE

PROBABLE

■ PSYCHOLOGICAL FACTORS
This diagnosis has some validity when physical disease can be excluded and gains strength if:
* There is a demonstrable psychological bonus from the behavior: typically, increased attention from others.
* The hysteric is not very disturbed by symptoms a "normal" person would find devastating, such as blindness.

Treatment is extremely difficult. It requires the hysteric to recognize that the cost of his or her behavior outweighs the short-term psychological gain. In most cases recovery occurs within a year or so with therapy.

POSSIBLE

■ UNDETECTED PHYSICAL DISEASE
Even the most blatantly hysterical symptoms should be given the benefit of the doubt, and a search should be made for physical disease.

RARE

■ BRAIN DISEASE
Hysteria may be an early symptom of dementia or a brain tumor. If symptoms specific to these diseases accompany the hysteria, seek medical advice. *See DEMENTIA,* and *page 394.*

INSOMNIA

Sleep is still a mystery; that we all need it is certain, but how much is very variable. Reported insomnia is often a mismatch between how much sleep someone thinks they need and how much their body really needs.

PROBABLE
TEMPORARY DISTURBANCE OF SLEEP PATTERNS

POSSIBLE
REDUCED NEED FOR SLEEP
DEPRESSION

PROBABLE

■ TEMPORARY DISTURBANCE OF SLEEP PATTERNS
Anxiety, pain, discomfort cause insomnia which frequently persists once these problems have passed. Stimulants such as coffee and alcohol may be to blame, as may day-time snoozes.
* A cause is usually obvious — after thinking carefully about it.
* Day-time sleepiness.
* Sleep eventually comes — because you are exhausted.

It is best to tackle insomnia by not going to bed until you feel tired, then following a set routine leading to bed. Sleeping tablets have a role only in the short-term treatment of insomnia.

THE BRAIN AND NERVOUS SYSTEM

POSSIBLE

■ REDUCED NEED FOR SLEEP
For many people, "eight hours" sleep and a daily bowel movement is Life's Golden Rule. Many people often cannot accept that they need far less of either.
* No obvious anxiety.
* No day-time sleepiness.
Chronic insomniacs should accept that they have gained extra hours in their day; that nature is telling them to do the ironing at 3.00 am and to leave the extra daylight hours for better things.

■ DEPRESSION
Insomnia is an important symptom of depression.
* Sleep comes easily but you wake after two or three hours.
* You have great trouble getting to sleep. *See page 389.*

IRRITABILITY

Functioning on a "short fuse"; quick with anger and hostility. No one need be in any doubt about normal irritability: it is a simple response to the stresses of workaday life:
* Fatigue.
* Frustration.
* Being fed-up.
Hunger and lack of sleep and feeling unwell often make people extra-irritable. The more sinister causes of irritability are:

POSSIBLE
ANXIETY
ALCOHOLISM

RARE
EARLY DEMENTIA
HEAD INJURY
MENINGITIS

POSSIBLE

■ ANXIETY
See page 377.
* Irritability out of proportion to circumstances.

■ ALCOHOLISM
Alcoholics often have poor emotional control, including irritability.

RARE

■ EARLY DEMENTIA
See page 386. As memory fades, irritability emerges in reaction to an increasingly bewildering world.

■ HEAD INJURY
An injury severe enough to cause unconsciousness is frequently followed by:
* Irritability.
* Difficulty in concentrating.
* Swings of mood.

■ MENINGITIS
* Anger at being touched or moved.
* In babies, crying at any contact;

bulging soft spot on skull.
* Intolerance of light.
* Headache.
* Stiff neck.
A rare but extremely serious possibility, which needs further tests in hospital.

MANIA

Manic behavior includes:
* Frantic activity, insomnia.
* Sudden switches of direction of thought.
* Ideas spilling out, but barely connected, grandiose.
* Rapid speech.
* Nervous, jittery activity.
* Hallucinations.
Full-blown cases of mania are rare. The milder hypomanic state is commonest.

PROBABLE
EMOTIONAL STRESS

POSSIBLE
OVER-ACTIVE THYROID GLAND
MEDICATION EFFECTS
DEMENTIA

RARE
MANIC DEPRESSION
SCHIZOPHRENIA

PROBABLE

■ EMOTIONAL STRESS
See also ANXIETY.
A hypomanic state:
* Understandable sources of stress.

POSSIBLE

■ OVER-ACTIVE THYROID GLAND
See page 378. It is as if the body's "thermostat" has been turned up.
* Trembling.
* Weight loss.
* Bulging eyes.

■ MEDICATION EFFECTS
Mania occurring in a previously sound personality may result from abuse of amphetamines or marijuana. Steroids, used widely in rheumatic disorders and asthma, may cause mania in some people with a sensitivity to these medications.

■ DEMENTIA
Mania arises from the loss of inhibition. A distressing combination. *See page 386.*

RARE

■ MANIC DEPRESSION
Mania and depression are opposite extremes; manic depressives swing between both moods.
* Recurrent mania.
* Recurrent depression.
* A combination of both.
Often needs hospital admission (for the individual's own safety),

followed by long courses of medication.

■ SCHIZOPHRENIA
See page 386. Acute schizophrenia may begin as a manic state, together with characteristic
* Delusions;
* Hallucinations.

POOR MEMORY

It is common to have an excellent memory for some types of information, for instance, names, but a poor memory for others, such as phone numbers.

PROBABLE
NORMAL AGING PROCESS
ANXIETY

POSSIBLE
ALCOHOLISM
HEAD INJURY
STROKE
VITAMIN B12 DEFICIENCY

RARE
DEMENTIA

PROBABLE

■ NORMAL AGING PROCESS
Every day, 10,000 of our brain cells die, more than 250 million over a 70-year lifetime. A dense web of additional cells and rich interconnections mask the effects of this loss; but eventually it catches up with us, and we notice our memories worsening.
* Memory for long-past events remains good.
* Difficulty learning new tasks.
* Personality generally unchanged.

There is some evidence that using your mind keeps it active.

■ ANXIETY
Interferes with concentration and memory. *See page 377.*

POSSIBLE

■ ALCOHOLISM
Affects memory by causing vitamin deficiencies. *See page 387.*

■ HEAD INJURY
See page 393.
* Poor memory.
* Irritability.
* Mood swings.

■ STROKE
See also CONFUSION, and page 404.
Sudden loss of memory together with:
* Loss of use of a limb.
* Interference with speech.

There is often recovery from a minor stroke over several months.

■ VITAMIN B12 DEFICIENCY
See page 406.

RARE

■ DEMENTIA
If the personality remains intact, it is very unlikely that memory loss is due to early dementia, *page 386*.

MENTAL IMPAIRMENT

A general lack of intelligence, as shown by:
* Poor learning ability.
* Difficulty handling complex situations.
* Poor language skills.
* Clumsiness.

Past illness and injury may be to blame, but many cases remain unexplained.

PROBABLE
CEREBRAL PALSY
CONGENITAL
STROKE

POSSIBLE
DEMENTIA
HEAD INJURY

RARE
DEGENERATION OF THE BRAIN
VITAMIN DEFICIENCIES
METABOLIC DISORDERS
SYPHILIS

PROBABLE

■ CEREBRAL PALSY
Injury or infection of the brain at birth.
* Child is floppy.
* Fails to thrive; *see page 412.*
* Spastic limbs.

■ CONGENITAL
A similar picture to that of cerebral palsy, *above*, but with specific features, giving a recognized condition such as Down's syndrome.

■ STROKE
See page 404. A reason for sudden deterioration in a previously normal person.

POSSIBLE

■ DEMENTIA
See page 386. General deterioration of brain function.

■ HEAD INJURY
See page 394. Has much the same effect as a stroke.

RARE

■ DEGENERATION OF THE NERVOUS SYSTEM
Can happen in several ways. Possible if:
* Intellect was previously normal.
* Gradual deterioration of thought processes.
* Associated trembling, weakness and paralysis.

Requires specialist diagnosis.

■ VITAMIN DEFICIENCIES
Affects the growing child and is a tragic cause of impaired intellect in undeveloped countries.
* Poor growth.
* Swollen belly, poor bone formation.
* Loss of hair, patchy pigmentation of skin.

Vitamin deficiencies are also found in alcoholics, the mentally ill and the poor.

■ METABOLIC DISORDERS
Such as liver and kidney disease. *See page 383.*

■ SYPHILIS
Can cause a general deterioration of brain function years after first infection. *See page 388.*

PARALYSIS, RAPID ONSET

Usually the inability to use an arm or leg, but less commonly affecting muscles of the eyes, swallowing and breathing. The manner of onset gives a clue to the cause.

Urgent medical attention is always needed.

PROBABLE
STROKE
SUBARACHNOID HEMORRHAGE
INJURY

POSSIBLE
ARTERIAL DISEASE

RARE
HYSTERIA

PROBABLE

■ STROKE
This is the overwhelmingly likely cause, being interference with blood flow to the brain usually from a suddenly damaged or blocked blood vessel. Normally in the middle-aged or elderly.
* Often a history of high blood pressure.
* Paralysis affects one side of the body.
* Face may droop.
* Speech is slurred.
* Confusion of variable degree, even coma.

Treatment consists of nursing and intensive physical therapy, plus attention to underlying causes, such as high blood pressure or heart disease. In many cases a return to near-normal function is achieved. Occasionally, investigations show up a brain tumor or abscess.

■ SUBARACHNOID HEMORRHAGE
A special type of stroke, caused by a bleeding blood vessel on the surface of the brain.
* Relatively common in those aged 55-60 but possible at any age.
* Sudden, severe headache, "like being hit in the back of the head".
* Collapse, neck stiffness, sensitivity to light.

Surgical intervention is sometimes necessary to stop bleeding and to prevent further occurrences.

■ INJURY
* A severe blow to the head.
* Probably coma and one-sided paralysis.

POSSIBLE

■ ARTERIAL DISEASE
Sudden paralysis of one leg, less commonly an arm, may be due to blockage of an artery if there is also:
* Sudden pain.
* Sudden paleness of the limb, developing into blueness. The limb is extremely cold.

To save the limb, the obstruction must be rapidly removed surgically.

RARE

■ HYSTERIA
See page 398. In exceptional cases, sudden apparent paralysis is a possible feature.

PARALYSIS, SLOW ONSET

PROBABLE
COMPRESSION OF A NERVE

POSSIBLE
BRAIN TUMOR
MULTIPLE SCLEROSIS
VITAMIN B12 DEFICIENCY

RARE
GUILLAIN-BARRE SYNDROME
MOTOR NEURONE DISEASE
POLIOMYELITIS

PROBABLE

■ COMPRESSION OF A NERVE
Common sites are the neck, affecting the arms; or a "slipped" disc in the back, affecting a foot.
* Persistent pain and tingling confined to one part of one limb.
* Partial weakness of the affected limb.
* Health otherwise good.

Investigations may show a reason for the compression and exclude general disease of the nervous system. Treatment depends on the cause.

POSSIBLE

■ BRAIN TUMOR
* Slow, progressive weakness of one side of the body.
* Headache.
* Change of personality.

The slow progression makes diagnosis difficult, but brain scans have improved the chance of reliable diagnosis.

■ MULTIPLE SCLEROSIS
A slowly degenerative disease of the young to middle-aged.
* Often begins with a sudden loss of vision in one eye.
* Numb patches, tingling, weakness of limbs, clumsiness.

THE BRAIN AND NERVOUS SYSTEM

* Symptoms come and go over months and years.

The outlook is very variable, often with years of relatively good health. An unfortunate minority become severely disabled.

■ VITAMIN B12 DEFICIENCY

* Pale skin.
* Tingling of hands and feet.
* Smooth, sore tongue.
* Stiff, weak legs.

The commonest cause is pernicious anemia (*see page 421*), easily treated with injections of Vitamin B12.

RARE

■ GUILLAIN-BARRE SYNDROME

A rare inflammation of the spinal cord that may follow a minor viral illness.

* Initially, tingling in the hands and feet.
* Paralysis of the limbs rapidly appears.
* May spread to involve muscles of swallowing and breathing.

This serious condition needs intensive nursing care and assistance with breathing. Although recovery may take months, 80 percent of sufferers recover completely.

■ MOTOR NEURONE DISEASE

An exceptionally rare, tragic disease of deterioration of muscle function in middle age.

* Begins with loss of bulk of the muscles of the hands.
* Muscle-wasting spreads more generally, with resulting paralysis.
* Widespread twitching of the muscles.
* Mental function remains intact.

There is no known cure.

■ POLIOMYELITIS

Rare now, because of vaccination programs.

* Mild, viral symptoms of sore throat, diarrhea, muscle aches.
* Sometimes symptoms of meningitis; *see page 444*.
* Then increasing muscle ache.
* Followed by paralysis, especially of leg and shoulder muscles.

Recovery can take a year; residual paralysis is common.

CHANGE OF PERSONALITY

PROBABLE
PSYCHOLOGICAL DISORDER(S)

POSSIBLE
ALCOHOL OR DRUG ABUSE
HEAD INJURY
STROKE

RARE
BRAIN TUMOR

PROBABLE

■ PSYCHOLOGICAL DISORDER(S)

It is hardly surprising that psychological factors underlie most changes of personality, since personality is the sum of our emotional state, mood, and intelligence and reflects our upbringing and experiences. Any psychological disease can affect personality.

Noticeable features include:
* Anxiety.
* Emotional instability.
* Irritability.
* Aggression or passivity.
* Delusional thought.
* Self-neglect.

These symptoms have to be judged against the background of:
* General health.
* Relationships.
* Pressures at work and at home.
* Age.
* Drug and alcohol consumption.

The symptoms are covered elsewhere in this section under individual headings. Stress and minor anxiety states will most often be to blame.

POSSIBLE

■ ALCOHOL OR DRUG ABUSE
Usually a self-evident diagnosis, suggested by:
* Self-neglect.
* Trembling, shaking.
* Emotional instability.
* Memory loss.

■ HEAD INJURY
See page 400.
Personality change is a common consequence, together with:
* Irritability.
* Poor memory.

■ STROKE
See page 404. The resulting brain damage can cause erratic behavior, irritability and emotionally instability.

RARE

■ BRAIN TUMOR
Although a rare reason for personality change, doctors bear it in mind if rapid change in personality is combined with:
* Recent severe headaches, which wake the individual at night.
* Double vision.
* Seizures suddenly occurring in adult life.
* Weakness of one side of the body.

Most brain tumors are secondary cancers, arising from cancer, often from the lung or breast. Brain scans have revolutionized diagnosis. Treatment depends on the exact type of tumor and may only be decided at the time of operation.

OBSESSIONS AND PHOBIAS

Meaning morbid fears or repeating the same ideas and thoughts over and over. Mild obsessions are common: for example, fear of spiders, or checking you have locked a back door three times before going on vacation. Severe forms can dominate your life: for example, agoraphobia, a fear of open spaces. Probably these symptoms reflect an inner insecurity, though often there is no obvious cause.

THE BRAIN AND NERVOUS SYSTEM

PROBABLE
PSYCHOLOGICAL FACTORS

POSSIBLE
SCHIZOPHRENIA

PROBABLE

■ PSYCHOLOGICAL FACTORS
In this situation, external factors causes stress, which leads to exaggerated feelings. These then become an obsession or phobia.
* Personality and thought is normal.
* The individual knows what is happening.

It is only when the particular focus of your obsession and phobia starts to make life unnecessarily difficult or impossible that you need professional help.

POSSIBLE

■ SCHIZOPHRENIA
* Strange obsessions.
* Hallucinations, delusions.

Presumably the obsession makes sense within the schizophrenic's distorted world-view.

SHOCK

In medical language, "shock" means a massive and rapid fall in blood pressure with its accompanying effects, and is a very serious condition that requires rapid treatment. This is totally different from the layman's use of the term in which shock is the emotional reaction to a serious psychological blow, such as terrible news or witnessing a serious accident. True medical shock is considered here in the context of the brain and nervous system because shock can appear to be a nervous reaction — indeed, the nervous system is in part responsible for its occurrence.

Anyone thought to be in shock needs emergency help as quickly as possible.

See also BLUISH SKIN, page 424, and COLLAPSE WITH SHOCK OR COMA, page 471.

Critical features of medical shock are the rapid appearance of:
* Collapse.
* Sweating.
* Pale skin.
* Weak, thready pulse.
* Confusion.

EMOTIONAL SHOCK
Features following a severe "fright reaction" include:
* Pale skin.
* Numbness of thought.
* Difficulty in concentrating.
* Life seems trivial.
* Nothing matters except the event.
* Tearfulness.
* Feelings of guilt.
* Loss of confidence.

Continuous support from relatives and friends is important. Talking about the event and getting emotions out, including crying, are helpful and necessary.

The Brain and Nervous System

PROBABLE
BLOOD LOSS
HEART ATTACK

POSSIBLE
SERIOUS INFECTION
DEHYDRATION
ALLERGIC SHOCK

PROBABLE

■ BLOOD LOSS
The source may be obvious, for example, after a stab wound or accident. Other symptoms of internal bleeding are:
* Black vomit.
* Black, tarry-looking stool following a severe blow to the abdomen.
* Ectopic pregnancy *(see page 355).*

■ HEART ATTACK
A combination of:
* Chest pain.
* Collapse.
* Breathlessness.

See page 228.

POSSIBLE

■ SERIOUS INFECTION
Danger arises when infection spreads into the bloodstream. Commonest in babies or the elderly.
* Usually a pre-existing illness, commonly of the chest or of the skin.
* Fever, sweats and rigors.
* Rapid collapse.
* Purple spots may appear on the skin.

■ DEHYDRATION
Loss of fluid from the body eventually causes:
* Thirst.
* Restlessness.
* Dry mouth, lax skin.
* Reduced output of urine.

Those especially at risk are babies and diabetics.

■ ALLERGIC SHOCK
Medical term is anaphylaxis. This is an unpredictable reaction to things like a bee sting, an injection, or some foods.
* Face and lips swell within minutes.
* Rapid appearance of red welts or patches on the skin.
* Breathing rapidly becomes wheezy.
* Collapse, possibly within a few minutes.

Those who know they are at risk should carry medication in their purse or automobile. This is usually an antihistamine or adrenaline shot.

"General" Symptoms

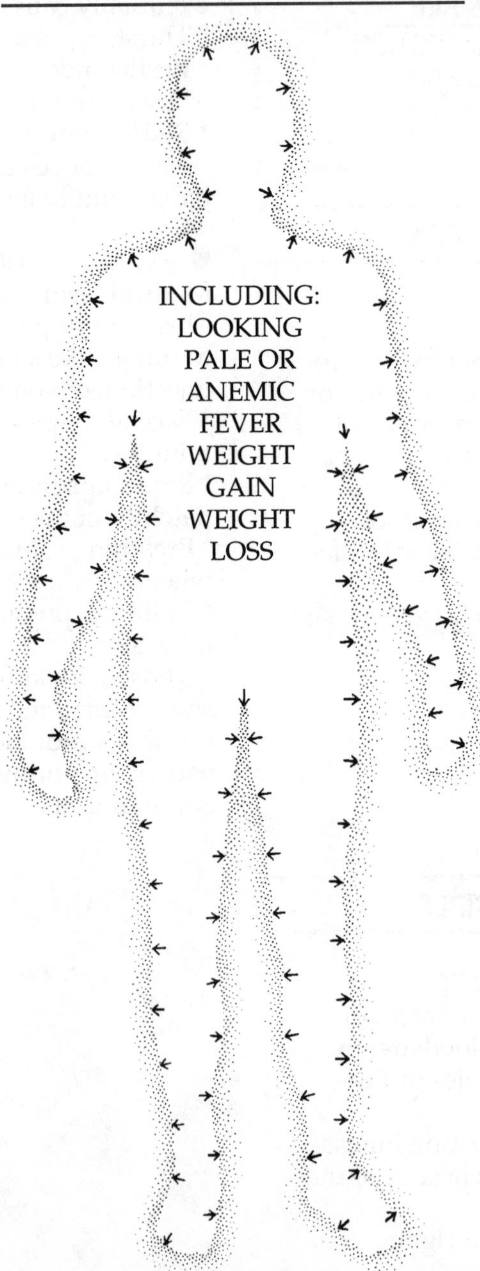

VERY SMALL BABY

Defined as less than 5lb (2.5 kg) birth weight. These babies tend to:
* Have difficulty feeding.
* Become jaundiced, with the possibility of effects on brain development.
* Have breathing problems immediately after birth.

Routine prenatal care aims to detect and to control problems in the mother such as high blood pressure, severe stress, smoking, alcohol or drug use which might result in a premature or a low birth weight baby. Frequently the reason for low birth weight is unknown and the baby goes on to develop into a normal child.

PROBABLE
DISADVANTAGED MOTHER
SMOKING IN PREGNANCY
PREMATURE BIRTH

POSSIBLE
MULTIPLE PREGNANCY
MATERNAL ILLNESS IN PREGNANCY
DRUGS
ABNORMALITY OF THE BABY

RARE
INFECTION IN THE MOTHER

PROBABLE

■ SOCIO-ECONOMIC DISADVANTAGE
The birth weight of a baby is linked to the mother's standard of living and probably reflects her general nutrition and self-care during pregnancy.

■ SMOKING
Babies born to mothers who smoke are, on average, about 1/2lb (0.25 kg) lighter than babies of mothers of similar socio-economic level who are non-smokers. The message is clear. If you really cannot stop smoking in pregnancy, try to cut back.

■ PREMATURITY
A baby born before 37 weeks gestation, for any reason. Sometimes doctors find it difficult to judge whether a baby is premature or has a low birth weight. The diagnosis depends on the overall appearance and behavior of the baby.

POSSIBLE

■ MULTIPLE PREGNANCY
The average birth weight of babies decreases in each pregnancy after the first three or four births. If there are twins or triplets, each baby often weighs less than average.

■ MATERNAL ILLNESS IN PREGNANCY
The most common in developed countries is high blood pressure. Worldwide, severe malnutrition is the major problem.

"GENERAL" SYMPTOMS

■ DRUGS
Mothers using drugs are likely to have small or premature babies. These babies may show signs of drug addiction and withdrawal and may be retarded in their development.

■ ABNORMALITY OF THE BABY
Many congenital abnormalities cause low birth weight, especially cerebral palsy, commonly known as brain damage.

RARE

■ INFECTION DURING PREGNANCY
Rubella is the commonest and is avoidable through vaccination.

No one can be certain of the long-term consequences of low birth weight, but there is strong evidence that babies born small can remain smaller than average at least up to puberty, and sometimes into adult life. Severely low birth weight babies must spend a long time in intensive care, and some will have delayed development or long-term affects on brain function.

BABY OR CHILD UNABLE TO PUT ON WEIGHT OR TO GROW ADEQUATELY

The medical term for this symptom is "failure to thrive", and applies to babies and young children who fail to reach the accepted milestones of development for their age. The baby will be checked for physical reasons, but it is well recognized that emotional neglect or severe family stress can also contribute to failure to thrive.

Feeding advice can be sought from pediatricians, family physicians, health departments, WIC programs and La Leche League.

PROBABLE
FEEDING PROBLEM
LOW BIRTH WEIGHT
NEGLECT

POSSIBLE
VOMITING
MALABSORPTION
INFECTION
FAMILY STRESS

RARE
HYPOTHYROIDISM

PROBABLE

■ FEEDING PROBLEMS
No neglect is implied, but simple problems such as:
* Feeds prepared incorrectly.
* Teat openings too small to allow adequate intake.
* An over-rigid feeding schedule.
* Difficulty with breast feeding.
* The baby rapidly catches up once the problem is identified. La Leche League, a national baby feeding organization, is available to give advice on the telephone.

"GENERAL" SYMPTOMS

■ LOW BIRTH WEIGHT
Severely premature babies, with low birth weight, may not to grow as well as normal babies at first. Babies born small but on time can be expected to grow at a normal rate, although they remain smaller compared to other children.

■ NEGLECT
This includes emotional neglect, as well as food deprivation.
* A withdrawn, unresponsive child.
* Fearful of strangers.
* Other signs of neglect such as injuries, bruising, dirtiness. This must be reported to social services.

POSSIBLE

■ VOMITING
All babies vomit, some more than others. It usually gets better over time and the baby's weight soon catches up. Pyloric stenosis is a not uncommon reason for persistent vomiting. It is caused by a blockage in the stomach and relieved by a minor operation:
* Much commoner in boys than girls.
* Vomiting begins after the first few weeks of life.
* The baby feeds normally, then vomits forcefully — called projectile vomiting.
* The baby is very hungry.

■ MALABSORPTION
The child has a normal intake of food, yet fails to grow. Suspicious symptoms would include:
* Chronic diarrhea, especially with bulky, greasy, foul-smelling stools.
* Recurring chest infections.

The commonest causes of malabsorption in developed countries are *CYSTIC FIBROSIS, page 146* and *CELIAC DISEASE, page 146*.

■ INFECTION
Repeated infection over time slows down growth. The most common causes are urinary and ear infections, causing fevers and belly pain. However, urinary infections may cause no symptoms at all, other than poor growth. They need to be investigated.

■ FAMILY STRESS
Although the baby is not neglected, severe stress, like divorce, spouse abuse, depression in the mother can affect the baby's development.

RARE

■ HYPOTHYROIDISM
An underactive thyroid gland. Appears in the first few weeks of life. Sometimes this goes undetected. If severe, symptoms could include:
* Prolonged jaundice in the days after birth.
* A lethargic baby, tending to constipation and poor feeding.
Routine screening tests are usually done in the hospital for this easily treated condition.

BIRTH ABNORMALITY PLUS FAILURE TO GROW

If the causes of failure to grow on *pages 412-3* have been excluded, malformation might be suspected. Specialists will test for: interference with swallowing, perhaps due to a cleft palate; cerebral palsy; heart disease; a *CHROMOSOMAL ABNORMALITY (see page 417)*; or (rare), a metabolic disorder or kidney failure. See relevant sections for further details.

DISTRESSED OR CRYING BABY

First, know your child. All mothers know that a child will cry in different ways, depending on whether he or she is hungry, angry or in pain. Daily experience of your child qualifies you to recognize when the child is crying in an unusual way. When this happens, check through the common causes. Remember also that a usually placid baby or child can become irritable in response to your own mood, or even to the way you handle it.

PROBABLE
HUNGER OR THIRST
DISCOMFORT
DESIRE FOR COMFORT

POSSIBLE
COLIC
INFECTION
PAIN

RARE
MENINGITIS

PROBABLE

■ HUNGER OR THIRST
* Due for a feed?
* Roots for the teat or nipple.
* Sucks eagerly.

■ DISCOMFORT
* A soiled diaper.
* Too hot: flushed, sweating.
* Cold: blue hands, cold to the touch.
* Noise, bright lights, smoke?

■ DESIRE FOR COMFORT
* Excited when you appear.
* Crying stops when cuddled, recurs when put down.

POSSIBLE

■ COLIC
* After a feed or in the evening.
* Draws up legs, whimpers.
* Relieved by winding or, in the case of evening colic, the problem simply stops after a few weeks.

■ INFECTION
* Runny nose, a *COLD (see page 454)* or a cough.
* Other signs of infection: increased sleepiness, fever, rash, will not eat normally.

■ PAIN
* Rubbing ear; teething?
* More of a scream than a cry.
* Only briefly relieved by comforting.

RARE

■ MENINGITIS *(see page 444)*. A serious infection of the brain which can appear quickly in a previously well baby or child. Because of the difficulty of diagnosis, see a physician immediately if you suspect meningitis. He or she will admit the child to hospital for tests and evaluation.
* The baby or child is initially irritable.
* Increasingly drowsy, lethargic and floppy.
* Vomiting.
* Soft spot on skull may be bulging.
* High-pitched cry.
* Fine purple skin rash.

SHORT STATURE

This is generally defined as height which is in the lowest three percent of the population for age. Although parents worry about it, regular measurements at three-month intervals will show whether a child is small, but growing at a normal rate.

PROBABLE
FAMILY PATTERN
SMALL-FOR-DATES BABY

Achondroplasia

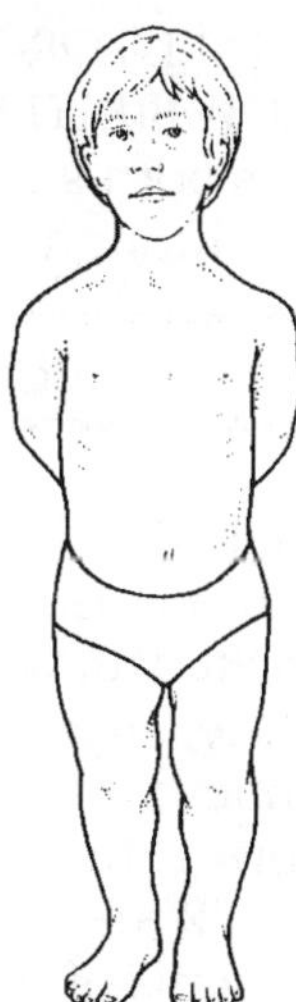

POSSIBLE
CHROMOSOMAL DISORDER
CHRONIC DISEASE
HYPOTHYROIDISM
ACHONDROPLASIA

RARE
GROWTH HORMONE DEFICIENCY

PROBABLE

■ FAMILY PATTERN
Short parents usually have children who will be short, although genetic mechanisms ensure that, on average, the children become taller than the parents. There are formulas, based on parental height, which can help to predict the final height of a child.

"GENERAL" SYMPTOMS

■ SMALL-FOR-DATES BABY
See LOW BIRTH WEIGHT, page 412.
Babies born small may remain small throughout life.

POSSIBLE

■ CHROMOSOMAL DISORDER
Common disorders are DOWN'S SYNDROME, with characteristic flat face; large hands; fold of skin on inner part of eyeball and other abnormalities. Another is TURNER'S SYNDROME; two symptoms of this condition are:
* Webbed neck.
* Infertility in later life.

■ CHRONIC DISEASE
Any long-term disease will stunt growth. Common culprits are kidney disease and heart disease.

■ HYPOTHYROIDISM
An under-active thyroid gland. *See page 460.* Most babies are screened for this condition. Treatment enables growth to resume at a normal rate.

■ ACHONDROPLASIA
A genetic disorder. The child is very small:
* Very short limbs.
* Large head, normal trunk.
* Normal intelligence.

RARE

■ GROWTH HORMONE DEFICIENCY
This unusual condition is now treatable by giving injections of the missing hormone.
* The child is normal, but grows slowly.
* Tendency to be overweight. Mental development is normal.

BLUISH-COLORED SKIN

See BLUISH SKIN, page 424.

BODY SIZE

See ACROMEGALY, page 275 and TALLNESS, page 428.

BRUISING

PROBABLE
ACCIDENT
PHYSICAL ABUSE

POSSIBLE
BLOOD DISORDER
SCURVY

PROBABLE

■ ACCIDENT
Bruises on exposed areas, such as shins, knees or elbows, which come and go.

■ PHYSICAL ABUSE
Suggested in particular if there is a history of family difficulties.
* Multiple bruises of varying ages, some old, some fresh.
* Inadequate explanation.
* Appearance of neglect — dirty, ill-fed.

* Bruising around ankles or wrists.
* The characteristic bruising of bite marks is not unusual on abused children. Must be reported to social services.

POSSIBLE

■ <u>BLOOD DISORDER</u>
Severe anemias and serious blood disorders.
* Purple spots or patches appear on skin.
* Spontaneous bleeding from gums, nose.
* Rapid onset in an already ill person.

A blood test is essential and should be taken as soon as possible. *See also BLEEDING — SPONTANEOUS AND GENERAL, page 426.*

■ <u>SCURVY</u>
Caused by lack of Vitamin C. *See page 426.*

PALE APPEARANCE, COMING ON SLOWLY

Some people are naturally pale, so the best way to check for a decrease in normal skin color is to look at the areas where blood flows close to the surface, for example beneath the finger-nails and under the eyelids.

PROBABLE
ANEMIA

POSSIBLE
HYPOTHYROIDISM

RARE
HYPOPITUITARISM

PROBABLE

■ <u>ANEMIA</u>
See also page 420. Inadequate supply of essential nutrients in the diet to make normal blood.

General features include:
* Tiredness; being easily fatigued.
* Breathlessness — gradual onset.
* Dizziness, especially on standing up.

In addition, there may be symptoms suggesting the underlying cause, such as:
* Weight loss.
* Swelling of belly.
* Self-neglect.
* Sores on skin and bruising.
* Heavy menstruation.
* Jaundice.

POSSIBLE

■ <u>HYPOTHYROIDISM</u>
See also page 460. An under-active thyroid gland causes a slow-down in all aspects of body function over several months. As well as pale skin, which is due both to a

"GENERAL" SYMPTOMS

mild anemia and to changes in the skin, you may notice:
* Sensitivity to the cold.
* Gruff voice, coarse skin, thinning hair.
* Constipation, slowness of thought.

This condition is readily treatable by taking thyroid medication once the diagnosis has been established by a physician.

RARE

■ HYPOPITUITARISM
A failure of the pituitary gland in the brain, crucial to controlling many hormones — the body's "chemical messengers". Pale skin can be a striking feature of this condition, plus other symptoms, such as:
* Hypothyroidism, as above.
* In women, menstruation ceases; loss of sexual drive.
* Loss of pubic hair, and hair under arms.
* Lack of stamina.

Usually treatable to some degree.

PALE APPEARANCE, COMING ON RAPIDLY

Over days, hours or minutes. Unless the individual has simply fainted, this may well signify a problem which requires urgent medical attention. The likeliest reason is blood loss.

PROBABLE
A FAINT
INTERNAL BLEEDING

POSSIBLE
HYPOGLYCEMIA
HEART RHYTHM DISORDER
GASTRIC UPSET
HEART ATTACK

RARE
ACUTE BLOOD DISORDER

PROBABLE

■ A FAINT
The many well-recognized causes of fainting include missing a meal; emotional shock; prolonged standing; excessive heat; pregnancy.
* Otherwise good health.
* Initial lightheadedness, sweating, dizziness.
* Collapse to ground or on to furniture.
* Cold, clammy skin; thin, slow pulse.

It is essential to leave someone who has fainted lying flat until they recover, which generally takes just a few minutes.

■ INTERNAL BLEEDING
Often there is a previous history of belly discomfort. The blood loss may be obvious:
* Bloody or black stools.
* Blood in urine.

* Vomit containing blood or with specks looking like coffee grounds.
* Excessive vaginal bleeding, especially after a delayed period.

Early symptoms are similar to those of anemia, *see page 420,* but of more rapid onset. As blood loss increases there will be:
* Severe dizziness.
* A feeling of being cold, with cold, sweaty extremities.
* Low urine output.
* Rapid breathing.
* Eventually, drowsiness and unconsciousness.

There may be signs of the cause of the bleeding. Previous dyspepsia (indigestion) suggests a duodenal or gastric problem. Bowel disturbance may signify inflammation of the bowel, a tumor or a perforation (hole) in the intestine. Aspirin and other anti-arthritic drugs can also cause bleeding into the bowel.

POSSIBLE

■ HYPOGLYCEMIA

A problem for diabetics, especially those on insulin, who must learn to recognize the early symptoms:
* Hunger, irritability, lightheadedness, progressing to:
* Sweating, confusion, slurring of speech, unconsciousness.

Taking sugar or glucagon gives relief in minutes.

■ HEART RHYTHM DISORDER

Very rapid, slow or irregular heart rhythms mean that blood is pumped around the body with reduced efficiency. Commonest in the 50-plus age group.
* You may be aware of a thumping or a fluttering in your chest.
* Onset is usually abrupt; symptoms often end abruptly, too.
* Pale face, breathlessness, dizziness.

■ GASTRIC UPSET

The early stages of a severe attack of gastroenteritis may start with:
* Nausea, vomiting, sweating, cramping belly discomfort.
* Pale skin.
* Diarrhea follows within a few hours.

■ HEART ATTACK

Looking pale will probably not be the only, or even the main, symptom. The classic picture is:
* Crushing pain in the central chest.
* Breathlessness, sweating, pale skin.

Heart attacks, especially in the elderly, may not be so clear-cut, causing just pale skin, fatigue and breathlessness.

RARE

■ ACUTE BLOOD DISORDER

Including leukemia and any breakdown in the blood's clotting mechanism. Commonest in children and young adults. Suggested by:
* A bad sore throat, vague ill health, then paleness.
* Nose bleeds, bleeding gums, blood in bowel or urine.
* Spontaneous bruising.

LOOKING PALE OR ANEMIC

When the body's red blood cells fall below the necessary level, or if hemoglobin, the oxygen-carrier in red blood cells, is somehow impaired or reduced, anemia develops. It results in:
* Pale skin — an important sign of anemia, but often a misleading one, since many people are naturally pale.
* Feeling tired much of the time.
* Fatigue on exertion.
* Faintness (in severe cases).
* Flat fingernails.

There are many possible causes of anemia.

PROBABLE
BLOOD LOSS IN MENSTRUATION
PREGNANCY
RAPID GROWTH (in childhood)
POOR DIET

POSSIBLE
PERNICIOUS ANEMIA
CHRONIC BLEEDING
SICKLE CELL ANEMIA

RARE
CANCER OR OTHER CHRONIC DISEASE
THALASSEMIA
WORM INFESTATIONS

PROBABLE

■ BLOOD LOSS IN MENSTRUATION
The two to three ounces of blood lost in normal menstruation is replaced by the body within a day or two. However, anemia is a risk if:
* Periods are very heavy, with clots.
* Menstruation is very frequent.
* Periods are prolonged, or there is bleeding in between.
* If you have a poor diet.

■ PREGNANCY
Anemia in pregnancy is detected by routine blood tests. In fact, it is so common in pregnancy that some degree of anemia is considered normal.

Iron and vitamin, including Folic Acid, supplements are usually given to pregnant women.

■ RAPID GROWTH
During childhood growth spurts, the body's need for iron and vitamins may outstrip the supply. The result can be slight anemia, just enough to make the child tire easily. A balanced diet should overcome this effect, so vitamin and iron supplements only make sense if your child's diet really is poor.

■ POOR DIET
That is, a diet deficient in iron or in the vitamins needed to make hemoglobin. The elderly, alcoholics or those on low incomes are at risk.

* Lack of meat, eggs or green vegetables.
* Cracked skin at corners of the mouth.
* Easy bruising, bleeding gums.

Leaving vegetables to soak, or boiling them for a long time, will destroy their vitamin and iron content. Steaming vegetables is preferable to boiling them; microwave cooking is excellent.

Dark leaf vegetables, fish, eggs, liver, meat and cereals are sources of iron.

POSSIBLE

■ PERNICIOUS ANEMIA
Caused by lack of Vitamin B12, because of failure to absorb the vitamin.
* Gradual onset, sometimes leading to very low levels of hemoglobin.
* Often, a family history.
* Sore, smooth tongue.
* Tingling, numbness of limbs.
* Unsteady walk.
* Slight jaundice is possible.

■ CHRONIC BLEEDING
Caused by disease, such as a bleeding peptic ulcer, or by drugs, of which aspirin and NSAIDs (anti-inflammatory agents) are the commonest. Also, don't underestimate the effect of chronically bleeding hemorrhoids.
* Passage of bloody or black stools.
* Blood in vomit.
* Excessive or prolonged menstrual bleeding (*see page 420*).

* Features of underlying disease, weight loss, anorexia, alteration of bowel habit.

■ SICKLE CELL ANEMIA
Blood cells have a genetic tendency to break down when there is a shortage of oxygen, or a fever. This happens as attacks of:
* Painful joints or muscles.
* Blood clots.
* Jaundice.
* Gallstones.
* Strokes
* Leg ulcers.

RARE

■ CANCER OR OTHER CHRONIC DISEASE
Anemia is unlikely to be the only symptom, except for cancers causing internal bleeding (*see CHRONIC BLEEDING, this page*). The same is true of chronic diseases such as kidney failure or rheumatoid arthritis.

■ THALASSEMIA
Occurs because of a failure of the mechanism which produces normal hemoglobin. It is familial.
* Generally causes a mild, chronic anemia, though more serious forms exist.

■ WORM INFESTATIONS
For example, tapeworm or hookworm; rare in many countries, but common causes of anemia in tropical countries. Detected from stool samples.

LOOKING PALE OR ANEMIC PLUS SKIN PROBLEMS

Rashes, sores and skin changes can be a feature of anemia, but usually only if the anemia is especially severe or if it is one of the rarer types which are a side effect of some other underlying disease.

PROBABLE
IRON DEFICIENCY ANEMIA

POSSIBLE
PERNICIOUS ANEMIA
SICKLE CELL ANEMIA

RARE
MEDICATION SIDE-EFFECT
AUTO-IMMUNE DISEASE

PROBABLE

■ IRON DEFICIENCY ANEMIA
See also anemia, page 420. General features of anemia, plus:
* Painful cracked skin at corners of mouth.
* Sore, smooth tongue.

POSSIBLE

■ PERNICIOUS ANEMIA
* Can cause a sore, smooth tongue.
See anemia, page 420, for more details.

■ SICKLE CELL ANEMIA
Can cause leg ulcers. *See page 421.*

RARE

■ MEDICATION SIDE-EFFECT
Any medication which causes anemia may also cause skin rashes, blotches, bruises and a sore mouth.

■ AUTO-IMMUNE DISEASE
A range of diseases in which the body attacks its own components resulting in general effects of feeling sick, rashes, joint pains.
* A butterfly-shaped rash across the cheeks is characteristic of *SYSTEMIC LUPUS ERYTHEMATOSUS, page 448.*

LOOKING PALE OR ANEMIC, PLUS LOSING WEIGHT

These symptoms are of concern in people of middleage and older. There is the possibility of underlying disease causing internal bleeding or possibly affecting the ability of the body to absorb the food, iron and vitamins needed to make red blood cells. In children, the combination is more likely to suggest poor food intake or a malabsorption condition.

PROBABLE
NEGLECT
MALABSORPTION

POSSIBLE
ANOREXIA NERVOSA
CHRONIC DISEASE
CANCER OF THE BOWEL
CANCER OF THE STOMACH

RARE
CHRONIC MYELOID LEUKEMIA

PROBABLE

■ NEGLECT
Typically self-neglect, with a diet so poor that individuals are literally starving themselves. In developed countries, it may be seen in the very poor, the frail elderly living alone, alcoholics and the mentally ill who are untreated and without support.

In children, there may be other signs of neglect by their guardians, such as:
* Unexplained bruising or injuries.
* Dirty appearance.
* Withdrawn behavior.
* No food in the house.

■ MALABSORPTION
The term covers a range of conditions which block digestion. Some clues which suggest malabsorption as the cause of anemia and weight loss are:
* Gradual appearance of symptoms
* Change in bowel habit, with persistent, loose stools or diarrhea.
* An apparently adequate intake of food.
* Appetite healthy until later stages of the illness.
* Co-existing, recurrent chest infections

Bowel cancer is common. Routine, annual bowel examinations and stool tests are increasingly used to test for signs of cancer. This is wise for people over the age of 50, or over the age of 40 if there is a family history of bowel cancer or other risk factors. Inspection of the lower bowel with a lighted flexible tube (sigmoidoscope) is also used to screen high-risk people for cancer or pre-cancer.

POSSIBLE

■ ANOREXIA NERVOSA
Although most common in young women, it is sometimes seen in men. Those with anorexia are often good athletes or high achievers at school. The signs are:
* Obsession with body image: the individual is convinced that she or he is overweight.
* Appearance may vary from very slim to outright starved.
* In women, menstrual periods cease.
* An excess of fine body hair may appear.
* Bouts of binge eating (bulimia).

"GENERAL" SYMPTOMS

■ CHRONIC DISEASE
Several chronic diseases, such as tuberculosis or long-term infection, can cause this combination of symptoms. The nature of the underlying disease will not necessarily be clear. Seek help from your physician if any symptoms persist.

■ CANCER OF THE BOWEL
This common cancer has an excellent outlook if diagnosed sufficiently early. Besides anemia and weight loss, the other warning signs are:
* Persistent change of bowel habit — for instance, the bowels open daily whereas they used to be open less often, or vice versa.
* Blood in stools.
* Mucus or slime from back passage.
* A feeling of not completely emptying the bowel.

■ CANCER OF THE STOMACH
Again, the earlier this is diagnosed, the better the outlook.
* Indigestion and acidity as a new symptom in middle age.
* Loss of appetite.
* Pains in upper abdomen.
* Vomiting of blood or passage of black stools.

RARE

■ CHRONIC MYELOID LEUKEMIA
A disease of gradual onset in middle age.
* Enlarged liver.
* Enlarged spleen.
* Diagnosis made on blood tests.

BLUISH SKIN

Otherwise known as cyanosis: a bluish-purple coloring, visible especially where blood flows close to the surface, for example the lips, the tongue and under the fingernails. It arises when blood becomes short of fresh oxygen from the lungs. Fingers commonly show cyanosis in cold weather due to sluggish blood flow. In more serious cases, the lips and tongue also become blue.

PROBABLE
TEMPORARY POOR CIRCULATION

POSSIBLE
CHRONIC BRONCHITIS OR EMPHYSEMA
INHALED FOREIGN BODY
HEART FAILURE

RARE
CONGENITAL HEART DISEASE (CHILDREN)
DRUG OVERDOSE

PROBABLE

■ TEMPORARY POOR CIRCULATION
Common at any age:
* Results from a drop in temperature.
* A slight degree of cyanosis confined to fingers and toes, which feel cold and numb.

* Disappears rapidly on warming the limb.
* Worse in winter, better in summer.

Occasionally, a blood clot may block the circulation to part of a limb, usually the lower leg or toes. This gives a quite different set of symptoms, typically found in an elderly person with pre-existing circulatory disease.
* Sudden onset of pain, coldness, numbness and paralysis of the limb.
* Limb may at first look pale, cyanosis setting in over a few hours.

This is an emergency: seek urgent medical help.

POSSIBLE

■ CHRONIC BRONCHITIS/EMPHYSEMA

See page 222. These are lung diseases causing persistent cough, wheeze and breathlessness. It is only after many years of disease that cyanosis becomes a regular feature, by which time the sufferer has long suffered breathlessness on the slightest exertion.
* Cyanosed nail beds, tongue and lips.
* Hands and feet can feel surprisingly warm.

■ INHALED FOREIGN BODY

The rapid appearance of cyanosis in someone who is breathless suggests a sudden obstruction to airflow. In children it may be caused by inhaling a small object.
* Typically occurs when eating steak or similar chunky food.
* Clutching at the throat, trying to gasp; clearly very distressed.

The Heimlich maneuver is a useful first aid procedure designed to relieve such obstructions.

For Heimlich Maneuver, *see page 235.*

■ HEART FAILURE

Mild heart failure is quite common, caused usually by diseased coronary arteries. It is readily and effectively treatable. Only in severe cases is cyanosis a prominent symptom together with:
* Constant breathlessness.
* Swollen legs.
* Breathlessness on lying flat.
* Coughing frothy fluid.

RARE

■ CONGENITAL HEART DISEASE (CHILDREN)

Usually produces a "blue" or cyanosed baby, because the blood is not pumped properly through the lungs.
Symptoms show at, or very soon after, birth.
* Breathlessness on feeding.
* Baby is distressed.
* The baby fails to gain weight normally during the first few weeks and months of life.
* Dizziness, headache and fatigue.
* Blood clots.

■ DRUG OVERDOSE

Suspected in an otherwise well young person who is:
* Unconscious.
* Breathing reduced to a point at which cyanosis appears.

BLEEDING

Everyone experiences surprise bleeding from time to time: blood on the tooth brush or perhaps bleeding from the rectum. Look up these symptoms in detail under the relevant sections for the part of the body involved.

APPETITE, LOSS OF

See NO APPETITE, page 473.

BLEEDING — SUDDEN AND GENERAL

Covered here is sudden bleeding from different parts of the body: the gums or nose; blood in the urine, in stools and from the vagina. It will almost certainly be accompanied by widespread bruising. The symptoms point to a general breakdown of the blood clotting process.

PROBABLE
SCURVY

POSSIBLE
ANTICOAGULANT OVERDOSE
THROMBOCYTOPENIA

RARE
HEMOPHILIA
SEVERE INFECTIONS

PROBABLE

■ SCURVY
Results from a diet lacking vitamin C, which is contained in fresh fruit and vegetables. So the problem is usually one of the elderly or the poor.
* Chronic feeling of being ill.
* Bleeding, especially from between the teeth.
* Sore gums, loose teeth.
* Easy bruising.

Readily treated by vitamin C supplements.

POSSIBLE

■ ANTICOAGULANT OVERDOSE
The drug warfarin is widely used for certain heart disorders, and also for thrombosis in a limb. Regular blood tests help to check that the dose is correct, but overdosage can happen easily.

See your physician immediately if you begin bleeding unexpectedly while taking warfarin. Nosebleeds can be the first sign of excessive dosage, which in some cases can even be fatal.

■ THROMBOCYTOPENIA
A general term for a fall in the numbers of platelets in the bloodstream. Platelets are crucial to blood clotting, so if they are in

short supply, widespread bleeding occurs. Many serious general illnesses can cause thrombocytopenia, the cause usually being obvious after just a few tests, for example:
* Aplastic anemia, with rapid appearance of weakness, pale skin and feeling sick.
* Childhood leukemia, as with aplastic anemia, but also sore throat.
* Adult leukemias: a slower onset than childhood leukemias, enlarged lymph nodes, sweats.
* Bone cancers, with pain, sickness, weight loss.

Thrombocytopenia can also be medication-induced. There is also a benign form, affecting children, which cures itself spontaneously. Treatment is aimed at the underlying cause, if known.

RARE

■ HEMOPHILIA
A bleeding disorder, caused by an inherited abnormality in the blood clotting system. Almost exclusively in males.
* A family history is common: two-thirds of cases are hereditary.
* Early symptoms are prolonged bleeding from, say, a small cut; spontaneous bruising; bleeding into joints, giving joint pain and swelling.

■ SEVERE INFECTIONS
Many serious infectious diseases cause chaos in the blood clotting system. These include septicemia (blood poisoning), malaria and typhoid fever.
* Sweats and chills.
* Generally very ill.

BLOOD SLOW TO CLOT

You may notice this as easy bruising; bleeding from the gums and teeth; blood in the urine or stools; or unusually heavy menstruation.

POSSIBLE
SCURVY
EXCESS OF ANTICOAGULANT MEDICATION

RARE
HEMOPHILIA

POSSIBLE

■ SCURVY
Vitamin C deficiency, associated with diets low in fresh fruit.
* Widespread, spontaneous bruising.
* Sore gums, loose teeth.
* Vague ill health.

Vitamin C treatment reverses the condition.

■ EXCESS OF ANTICOAGULANT MEDICATION
See page 426.

RARE

■ HEMOPHILIA
See this page.

"GENERAL" SYMPTOMS

TALLNESS

Meaning (for a given age) height greater than that of the tallest three percent of the population. Only rarely is tallness due to disease.

PROBABLE
NATURAL TENDENCY
EARLY PUBERTY

POSSIBLE
HYPERTHYROIDISM

RARE
EXCESS GROWTH HORMONE
MARFAN'S SYNDROME

PROBABLE

■ NATURAL TENDENCY
Tall parents usually have tall children. There are formulas which can predict a child's height, based on the heights of the parents.

■ EARLY PUBERTY
The complex hormonal changes of puberty can make a child leap up in height. In later puberty, growth slows, so the child who was unusually tall may finish smaller than his or her peers who reach puberty later. The familiar signs of puberty are:

* Growth of body hair around genitals and in the underarms.
* Breast development.
* Deepening voice.

POSSIBLE

■ HYPERTHYROIDSM
This will enhance growth in childhood. *See page 479.*

RARE

■ EXCESS GROWTH HORMONE
In children, this causes excessive height and size. In adults it causes acromegaly with progressively coarse, heavy features.
* Enlargement of hands and feet.
* Protrusion of lower jaw.
* Possibly heavy sweating and diabetic symptoms.

■ MARFAN'S SYNDROME
This hereditary condition affects about two people per 100,000; it causes:
* Long thin bones, spider-like fingers and toes.
* An unusually high arch to the palate.
* Heart valve problems, which may cause breathlessness.
* Visual disturbance through dislocation of the lens of the eye.

SWOLLEN BODY

Three categories of disorder cause generalized body swelling: heart failure, kidney disease and low-protein states.

The mechanics of swelling are complex. Because fluid sinks to the lowest level of the body, the early signs are swollen ankles in the evening or a puffy face on waking. As more fluid accumulates, swelling spreads up the legs and builds up inside the belly and chest.

PROBABLE
PRE-MENSTRUAL SWELLING
PRE-ECLAMPSIA
HEART FAILURE

POSSIBLE
NEPHRITIS
LIVER DISEASE
MALNUTRITION
MALABSORPTION

RARE
NEPHROTIC SYNDROME
VITAMIN B1 DEFICIENCY

PROBABLE

■ PRE-MENSTRUAL SWELLING
Hormone changes in the few days before menstruation cause a mild degree of fluid retention:
* A regular pattern each month; health otherwise normal.
* Breasts, abdomen, ankles all become slightly enlarged.
* Weight gain of a few pounds.
* Disappears within days of the start of menstruation.

■ PRE-ECLAMPSIA
Rapid swelling due to fluid retention in late pregnancy. Checks may also show a rise in blood pressure and protein in the urine. Requires hospital treatment. Commonest in first pregnancies.
* Rapid weight gain over a few days.
* Swollen fingers and feet.
* Headaches, dizzy spells, nausea.
Treatment of pre-eclampsia is necessary to prevent progression to eclampsia — dramatic rise in blood pressure, epileptic seizures, danger to the baby.

■ HEART FAILURE
A common cause of persistent swelling of the legs in later life.
* Often high blood pressure, angina or other heart disease.
* At first, swelling of ankles, tiredness.
* Later, breathlessness on activity, or when lying down.
* Attacks of breathlessness at night, coughing frothy sputum.
Modern medications can usually provide effective treatment, although the swelling may not clear completely.

POSSIBLE

■ NEPHRITIS
Actually a group of diseases, all of which involve some degree of inflammation of the kidneys. This causes swelling of the body, partly due to loss of protein in the urine and partly due to failure to produce sufficient urine. In children, nephritis presents with:
* Sudden onset, often after a

"GENERAL" SYMPTOMS

minor throat infection.
* Low urine output.
* Blood in urine.
* Puffiness, especially of the face.
The outlook for recovery is good. In adults it tends to present more slowly, with:
* Progressive swelling of the legs.

Assessment involves blood tests and biopsy of the kidney.

■ LIVER DISEASE
One of the liver's many functions is to make proteins. These circulate in the blood stream, and if their levels fall, body swelling follows.
* Often a history of alcohol abuse, hepatitis, medications toxic to the liver.
* Easy bruising, blood-stained vomit.
* Tiredness, loss of sexual drive, clubbed fingers.
* Tiny, spider-like red veins on face, upper body.
* Red palms.
* Swelling of the belly, caused by fluid.
* Jaundice is a late symptom, as is confusion, coma.

■ MALNUTRITION
Globally, this is a major cause of swelling in children:
* Swollen belly.
* Patchy pigmentation of body.
* Apathy, coarse skin, lack of resistance to infection.

■ MALABSORPTION
A possibility in those with chronic bowel disease, for example celiac disease or ulcerative colitis — which interfere with absorption of nutrients. Some general symptoms include:
* Failure to thrive (children); diarrhea, greasy stools.
* Bleeding from bowel.
* Chronic belly pain.
* Recurrent, severe chest infections.
* Clubbing of finger-nails.

RARE

■ NEPHROTIC SYNDROME
The term describes generalized swelling associated with low blood protein and heavy loss of protein in the urine. There are many causes, including medications and chronic infections, as well as kidney disease. It produces a characteristic, gradually developing picture of:
* Puffy face, swollen eyelids.
* Belly distended with fluid.
* Breathlessness, tiredness.

Recovery depends on the cause. Children usually recover completely.

■ VITAMIN B1 DEFICIENCY
Also called beri-beri. Vitamin B1 (thiamine) is found in whole-grain cereals including rice, and in liver. In developed countries, the deficiency is likely only through severe malnutrition or alcohol abuse.
* Early symptoms are sore legs and vague weakness.
* Then swelling of legs, palpitations.
* Eventually, general swelling, exhaustion, rapid pulse.

Treatment with B1 gives dramatic improvement within hours. Many manufactured foods and cereals contain added levels of this vitamin.

SWOLLEN PART OF BODY

PROBABLE
INJURY
INFECTION
DEPENDENT EDEMA

POSSIBLE
LYMPHATIC OBSTRUCTION
VENOUS THROMBOSIS

RARE
ALLERGY
CANCER

PROBABLE

■ INJURY
Tissue swelling is the normal reaction to moderate injury, together with reddened, warm skin.

■ INFECTION
Including insect bites and minor cuts.
* Throbbing pain, redness.
* Swelling of local lymph glands.
* Pus may be visible.

■ DEPENDENT EDEMA
One of the commonest reasons for a mild degree of ankle swelling is inactivity such as on long airplane flights. Older people who sit all day at home or at work may notice it.
* General health good.
* Swelling lessens if activity is increased.

No need for treatment unless it is a nuisance.

POSSIBLE

■ LYMPHATIC OBSTRUCTION
Also known as lymphedema. Results from interference with the lymphatic channels, which drain away tissue fluid. Commonest after surgery in the groin or underarm — typically to treat breast cancer. In rare cases it can be present from birth.
* Swelling of limb.
* Swelling becomes hard; does not "pit" when pressed.

■ VENOUS THROMBOSIS
Sudden swelling of a limb, nearly always a leg, suggests thrombosis. It occurs when clotted blood obstructs a blood vessel.
* Acute onset of pain in lower leg.
* Swelling and warmth of lower leg.

If confirmed, needs anti-coagulants to reduce the risk of a clot in the lung *(see page 225)*.

RARE

■ ALLERGY
In reaction to an insect bite or injection.
* Limb swells dramatically in a few seconds.
* Swelling may spread to body, lips, throat.
* At worst, difficulty breathing, collapse *(see page 468)*.

Needs medical attention urgently.

■ CANCER
Suspected in otherwise unexplained swelling of a limb. Long bones are the likeliest sites.
* Persistent pain, tenderness.
* Enlarged local lymph nodes.

Cancer may also obstruct the drainage of fluid from a limb: for example, pelvic cancers may cause swelling in the legs.

WEIGHT LOSS WITH ANEMIA

See LOOKING PALE OR ANEMIC, PLUS LOSING WEIGHT, page 422.

WEIGHT LOSS AND LACK OF APPETITE

See NO APPETITE, LOSING WEIGHT, page 475.

WEIGHT LOSS — PROGRESSIVE

Persistent, progressive weight loss ranks as one of the major symptoms of disease. Medical assessment is essential for this symptom.

The following are some of the possibilities for which there are few other symptoms to point the way. Many of these possibilities are considered in more detail elsewhere in the book.

PROBABLE
DIABETES MELLITUS
ANXIETY
CANCER OF THE STOMACH

POSSIBLE
CHRONIC INFECTION
ANOREXIA NERVOSA
HYPERTHYROIDISM
PYLORIC STENOSIS
TUBERCULOSIS
CANCER — GENERAL

RARE
MALABSORPTION
PARASITE INFECTION
KIDNEY DISEASE
HIV INFECTION/AIDS

"GENERAL" SYMPTOMS

PROBABLE

■ DIABETES MELLITUS
In young adults and children, the onset of diabetes tends to be dramatic: rapid weight loss is prominent, along with thirst and excessive urine output. *See page 484.*

■ ANXIETY
A modest, slow weight loss could reasonably be put down to anxiety or stress in the absence of other symptoms, and where there is no other clear physical cause. Anxiety should not divert attention from the significance of a steady weight loss, particularly in adults, where other causes must be checked out.

■ CANCER OF THE STOMACH
Early detection of this cancer gives the best hope of cure. For this reason, the possibility is considered in any adult with weight loss, especially if there is also:
* Loss of appetite.
* Blood in vomit or in stools.
* Pain in upper belly.
* Feeling of fullness after eating only a small amount.
* Indigestion appearing for the first time in someone over the age of 40.

POSSIBLE

■ CHRONIC INFECTION
This includes chronic abscesses — *see page 447.*

■ ANOREXIA NERVOSA
Excessive dieting, usually in young women who have a distorted body image. *See page 423.*

■ HYPERTHYROIDISM
Weight loss alone is unusual, unless the accompanying tremor and sweating have been overlooked. Described on *page 479.*

■ PYLORIC STENOSIS
A childhood condition: part of the intestine is obstructed, causing profuse vomiting and rapid weight loss a few weeks after birth. *See page 144.*

■ TUBERCULOSIS
The poor, alcoholics and people from underdeveloped countries might have this serious but curable infection. *See page 447.*

■ CANCER — GENERAL
Lay persons and physicians think of cancer to explain weight loss in the 40-plus age group. It is by no means the only explanation, yet it remains true that, occasionally, an advanced cancer, which has spread around the body, produces only vague symptoms until a late stage. So, be aware of your body: report to your physician any unusual changes such as bleeding, swellings, weight loss, pain or prolonged cough.

RARE

■ MALABSORPTION
This causes weight loss by preventing the absorption of food. Associated symptoms are:

"GENERAL" SYMPTOMS

* Difficulty in swallowing.
* Anemia.
* Recurrent belly pains, intermittent diarrhea, greasy stools.
* Blood in stools.

Underlying causes include cancer of the esophagus, which causes very rapid weight loss, ulcerative colitis, Crohn's disease, coeliac disease and chronic pancreatitis.

■ PARASITE INFECTION
Diagnosis is confirmed by identifying cysts in stools.

■ KIDNEY DISEASE
This needs to be confirmed by blood and urine tests. *See page 467.*

■ HIV INFECTION/AIDS
Now to be considered in any case of vague ill-health, weight loss, fevers and cough, particularly when an individual is at increased risk: homosexuals, bisexuals, intravenous drug users.

Heterosexuals, too, are increasingly affected by the HIV virus.

LOSING WEIGHT PLUS JAUNDICE

The combination points to disease of the liver and related parts of the digestive system. Appearance in adults must trigger a careful search for a primary cancer, which may have spread to involve the liver. The jaundice results from obstruction to bile flow from the liver.

PROBABLE
CANCER OF THE PANCREAS
SECONDARY CANCER OF LIVER

POSSIBLE
CANCER OF THE STOMACH
PERNICIOUS ANEMIA

RARE
CANCER OF GALL BLADDER

PROBABLE

■ CANCER OF THE PANCREAS
The pancreas lies at the back of the abdomen, partly surrounding the bile duct. The tumor blocks the bile duct, producing jaundice.
* Initially, vague upper belly pain.
* Weight loss.
* Painless jaundice.

■ SECONDARY CANCER OF LIVER
Cancers of many kinds can spread around the body from their original site. The liver is a common secondary site. The primary cancer is likely to have shown itself already, with symptoms such as:
* Weight loss.
* Pain.
* Swelling.
* Unusual bleeding.

POSSIBLE

■ CANCER OF STOMACH
See STOMACH DISEASE, page 164.

■ PERNICIOUS ANEMIA
The combination of anemia and a yellow tinge to the skin gives an impression of jaundice. The diagnosis is based on blood tests. *See page 421*. Treatment reverses symptoms.

RARE

■ CANCER OF GALL BLADDER
A disease causing symptoms similar to gall stones.
* Jaundice, sometimes without any other symptoms.
* Recurrent pains in the right upper abdomen.

BODY APPEARS STIFF AND HUNCHED

PROBABLE
AGING

POSSIBLE
ANKYLOSING SPONDYLITIS
PARKINSON'S DISEASE
PAGET'S DISEASE

RARE
TUBERCULOSIS OF THE SPINE
RICKETS
SCOLIOSIS

PROBABLE

■ AGING
With age, bone density is lost and there is shrinkage of the discs between the vertebre — the bones which link together to form the spine. In some post-menopausal women, rapid thinning of bone, or osteoporosis, takes place, leaving the vertebre somewhat delicate and liable to collapse.
* Spine becomes hunched over several years.
* Collapse of a vertebra causes a sudden change of posture plus pain.

Calcium and hormone replacement therapy are being used increasingly to help delay and alleviate this process.

POSSIBLE

■ ANKYLOSING SPONDYLITIS
A disease that begins in early adult life, especially affecting men. Over many years, the normal joints and ligaments of the spine are replaced by inflexible bone. Genetically transmitted.
* First, just back pain, and morning stiffness of the spine.
* The back becomes increasingly rigid, with a stooped posture.
* Eventually, spine movements are severely restricted.

The stooped posture, though not totally avoidable, need not be as severe a problem as in the past, thanks to improvements in treatment.

"GENERAL" SYMPTOMS

■ PARKINSON'S DISEASE
See page 438. A neurological disease rarely present before the age of 50. The main symptoms are:
* Trembling of the hands at rest.
* Stooped, rigid posture.
* Shuffling gait.
* Immobile facial expression.

■ PAGET'S DISEASE
A disorder of bone formation, quite common in a mild form in later life and frequently causing no symptoms.
* Pain in bones.
* Legs becomes bowed, back stoops; head may enlarge (hat size may increase).
* Deafness.

Advanced cases are generally easy to recognize, but usually X-rays and blood tests are needed to confirm the diagnosis.

RARE

■ TUBERCULOSIS (TB) OF THE SPINE
This used to be common. The infection destroys bone.
* Increasing pain and stiffness in part of the spine.
* Other features of TB such as feeling sick, weight loss, cough, night sweats.

■ RICKETS
A bone disease caused by a disturbance in the way calcium is incorporated. Other symptoms include some bone pain, bow legs and weakness. Associated with poor diet and living conditions. Cured by taking vitamin D.

■ SCOLIOSIS
A sideways bending of the spine develops in childhood. It tends to give an S-shape to the spine. In race cases a severe deformity develops in adult life.

LOOKING OLD BEFORE YOUR TIME

POSSIBLE
SMOKING
HYPOTHYROIDISM
SUN DAMAGE (HOT CLIMATES)

POSSIBLE

■ SMOKING
This is known to accelerate the development of lines on the face and coarsening of the skin.

■ HYPOTHYROIDISM
See page 460. This common condition makes the skin thicken and coarsen.

■ SUN DAMAGE
In hot, sunny climates, where people spend a lot of time outside, sun damage is the most common cause of a prematurely aged appearance.

BODY SIZE, SHRINKING

PROBABLE
OSTEOPOROSIS

RARE
PAGET'S DISEASE OF BONE

PROBABLE

■ OSTEOPOROSIS
See page 276.

RARE

■ PAGET'S DISEASE OF BONE
Also known as osteitis deformans. Abnormal turnover of bone causing thickening and deformity of bones, particularly the skull, and the long bones. The bone, despite appearing thicker, is weaker than normal bone. The disease affects men and women equally, but rarely affects people from Asia, Africa and the Middle East. It normally appears after the age of 40. Although often symptom-free, there may be:
* Bony deformities. The skull may appear large; often, only one bone is affected.
* Fractures.
* Kyphosis *(see page 288)*, causing apparent height loss.
* Heart failure, due to increased workload on heart.
* Vision and hearing deteriorate as deformed bone damages nerves.

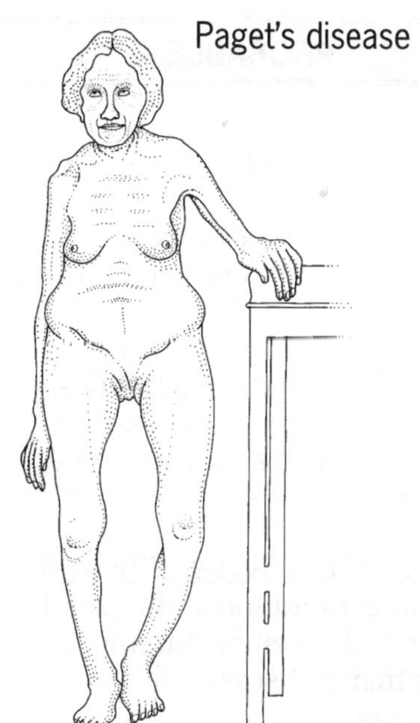

Diseased bone can, very rarely, develop into a malignant bone tumor — osteosarcoma. Diagnosis is confirmed by blood tests.

TREMBLING OR SHAKING

PROBABLE
NATURAL PHYSIOLOGICAL CAUSE
BENIGN ESSENTIAL TREMOR

POSSIBLE
HYPERTHYROIDISM
PARKINSON'S DISEASE
ALCOHOL ABUSE

RARE
BRAIN DISEASE
SYPHILIS

"GENERAL" SYMPTOMS

PROBABLE

■ NATURAL PHYSIOLOGICAL CAUSE
How steady are your hands? Everyone has tremor (trembling or shaking) to some degree.
* Mostly causes no interference with delicate manual activities.
* Worsened by anxiety, alcohol, stimulants such as coffee, some medications.

■ BENIGN ESSENTIAL TREMOR
An exaggerated form of normal tremor and an embarrassment rather than a disease.
* Hereditary.
* Slow tremor, affecting upper limbs and head.
* Gradually worsens with age.

POSSIBLE

■ HYPERTHYROIDISM
See page 479. An over-active thyroid gland causes an exaggeration of normal tremor.

■ PARKINSON'S DISEASE
Trembling movements of the thumb and forefinger:
* An early symptom is loss of normal swinging of arms when walking.
* Limbs held rigid, slowing of all movements.
* Tremor at rest, improves with activity.
* Immobile, "mask-like" facial appearance.
* Handwriting becomes increasingly small.

There are now many useful treatments for this common disorder.

■ ALCOHOL ABUSE
Heavy, chronic alcohol intake and especially withdrawal can produce trembling.

RARE

■ BRAIN DISEASE
Brain tumors, strokes, multiple sclerosis and head injuries may all cause tremors. Associated symptoms might include:
* Paralysis of one side of the body.
* Progressive headache, blurring of vision.
* Change of personality.
* Deterioration of memory, slurring of speech.
* Noticeable flickering movements of the eyes.
* Difficulty in walking.

■ SYPHILIS
Syphilis has become more common again and its effects can appear many years after infection, so it is still routinely considered as a possible cause of dementia.
* Dementia.
* Tremor of the head and the lips.
* Stiff legs.

TWITCHING

Uncontrollable, short-lived muscle jerks. There is rarely any reason to suspect disease in the absence of other symptoms.

PROBABLE
HABIT
SPASMODIC TORTICOLLIS

POSSIBLE
BENIGN FIBRILLATION
EPILEPSY

RARE
CHOREA
GILLES DE LA TOURETTE SYNDROME
MOTOR NEURONE DISEASE
KIDNEY FAILURE

PROBABLE

■ HABIT
Blinking and similar grimaces, normal in everyone to a degree, which sometimes become excessive.
* Frequency increases under stress.
No satisfactory treatment.

■ SPASMODIC TORTICOLLIS
Recurrent jerking of the neck to one side.
* A disorder of the middle-aged.
* The individual is otherwise perfectly well.

Treatment with botulinum toxin looks promising.

POSSIBLE

■ BENIGN FIBRILLATION
A part of a muscle that twitches spontaneously; the thigh and around the eye are common sites.
* Other muscles unaffected.
* Muscle strength normal.
* Disappears after a few days.

■ EPILEPSY
Spasmodic jerking of limbs is a feature of most forms of epilepsy:
* Same limb is affected each time.
* Brief warning before the jerking episode starts.
* May progress to a generalized seizure, with loss of consciousness, incontinence, foaming at mouth. There is usually very little doubt that epilepsy is the cause.

RARE

■ CHOREA
Irregular movements of limbs. Rheumatic fever was once a common cause; *see page 448*. Other neurological conditions with twitching as a feature include Huntington's chorea:
* A strong family history.
* Disintegration of personality in middle age.
* Eventually, dementia, epilepsy, paralysis.

"GENERAL" SYMPTOMS

■ GILLES DE LA TOURETTE SYNDROME
A disorder with a reputation out of all proportion to its rarity.
* Onset in adolescence.
* Multiple tics.
* Abrupt cursing, grunting.
* Echoing other people's words.

■ MOTOR NEURONE DISEASE
Exceptionally rare, tragic disease causing deterioration of muscle function in middle age.
* Begins with loss of bulk of muscles in hands.
* Muscle-wasting spreads generally.
* Widespread twitching of muscles may be seen.
* Mental function remains intact.
* Eventually, paralysis.

■ KIDNEY FAILURE
A late symptom in someone already known to have kidney disease:
* Nausea, vomiting.
* Twitching of muscles.
* Clouded consciousness.
* Spontaneous bleeding.
* Low urine output.

FEVER, INTRODUCTION

Just why the body produces fever in response to illness is still not fully understood. Generally it is thought that the white blood cells produce chemicals called pycogens that stimulate the metabolism.

Fevers often tell us much about the illness itself, as certain illnesses have special patterns of fever.

Common causes of fever not related to disease include: exercise, heat stroke, wearing too many clothes (especially in children), dehydration and some medications.

WHEN TO GET CONCERNED?
In the very young and in the elderly, fever calls for a careful assessment of health; but in older children and for much of adult life a day or two of raised temperature will usually be the prelude to one of the minor illnesses considered in the following pages. Of course, there are more dangerous possibilities, but they are rare, and fever alone is not automatically a cause for alarm.

Before getting concerned, look at the person's overall condition, assessing:
* Risk factors for unusual disease, for example, foreign travel, poor sanitation, local epidemics.
* Rapid onset of a high fever — greater than 104°F (40°C).
* Severe headache or delirium.
* Pain.
* Night sweats.
* A rapid pulse or fast breathing, remembering that:
* Pulse rate rises by about ten beats per minute for every 0.5 degree Centigrade rise in temperature.
* A baby's normal pulse rate is about 120 per minute, even at one year of age.

TAKING TEMPERATURE
An adult's normal temperature is conventionally taken to be between 35°C - 37°C/96°F - 98.6°F, based on a mouth reading. Body

temperature is usually low in the morning and higher in the evening. Fever occurs if temperature is more than a 100°F (37.7°C). High fevers in babies and small children can cause seizures. *See page ... for Febrile Seizures.*

In children, temperature can be measured under the arm (36.5°C/97.7°F is the norm).

Take into account:

* Mouth breathers, whose mouth temperature is lower than normal.
* The amount of clothing worn may raise or lower temperature.
* Warm or cold drinks alter temperature in the mouth for about 15 minutes.

Feeling the forehead offers comfort, but is not very reliable, especially if there is a low-level fever, with sweat on the forehead that cools the skin.

FEVER: THE POSSIBILITIES

To list all the hundreds of possible reasons for fever would simply be confusing. Instead, we look, on the following pages, at fevers of different durations. We believe that this is how you will usually meet the problem.

The possibilities listed are generally those expected in a developed country. There is a separate section (*see page 450*) on what to do about diseases that may be brought back home after foreign travel. We remind you again that fever in the very young and very old demands special attention, and that it is reasonable to get professional advice, even if the fever itself is minor.

FEVER, THE FIRST 48 HOURS, this page.
FEVER, 3 TO 14 DAYS, page 444.
FEVER LASTING TWO WEEKS OR MORE, page 446.
FEVER, RECURRENT ATTACKS, page 449.
FEVER AFTER VISITING OTHER COUNTRIES, page 450.

FEVER, THE FIRST 48 HOURS

See also FEVER, INTRODUCTION page 440. Along with the fever there will be some combination of chills, muscle aches, sweating, a mild headache and tiredness.

PROBABLE

VIRAL ILLNESS
GASTROENTERITIS
EAR INFECTION
TONSILITIS
CHEST INFECTION
SINUSITIS

POSSIBLE

URINARY INFECTION
CHICKENPOX
RUBELLA
MUMPS
SCARLET FEVER

RARE

MENINGITIS

"GENERAL" SYMPTOMS

PROBABLE

■ VIRAL ILLNESS
Including the build-up to a common cold; *see page 454.*
* Mild, sore throat.
* Symptoms vary between mild and irritating within hours.
* Sniffing and sneezing begins after a couple of days.
* Cough.
* Aches and pains in muscles.

■ GASTROENTERITIS
Usually caused by a virus or food poisoning.
* Belly cramps.
* Diarrhea, sometimes with blood.
* Nausea – occasionally vomiting.

Improves rapidly, if not seek medical help.

■ EAR INFECTION
Very common in children, sometimes with no other symptoms.
* Typically, the child already has a cold.
* Abrupt onset of pain in ear, often at night.
* Babies just begin crying and will not settle, even with comforting. They may shake their head, or rub an ear.
* Occasionally progresses to a burst ear drum, causing a green/yellow, possibly bloodstained discharge for a few days. Healing over a couple of weeks is normal.

Painkillers will help the symptoms. Needs medical assessment.

Mumps

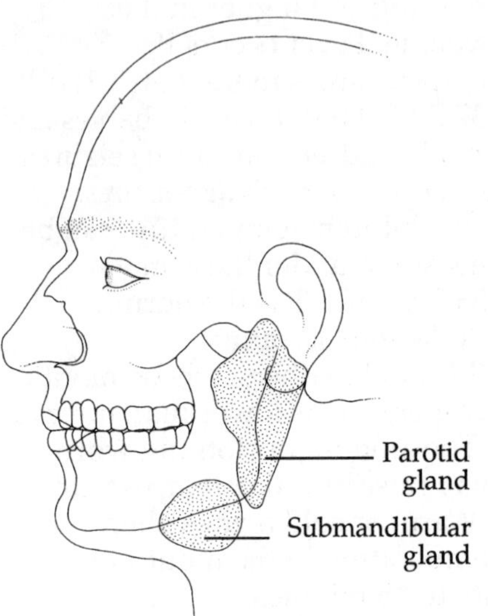

■ TONSILITIS
The picture presented is usually clear.
* Pain in the throat, worse on swallowing.
* Swollen neck glands.
* Nasal twang to speech.
* Breath smells foul.
* White spots on the tonsils.

A quick test can reveal whether it is a virus or strep throat, which needs penicillin.

■ CHEST INFECTION
Again, the picture is usually clear.
* Cough.
* Mucus, often yellow or green.
* Chest pain when breathing deeply.

■ SINUSITIS
Usually improves within a few days, if not seek medical attention. *See page 454.*

POSSIBLE

■ URINARY INFECTION
* Pain or burning sensation when passing urine.
* A need to pass urine frequently.
* Aching over the kidneys.
* In severe cases, chills, blood in the urine.
* In babies, there may be no symptoms other than fever and irritability, hence the need to test urine in a feverish infant.

■ CHICKENPOX
A viral illness causing small blisters over the body, in the mouth and in the scalp. Usually occurs in epidemics. Incubates for about 14-21 days after contact with another carrier.
* Itchy rash appears within 48 hours of fever.
* Rash lasts for two or three weeks.

The rash consists of spots, which tend to appear in crops and soon become blisters; they dry out and become scabs.

Usually a mild, though miserable, illness calling for plenty of care and attention.

■ RUBELLA — GERMAN MEASLES
Mild in itself but notorious because of the risk to the developing baby if the mother catches it during early pregnancy. For this reason there are public health vaccination programmes which have made the disease less common.
* A fine, red-brown rash appearing after 24-48 hours of fever.
* Rash with no particular pattern to its spread appears all at once.
* Swollen tender glands at the back of the skull.
* In adults, often accompanied by mild arthritis lasting for some weeks.

■ MUMPS
An infection of the salivary glands, increasingly uncommon thanks to vaccination programs. The incubation period is two to three weeks.
* Non-specific fever and chills for 24-48 hours..
* Then the salivary glands enlarge at the angles of the jaw and just in front of the ears.
* The illness settles in five to ten days.
* Complications can give pain in the testicles and the abdomen, and cause deafness, but these are rare.

■ SCARLET FEVER
Onset is sudden with high fever, sore throat or even tonsillitis; *see above.*
* A very fine generalized red rash after 24-48 hours.
* The rash spares the area around the mouth, giving it a contrasting, white appearance.
* Furred tongue goes from whitish to raw over a few days.

Scarlet fever was once much feared because it could cause rheumatic fever *(see page 448)* and nephritis *(see page 429)*. These complications are now extremely rare. However, penicillin is still necessary if scarlet fever is diagnosed.

"General" Symptoms

RARE

■ MENINGITIS
Mentioned here as a reminder that it should be considered in any feverish child, especially if the child shows:
* Drowsiness.
* Stiff neck.
* A wish to avoid bright lights.
* Sudden appearance of a fine purple rash.
* And, in a baby, a bulging soft spot (fontanelle) on the top of the head.

If suspected, this is an emergency and medical help must be sought.

FEVER, 3 TO 14 DAYS

See also FEVER, INTRODUCTION page 440. Minor viral illness is still likely to underlie this symptom, just as with fever lasting 48 hours *(see page 441)*. However, the need to consider less common illnesses arises.

PROBABLE
VIRAL ILLNESS
MEASLES
ROSEOLA

POSSIBLE
GLANDULAR FEVER
PNEUMONIA
ABDOMINAL INFECTION
INFECTIOUS HEPATITIS
ROCKY MOUNTAIN SPOTTED FEVER
DYSENTERY

RARE
TYPHOID/PARATYPHOID FEVER
SEPTICEMIA
ENDOCARDITIS

PROBABLE

■ VIRAL ILLNESS
No rash, no progression, and no other symptoms apart from sweats, aches and generally feeling unwell. But although the cause is probably a virus, it is prudent to review the diagnosis every few days, considering the possibility of any of the following:

■ MEASLES
"Measles is misery" sums up this childhood illness, now avoidable thanks to vaccination. It usually occurs in epidemics, with an incubation period of 10 to 14 days from being infected by another carrier.
* A miserable, snuffly, coughing child with bloodshot eyes who wants to avoid bright lights.
* Delirium at night is common.
* White spots may be seen in the mouth by the back teeth.
* A blotchy red rash appears after

four days of fever, spreading downwards, from face via chest to the limbs.
* The child continues feverish for several more days as the illness subsides.

Measles is a serious problem in underdeveloped countries, but in developed countries its complications, such as pneumonia or encephalitis, are rare.

■ ROSEOLA
A fairly common, harmless viral illness which can fool physicians into suspecting measles.
* High fever for three to four days; the child is snuffly.
* A pinkish rash appears over the body.
* The fever stops, and the child improves.

POSSIBLE

■ GLANDULAR FEVER (MONO)
(see also page 462).
* Bad sore throat or tonsillitis.
* Fever and fatigue persisting for weeks or months.
* Swollen lymph glands.

The problem usually clears up.

■ PNEUMONIA
Certain forms of pneumonia are known for causing fever alone, without the other, more dramatic symptoms of pneumonia.
* Slight cough.
* Feeling vaguely unwell; fatigue, night sweats.

A chest X-ray confirms the diagnosis and treatment is straightforward.

■ ABDOMINAL INFECTION
Suspect this if fever starts soon after abdominal surgery, or after abdominal pain. Prolonged fever can signal an abscess in any of the abdominal organs, the commoner ones being:

The appendix, preceded by a few days of pain, which may start centrally but then settles low down on the right.

The large intestine: pain in the left lower side, possibly bleeding from the rectum, intermittent diarrhea.

Infected ovaries or fallopian tubes: lower abdominal pain, vaginal discharge.

■ INFECTIOUS HEPATITIS
This is now known to be caused by several different viruses, hepatitis B being the dangerous form, spread by shared needles used for intravenous drug abuse and by unprotected homo- and heterosexual intercourse. The incubation period of hepatitis A is a few weeks, of hepatitis B a few months.
* Fever, chills, joint pains, back aches; generally feeling unwell for a week.
* Jaundice — yellowish discoloration of the skin — first spotted in the whites of the eyes; then the skin turns yellow.
* Darkening of urine, light stool color.

There is no treatment other than rest. With hepatitis B there is a risk of long-term liver damage. Those at risk, including people exposed to blood in their work, should be vaccinated against hepatitis B.

"GENERAL" SYMPTOMS

■ ROCKY MOUNTAIN SPOTTED FEVER
A tick-borne infection occurring in many parts of North America.
* High Fever.
* Nausea.
* Headache.
* Belly pain.
* Rash on hands and feet, spreading inward.
* Muscle aches.

Immediate evaluation and treatment needed.

■ DYSENTERY
Caused by bacteria. Results from poor sanitation and infected drinking water.
* Belly cramps.
* Diarrhea, often with blood.
* Comes and goes.

Needs medical attention.

RARE

■ TYPHOID OR PARATYPHOID FEVER
Infections spread via food and water in conditions of poor sanitation. Profuse diarrhea is a major feature.
* Fever, gradually rising to a peak over a couple of weeks.
* Cough, headache, limb pains.
* After a week, a non-itchy rash appears on the stomach, chest and lower back. In typhoid, it is sparse and rapidly fading; in paratyphoid, more widespread.
* Diarrhea begins after a week or so, becoming profuse.

Typhoid is still a very serious illness, despite modern antibiotic treatment. Paratyphoid, though less serious, is nevertheless very unpleasant.

Immunization is recommended for many parts of the world.

■ SEPTICEMIA
This means infection spreading in the blood stream. It is usually a rapidly developing illness causing chills and collapse.

■ ENDOCARDITIS
See page 462. An infection of the valves of the heart, causing chronic illness including fever, anemia and clubbed finger-nails.

FEVER LASTING TWO WEEKS OR MORE

See also FEVER, INTRODUCTION, page 440. By now, fever is a diagnostic challenge. It is likely that someone who is ill as well as feverish for as long as this would be admitted to hospital for investigation.

However, in some people, fever shows itself only with the feeling of being vaguely unwell (malaise) together with night sweats and other symptoms pointing to nothing in particular. Causes now include not only infections, but also rheumatic diseases, connective tissue disease, cancers and drug side effects. But remember that many of the illnesses noted in *FEVER, 3 TO 14 DAYS, page 444,* could still be suspected, along with the following:

"GENERAL" SYMPTOMS

PROBABLE
CHRONIC INFECTION
TUBERCULOSIS

POSSIBLE
ULCERATIVE COLITIS
CANCER, LEUKEMIA
HODGKIN'S DISEASE
RHEUMATOID ARTHRITIS
RHEUMATIC FEVER
SYSTEMIC LUPUS
ERYTHEMATOSUS (SLE)

RARE
SYPHILIS
MEDICATION SIDE-EFFECT
BRUCELLOSIS
AIDS
BRAIN TUMORS
HYPERTHYROIDISM

PROBABLE

■ CHRONIC INFECTION
This is still the likeliest reason for prolonged fever. Recent surgery, together with abdominal pain, could be pointers. Pelvic inflammatory disease from gonorrhea is a common cause. Less common causes might include:

Prostatitis *(see page 362*: in men, pain in the lower belly above the genitals, burning urine.

Osteomyelitis *(see page 275)*: pain and tenderness in a bone; usually in children. The long bones, typically of the leg, are most commonly involved.

Bronchiectasis *(see page 223)*, causing persistent cough, sweats, possibly breathlessness, finger clubbing.

■ TUBERCULOSIS
A significant possibility, causing chronic illness, weakness and infection:
* A low-grade fever.
* Weight loss.
* Cough.
* Night sweats.
* Possibly bloodstained sputum.

POSSIBLE

■ ULCERATIVE COLITIS
A chronic inflammation of the bowel. The early symptoms can be limited to:
* Persistent diarrhea.
* Weight loss.
* Low-grade fever.
* Vague ill health.

Once suspicion is aroused, this illness can be rapidly confirmed and treated.

■ CANCER, LEUKEMIA
Fever otherwise unexplained and lasting for months brings these to mind. There may well be other suspicious symptoms such as:
* Weight loss.
* Unusual pains.
* Unusual bleeding from bowel, bladder, vagina, stomach.
* Chronic cough.

These symptoms may allow the cancer to be tracked down. Blood tests will screen for leukemia. Cancer of the kidney is one tumor well known to cause persistent fever.

"GENERAL" SYMPTOMS

■ HODGKIN'S DISEASE
Young people are at most risk of this disease of the lymph glands. As well as fever there will be:
* Persistently swollen, painless glands in the neck, groin or armpits.
* Night sweats.
* Anemia.

The sooner it is diagnosed, the greater the chance of a complete cure.

■ RHEUMATOID ARTHRITIS
Persistent fever and vague ill health can continue for several weeks. *See page 279.*

■ RHEUMATIC FEVER
Thankfully, a rarity in developed countries but, sadly, common elsewhere.
* Usually begins after a sore throat.
* Fleeting pains in knees, ankles, elbows.
* Rashes can occur.
* Jerkiness of movement, involuntary movements.

The heart valves are damaged, leaving the child prone to future heart disease.

■ SYSTEMIC LUPUS ERYTHEMATOSUS (SLE)
One of a group of connective tissue disorders in which the body reacts against its own tissues. It can be a very vague illness at first. Commonest in women aged between 30 and 50.
* Rashes, joint pains, feeling sick.
* A butterfly rash across the cheeks is typical.

Early diagnosis is important to prevent progression to the kidneys or the brain.

RARE

■ SYPHILIS
Characteristically, six to 12 weeks after the initial infection, syphilis causes:
* A rash over hands and feet, including the palms and soles.
* Fever, enlarged lymph nodes, aching joints.
* Wart-like swellings around genitals and anus.

Treatable with antibiotics.

■ MEDICATION SIDE-EFFECT
A number of medications may be suspected as the cause of a persistent fever. The body becomes allergic to them – for instance, antibiotics, phenothiazines.

■ BRUCELLOSIS
A disease spread through cow's and goat's milk, and therefore a risk for workers in the dairy industry.
* Gradual onset, with fevers, joint pains, cough, loss of appetite, night sweats.
* Bouts of fever every few days or every few weeks.
* Often cures itself.

■ AIDS
A risk mainly for drug abusers and homosexuals; but also increasingly present in the heterosexual population.
* Weeks or months of fever and night sweats.
* Diarrhea, slight swelling of lymph nodes.

* Loss of weight.

The change from being HIV positive to developing AIDS may be signalled by many different symptoms. Prolonged fever is just one of these.

■ BRAIN TUMOR
This can affect the temperature regulating mechanism in the brain, causing fever. Other symptoms usually present. *See page 394.*

■ HYPERTHYROIDISM
Over-active thyroid gland increases the metabolism of the body, raising the temperature. *See page 479.*

FEVER, RECURRENT ATTACKS

See FEVER, INTRODUCTION, page 440. Apart from brucellosis, most of these infections are somewhat unusual in developed countries. Their symptoms return after a period of apparent recovery. This is in contrast to the far more conventional pattern of infections in which there is fever by day or by night, whose disappearance can be taken as a reliable sign of recovery.

POSSIBLE
BRUCELLOSIS
MALARIA
TYPHOID

RARE
DENGUE
RELAPSING FEVER
TRYPANOSOMIASIS
YELLOW FEVER

POSSIBLE

■ BRUCELLOSIS
A disease spread through unpasteurised milk or cheeses, or through contact with cows and goats. It gives rise to bouts of fever for days at a time, which appear to settle, only to recur after weeks or months. *See also page 446.*

■ MALARIA
See page 453. Anyone who has returned from abroad, and who has been in an area where malaria is present, and who develops a high temperature and chills should be suspected of having this dangerous illness particularly if they have not been taking anti-malaria tablets. Depending on the type of malaria, the episodes of fever and shaking return every three or four days.

The fever may recur some months after foreign travel.

■ TYPHOID
A feverish illness causing severe diarrhea, spread through poor sanitation or contaminated water, or food — mainly shellfish products. *See page 446.* The illness takes three to four weeks to run its course.

"General" Symptoms

RARE

Meaning rare in developed countries. Elsewhere these are fairly common diseases, but they pose a relatively small risk for tourists. Check with the local "traveler's clinic" or call the Center for Disease Control International Traveler's Hotline at (404) 332-4559 about areas where these diseases might be a hazard, and for prevention advice. If you develop feverish illness soon after returning from a danger area, report it to a physician without delay, being ready with details of where you have been.

■ DENGUE
A mosquito-borne infection of south-east Asia and Africa.
* Begins with sudden fever, aches and rash.
* Severe pains in the bones are particularly characteristic.
* Improvement over about a week.
* Relapse after another few days, with a more widespread rash.

Recovery takes several weeks.

■ RELAPSING FEVER
Spread by ticks. Common in Africa, India, South America and parts of the Mediterranean.
* Abrupt high fever and confusion lasting for about a week.
* Then apparent recovery, followed by relapse after another week or so.
* Several further relapses may occur.

Effective treatment exists.

■ TRYPANOSOMIASIS
Sleeping sickness. Different forms exist in Africa and South America. Treatment, started early, is quite effective. After an insect bite there is typically:
* Painful swelling at the site of the bite.
* Then relapsing fevers, enlarged lymph nodes.
* Eventually, after months or years, lethargy, continuous mild confusion, headaches, drowsiness.

■ YELLOW FEVER
Especially prevalent in Africa, Central and South America. There is no specific treatment for this serious illness, but vaccination is effective.
* Abrupt fever, rigors, jaundice.
* Signs of improvement by fourth or fifth day.
* Relapse during the next week with more fever, jaundice.

FEVER AFTER VISITING OTHER COUNTRIES

Unusual disease should always be considered in someone who becomes feverish soon after returning from a "Third World" country or certain parts of "developed" countries where they are a known risk.

Protective measures and vaccinations exist for many of these diseases and anyone likely to be at risk should see their physician to arrange these before travelling. Some of the measures require time to become effective.

You may also check with the

Center for Disease Control, in Atlanta, GA, for up-to-the-minute information. Tel: (404) 332-4559.

ABNORMALLY LOW TEMPERATURE

Defined as a fall in "core" body temperature to below about 35°C/95°F when measured in the rectum. Technical term: hypothermia. Below about 32°C/89.5°C, there will be drowsiness, apathy, coma and eventually death.

Those at risk are the elderly without adequate heating and the new-born. Cold new-born babies do not shiver: they become lethargic, with cold limbs.

Hypothermia is an emergency, requiring immediate warmth and warm fluids. Severe hypothermia requires gradual, carefully monitored rewarming. Rapid heating up is dangerous.

Elderly people who suddenly become confused in the winter may be suffering from hypothermia.

Do not give alcohol to an elderly person whom you suspect is suffering from hypothermia. It may worsen their condition.

PROBABLE
EXPOSURE TO COLD

POSSIBLE
EXCESS ALCOHOL

RARE
HYPOTHYROIDISM
MEDICATION SIDE-EFFECT

PROBABLE

■ EXPOSURE TO COLD
* Shivering, feeling cold.
* Then apathy, slurred speech, difficulty in concentrating.
* Finally confusion, coma.

Remember, babies cannot control their temperatures as adults do. They are at risk in low temperatures, unless kept warm.

POSSIBLE

■ EXCESS ALCOHOL
By dilating blood vessels, alcohol increases heat loss. Add confusion (if not unconsciousness) following a heavy drinking bout, plus cold conditions, and there is potential for serious danger.

RARE

■ HYPOTHYROIDISM
A grossly underactive thyroid gland can cause severe hypothermia. It is rare nowadays for this degree of underactivity not to be noticed. *See page 460.*

■ MEDICATION SIDE-EFFECT
Anti-depressants and tranquillizers can make temperature drop. Usually this is a trivial effect, unless the

"General" Symptoms

medications are taken in overdose or combined with self-neglect, alcohol and exposure to the elements.

SHIVERS OR CHILLS PLUS FEVER AND HEADACHE

In adults, this combination of symptoms, in a mild form, is not unusual and is often the earliest sign of a viral illness. In children this is by far the most likely reason, but other possibilities need to be considered, especially if the headache seems to be the major feature.

PROBABLE
COMMON COLD
INFLUENZA
SINUSITIS

POSSIBLE
CHEST INFECTION
INFECTION ELSEWHERE

RARE
MENINGITIS
WEIL'S DISEASE
MALARIA
OTHER TROPICAL DISEASE
TYPHUS
ROCKY MOUNTAIN SPOTTED FEVER

PROBABLE

■ COMMON COLD
See page 454.

■ INFLUENZA
See VIRAL ILLNESS, page 442.

■ SINUSITIS
Infected sinuses commonly produce headache and if severe, a fever. Antibiotic therapy is needed. *See page 454.*

POSSIBLE

■ CHEST INFECTION
These three symptoms in combination can be a feature of severe bronchial or lung infections.

■ INFECTION ELSEWHERE
An infection in any part of the body may give this combination of symptoms.
Consider whether you have any other noticeable symptoms and look those up too.

RARE

■ MENINGITIS
An infection of the brain and surrounding tissues. Meningitis is mainly a disease of childhood. The condition is checked for as a matter of routine if a baby appears to be seriously ill.
* The illness may develop rapidly over a few hours.
* Light hurts the eyes.

* Pain or stiffness in the neck on trying to lift the head.
* Nausea and vomiting.
* Drowsiness, delirium or coma.

Outbreaks of bacterial meningitis occur from time to time, usually affecting school-aged children. If there are reports in your area, watch for:
* Excessive irritability, or worsening of an existing condition.
* Temperature rises higher than expected.
* Pain on being moved about.
* Inability to feed or drink adequately.
* Fine purple rash.

Always seek medical help at an early stage. If later still in doubt, check again with your physician. If suspected, immediate medical attention is required.

■ WEIL'S DISEASE

Rats spread this disease by infecting lakes, canals, sewers and mines. Swimmers, sailors and canoeists should be aware of this, as should sewage workers, miners or anyone working in a rat-infested area.
* Rapid onset of fever, headache and backache.
* Red eyes.
* A mild degree of jaundice is usual.
* Spontaneous bleeding from mouth, nose may occur.

■ MALARIA

Caused by a parasite spread by mosquitoes. A risk in tropical and sub-tropical regions. Modern air travel means that malaria can be transported to anywhere in the world, so the possibility is worth considering in someone recently returned from Africa, Asia or India, even if they have been taking anti-malaria tablets.
* Attacks every two or three days.
* Attack begins with an hour or two of severe shivering and headache.
* High fever starts as shivering finishes, and lasts for several hours.
* Heavy sweating.
* In between attacks, the infected person may feel quite well.

If malaria is suspected, seek medical help urgently.

■ OTHER TROPICAL DISEASE

If someone recently returned from the tropics becomes ill with high fever, it is safest to suspect tropical disease first. Which one it is will depend on where they have been staying, and on the features of their illness. Seek medical help urgently.

■ TYPHUS

A general term for a variety of diseases spread by fleas and lice.
* Illness develops over seven to 14 days.
* Tenderness and redness of the eyes is typical.
* A rash eventually appears.
* Joints and muscles may be painful.

The illness varies from mild to severe, depending on the cause.

Needs immediate treatment.

■ ROCKY MOUNTAIN SPOTTED FEVER

See page 247.

"GENERAL" SYMPTOMS

A COLD?

Runny nose, itching eyes and aching across the face? It is usually caused by an infection of the upper respiratory tract, which includes nose, larynx and pharynx. Hence the medical term for a common cold — upper respiratory infection, or "URI". Any of more than 100 different viruses may be responsible.

However, a cold might be more than just a cold if the symptoms are recurrent or persistent.

PROBABLE
COMMON COLD

POSSIBLE
HAY FEVER
SINUSITIS
ALLERGY
NASAL POLYPS
FOREIGN BODY IN NOSE

RARE
HEAD INJURY COMPLICATION
NASAL TUMOR

PROBABLE

■ COMMON COLD
Probably a Nobel prize awaits the medical researcher who finds a cure for this condition.
* Begins with a sore or raw throat.
* Increasingly runny nose and sneezing with clear mucus.
* Mucus may turn yellow or green.
* Two or three days of loss of smell and taste.
* Occasionally progresses to a chest infection (*see page 223*).
* The illness runs its course over five to seven days, usually requiring no more than fluids, rest and warmth.
* Antibiotics reserved for those at risk of the cold progressing to a chest infection.

POSSIBLE

■ HAY FEVER
An allergic reaction of the lining of the nose in response to pollens, grass and other irritants.
* Sneezing at specific times of year or in specific environments.
* Persistent sniff and blocked nose.
* Itching, watery eyes.
* Sufferers frequently also have eczema or asthma.

■ SINUSITIS
* Persisting common cold symptoms (*see this page).*
* Passage of large quantities of yellow or green mucus.
* Aching across face, above and below the eyes, especially on leaning forward.
* Nasal tone of voice.

■ ALLERGIC RHINITIS
A general term which includes hay fever and perennial rhinitis — "allergic" runny or streaming nose.
* Reactions as for hay fever.

"GENERAL" SYMPTOMS

Upper respiratory tract

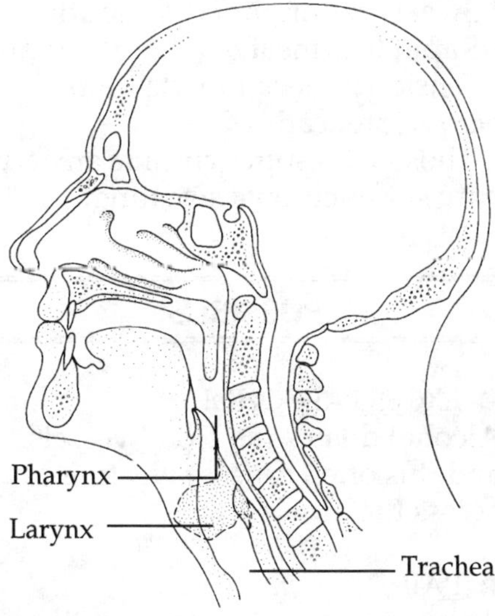

■ NASAL POLYPS
Common in people who suffer from allergic rhinitis.
* May be visible as fleshy lumps inside the nostrils.
* Constant feeling of blocked nose.
* A persistent sniff with clear nasal discharge.
* Can be removed, but they frequently recur.

■ FOREIGN BODY IN NOSE
Small children often put small, round objects into their noses and ears.
* Persistent infected discharge from one nostril.
* Discharge may be blood streaked.
* The foreign body, typically a bead, is often visible.

RARE

■ HEAD INJURY COMPLICATION
Leakage of cerebro-spinal fluid, the liquid which surrounds the brain, might be suspected if, after a head injury, there is a persistent, clear watery discharge from the nose.

■ NASAL TUMOR
* Persistent, one-sided bloody or foul-smelling discharge.

COLD SYMPTOMS PLUS FEVER

See FEVER LASTING 3 TO 14 DAYS, page 444.

SWEATING

Sweating is one of the body's ways of balancing heat loss against heat gain — an unglamorous, but still sophisticated mechanism. Normally, it goes on as a background activity with barely noticeable perspiration. Some people sweat excessively without the presence of disease.

PROBABLE
EXERCISE
FEVER
STRESS

"GENERAL" SYMPTOMS

POSSIBLE
EXCESS ALCOHOL
PAIN

RARE
DRUG-RELATED
TUBERCULOSIS
HIV INFECTION (AIDS)

PROBABLE

■ EXERCISE
It is of course normal that one should sweat when exercising vigorously. If you haven't exercised in a long time, and you are also overweight, you may be unpleasantly surprised at how much sweat you produce — but it is normal.
* Perspiration from brow, under arms and back.
* Clearly related to increased levels of activity.
* Decreases over a few minutes once exercise is stopped.

■ FEVER
Most fevers are accompanied by sweating. There will be the familiar symptoms of feverish illness such as:
* Aching muscles, headache, feeling sick, shivering.
* Commonly progressing to a sore throat, cough, earache.

Sweating as part of a feverish illness is less noticeable in the very old and the very young, whose temperature control mechanisms are less efficient than those of adults.

■ STRESS
Or anxiety produce:
* Sweaty palms, but dry mouth.
* Rapid heartbeat.
* Tension in neck muscles and across forehead.

Those who suffer chronic anxiety may suffer chronic sweating.

POSSIBLE

■ EXCESS ALCOHOL
Alcohol dilates the blood vessels, and this often causes sweating across the brow.

■ PAIN
Any severe pain causes sweating through nervous reflexes that also cause:
* Pale skin, restlessness.
* Rapid pulse.
* Collapse — in severe cases.

Thus sweating would be expected in any of the conditions causing *COLLAPSE* *(see page 468)*, including heart attacks, fracture and severe abdominal pain. But if there has been so much blood loss that the circulation is beginning to fail, clamminess replaces sweating.

RARE

■ DRUG-RELATED
Reactions due to abrupt withdrawal from alcohol or narcotic drugs cause sweating plus:
* Restlessness, muscle pains, drowsiness.
* Runny nose, dilated pupils, abdominal pains (narcotics).

* Shakes, disorientation, hallucinations (alcohol withdrawal).

Several medications, including anti-depressants, can cause unusual sweating and need to be considered in otherwise unexplained cases.

■ TUBERCULOSIS
Frequent night sweats may be the first indicator of this serious infection. You should seek a physician's advice as soon as possible. *See page 447.*

■ HIV INFECTION (AIDS)
AIDS causes sweating as an early symptom. *See page 448.*

HEAVY SWEATING

Covered here are causes of sweating *other* than infectious diseases, for which *see FEVER, pages 440-51.*

PROBABLE
NATURAL TENDENCY

POSSIBLE
HYPERTHYROIDISM
MENOPAUSE

RARE
CARCINOID SYNDROME
PHEOCHROMOCYTOMA
ACROMEGALY

PROBABLE

■ NATURAL TENDENCY
In other words, the way you are made. Though frequently just a nuisance, it becomes a significant problem if it ruins clothes, causes unpleasant body odor or interferes with your job. May also lead to social problems such as a reluctance to shake hands. The problem starts after puberty.
* Hands, underarms or feet pour sweat.
* Symptoms tend to be unrelated to exertion, temperature.

Several effective roll-on and lotion treatments are now available. As a last resort, it is possible to operate on the nerves near the spinal cord which control sweating of the hands or feet.

POSSIBLE

■ HYPERTHYROIDISM
See page 479. The thyroid gland could be described as the body's thermostat. Overactivity "turns up" all aspects of body function. Profuse sweating plus:
* Hyperactivity, jitteriness.
* Staring eyes.
* Weight loss, hunger, diarrhea.
* Trembling hands.
* Fatigue.

Effective therapy is available. Tends to recur.

■ MENOPAUSE
Even before menstruation ceases, women may be aware of flashes and sweating.

"GENERAL" SYMPTOMS

* Usually in the 40 to 55 age range.
* Menstrual pattern changes and eventually menstruation ceases.
* Associated with increased wrinkling (loss of elasticity) of skin, irritability or mild depression.
* Sudden sweats at any time, especially at night.
* Tiredness, headache, palpitations.

Modern treatment consists of hormone replacement therapy, which alleviates the symptoms and reduces thinning of the bones. All women should at least be offered the opportunity to consider taking hormone replacement therapy.

RARE

■ CARCINOID SYNDROME

Another hormone disorder. The nervous reactions that accompany changes in mood become grossly exaggerated. Caused by a hormone-secreting tumor in the intestine or liver. The full picture may take years to develop.
* Bouts of profuse watery diarrhea with excessive bowel sounds.
* Facial flushing and sweating, especially after alcohol.
* Asthma.

■ PHEOCHROMOCYTOMA

A tumor, which may occur near the kidneys, though not exclusively, causing high blood pressure and sudden, severe bursts of anxiety. It is usually treatable, and though relatively rare, physicians often run tests for it if there are:
* High blood pressure, sometimes highly variable.
* Abrupt episodes of headache, sweating, pallor, palpitations.

Tracking the tumor down can be like detective work. Requires surgical removal.

■ ACROMEGALY

See page 275.

HEAVY SWEATING AT NIGHT

Of concern if this persists for more than a few nights.

PROBABLE
FLU-LIKE ILLNESS

POSSIBLE
ABSCESS
SUBPHRENIC ABSCESS
ENDOCARDITIS

RARE
TUBERCULOSIS (TB)
BRUCELLOSIS
HODGKIN'S DISEASE
HIV DISEASE/AIDS

PROBABLE

■ FLU-LIKE ILLNESS

* Muscle aches.
* Mild headache.
* Sweating can be profuse.

After a few days, symptoms die away, with the possible emergence of a sore throat, cough or similar mild illness.

POSSIBLE

■ ABSCESS
An abscess is a collection of pus; it can form anywhere in the body and can cause pain and fever. Although the symptoms should raise suspicion, blood tests are the only reliable proof of continuing infection. Pain or recent surgery may point to a probable site of infection. When all else fails, modern imaging techniques, such as ultra-sound scan or CT scan can find the abscess.

■ SUBPHRENIC ABSCESS
A collection of pus underneath the diaphragm. Could be a possibility after abdominal surgery or peritonitis. There may be no more than non-specific features, such as:
* Feeling sick, sweats, anemia.
* Recurrent fever.
* Shoulder tip pain is a more tell-tale sign, caused by irritation of the diaphragm.

Treatment involves drainage and intensive antibiotic therapy.

■ ENDOCARDITIS
Infection of the valves of the heart. There is usually a previous history of heart valve problems. Both adults and children are susceptible. Onset can be gradual, with:
* Anemia.
* Feeling sick, recurrent sweats.
* Eventually, clubbed finger-nails, enlarged spleen.
* Splinter-like marks under the finger-nails.

Treatment takes several weeks, with monitoring of the heart valves by ultrasound devices.

RARE

■ TUBERCULOSIS
Tuberculosis is increasing again after many years. All ages and all income groups can be affected.
* Cough, which may be blood stained.
* General malaise, weight loss, debility.

Modern treatments cure the disease if continued over several months.

■ BRUCELLOSIS
See page 448.

■ HODGKIN'S DISEASE
See page 489.

■ HIV DISEASE/AIDS
See page 448.

TIREDNESS

PROBABLE
OVER-EXERTION
ANXIETY
ANEMIA

POSSIBLE
POST-VIRAL SYNDROME
DEPRESSION
HYPOTHYROIDISM
HYPERTHYROIDISM
DIABETES

"GENERAL" SYMPTOMS

RARE
HEART DISEASE
CANCER
MALNUTRITION
KIDNEY DISEASE
OTHER: ADRENAL INSUFFICIENCY
MYASTHENIA GRAVIS

PROBABLE

■ OVER-EXERTION
A few remarkable people never need relief from constant pressure and stress and can make do with short periods of sleep. But even they usually have some compensatory mechanism. The rest of us suffer from fatigue, which commonly goes with:
* Irritability.
* Tense feelings in neck and head.
* Diminished enthusiasm for life.

■ ANXIETY
As well as the symptoms given above for over-exertion:
* Palpitations, muscle tremors.
* Sweating.
* A constant fear that something unpleasant is going to happen.

At worst, anxiety is a truly disabling disorder needing treatment with a combination of psychological counseling and medication.

■ ANEMIA
See page 420.

POSSIBLE

■ POST-VIRAL SYNDROME
After a viral illness such as influenza *(see page 442)*, it is common to get easily fatigued for a few weeks, occasionally for longer. Psychological support and an undemanding lifestyle are the best advice that physicians can offer at present.

In a few cases, this develops into a chronic problem, causing severe exhaustion – called Chronic Fatigue Syndrome. Its cause is unknown.

■ DEPRESSION
Commonest in adult life, appearing over several weeks.
* Poor sleep.
* No enjoyment of anything, lack of motivation.
* Poor self-image.
* Crying.
* Changes in body weight.
* Poor concentration.

■ HYPOTHYROIDISM
This means an underactive thyroid gland. A disease of middle and later life, progressing so slowly that even the close family may not spot anything wrong, putting the symptoms down to aging.
* The skin becomes dry and rough.
* You "feel the cold".
* Your voice becomes gruff, your features coarse.
* Weight gain, constipation, slow speech, slow thought.

It is important to recognize this combination of symptoms because the problem is so easily treated.

■ HYPERTHYROIDISM
An over-active thyroid gland can also cause tiredness. This is usually a rather dramatic disease appearing over a few weeks with:
* Nervousness, fine trembling of the hands.
* Sweating, weight loss, increased appetite.
* Muscle ache.
* Staring eyes.
* Diarrhea.
* Rapid heart rate (tachycardia).
Treated with medication.

■ DIABETES
Fatigue can be an early symptom of diabetes when there are no other obvious features. As diabetes is such a common disease, anyone with unusual fatigue should be tested for it. For more details, *see page 485*.

RARE

■ HEART DISEASE
In heart failure, especially in the elderly, fatigue may be the only early symptom. Look also for:
* Breathlessness on mild effort, and when lying flat.
* Swollen ankles.

■ CANCER
Fatigue is of concern if found together with other symptoms suggesting cancer, such as:
* Weight loss, loss of appetite.
* Unusual pains.
* Unusual swellings.
* Blood in sputum, vomit, urine, stools or from the vagina (see under individual entries for these symptoms).

■ MALNUTRITION
Common worldwide. The fatigue is due to lack of vitamins, protein and energy supplies. In the developed countries, may be seen in those with malabsorption *(see page 423)* or alcoholics who eat poorly.

■ KIDNEY DISEASE
Fatigue is an early symptom along, with the increased output of urine day and night.

■ OTHER
Severe, unexplained fatigue also raises the possibility of two rare disorders: adrenal insufficiency and myesthenia gravis, a disease of gradual onset in which muscles seem to work normally but rapidly tire, with exceptional weakness. Drooping eyelids are typical.

TIREDNESS AND LOOKING PALE

Anemia is a common and significant cause of fatigue. Even mild anemia can cause fatigue and may not be obvious. Those most likely to be affected are:
– Children during growth spurts.
– Women during the years of menstruation.
– Women during pregnancy.
– People on low incomes with a poor diet, lacking iron and vitamins.

"General" Symptoms

TIREDNESS PLUS FEVER

A minor degree of fatigue always accompanies feverish illness such as the common cold.

PROBABLE
VIRAL ILLNESS SUCH AS FLU
OTHER ACUTE INFECTIONS

POSSIBLE
GLANDULAR FEVER
CHRONIC INFECTION

RARE
RHEUMATOID ARTHRITIS
ENDOCARDITIS
CANCER

PROBABLE

■ VIRAL ILLNESS
Including influenza, the common cold and other minor illnesses common during the winter months.
* A sore throat for two or three days.
* Aching muscles.
* Mild headache, shivering.
* Cough, hoarseness.
* The illness runs its course over a week or so.

■ OTHER ACUTE INFECTIONS
A wide range of acute viral and bacterial infections are associated with tiredness.

POSSIBLE

■ GLANDULAR FEVER (MONO)
A viral infection which usually starts as a particularly bad sore throat with excessive fatigue. The fatigue decreases over a few weeks, but can persist for months. Mainly an illness of young adults.
* A fine rash can be found.
* Can cause a mild degree of jaundice.

It is checked for with a simple blood test, called a "monospot".

■ CHRONIC INFECTION
Persistent fatigue and fevers would lead to a search for a smouldering infection in a common site such as the lungs, abdomen or urine; or a tooth abscess.

RARE

■ RHEUMATOID ARTHRITIS
This illness of the joints, most common in middle-aged women, can be preceded by a period of otherwise unexplained fever and fatigue along with:
* Transient aches and pains.
* Feeling unwell.
* Varying stiffness and swelling of the small joints.

Eventually, the full-blown illness shows itself with severe pain and swelling of the joints.

■ ENDOCARDITIS
An infection of the valves of the heart, most likely in someone known to have a valve problem,

caused, for example, by previous rheumatic fever.
* Anemia.
* Clubbed finger-nails.
* Tiny splinter-like streaks of bleeding under the nails.

■ CANCER
Certain cancers such as Hodgkin's disease and leukemia have these symptoms. There will usually be other symptoms and signs of the problem.

TIREDNESS PLUS HEADACHE

This is such a common combination of symptoms that only rarely should it cause concern about underlying disease. Often, the cause is tension.

PROBABLE
TENSION HEADACHE
PRE-MENSTRUAL TENSION

POSSIBLE
MIGRAINE
DEPRESSION

RARE
CARBON MONOXIDE POISONING
RAISED BLOOD PRESSURE

PROBABLE

■ TENSION HEADACHE
Ninety-eight percent of headaches are caused by tension. This starts in the neck muscles and spreads across the scalp.
* Headache like a band around the head.
* Cause may not be obvious.
* Usually work or family-related pressures are to blame.

■ PRE-MENSTRUAL TENSION
Fairly common in the week before menstruation.

POSSIBLE

■ MIGRAINE
Prolonged tiredness can trigger a migraine. Full symptoms include feeling sick and, sometimes, visual disturbance. *See page 113.*

■ DEPRESSION
Insomnia, feeling blue, aches and pains and headache are often associated with tiredness. *See page 486.*

RARE

■ CARBON MONOXIDE POISONING
Probably more common than is recognized, and caused by fumes from inefficient gas appliances. The early symptoms are vague.
* Symptoms disappear rapidly once the individual breathes fresh air.
* Drowsiness or coma.

■ RAISED BLOOD PRESSURE
Usually only severely raised blood pressure, under exceptional circumstances, causes a headache.

FEELING WEAK OR FEEBLE

Weakness is such an unspecific symptom that few medical textbooks even recognize it as a topic in its own right. However, people do report weakness to their physician and expect him or her to discover associated symptoms that will point to a diagnosis.

If you are in search of symptoms associated with weakness, this book is full of them: perhaps the most significant are *BREATHLESSNESS, pages 207-18* and *FEVER, pages 440-51*.

In the following pages we concentrate on those conditions which can cause weakness without many other significant symptoms. The terms weakness and tiredness are used interchangeably.

WEAKNESS, RAPID ONSET

PROBABLE
OVERWORK
VIRAL INFECTION
ANXIETY

POSSIBLE
HEART RHYTHM IRREGULARITY
LOW BLOOD SUGAR
PREGNANCY

RARE
HEMORRHAGE
DEHYDRATION
HEART DISEASE
INFECTIOUS HEPATITIS
GUILLAIN-BARRE SYNDROME

PROBABLE

■ OVERWORK
This may be obvious to others, but it is surprising how often an overworked individual is simply unaware of the pressures on him or her. Very often, people overlook this cause of weakness and tiredness because they tend to find "medical" reasons for the symptom. Try to take an honest look at your own life style and pressures. Is there a link between periods of maximum pressure and episodes of weakness?
* Tension in neck, shoulders.
* Slight headache.
* Irritability.
* Sheer fatigue.

■ VIRAL INFECTION
Tiredness or weakness frequently precedes infection by a day or two. You suspect that you are about to "come down with something". Soon there will be:
* Fever, muscle aches.
* Joint pains, headache.

* Cough, cold or sore throat.
See also POST-VIRAL SYNDROME, page 460.

■ ANXIETY
The source may be obvious: conflicting demands on your time, emotional stress, or anxiety may just be a feature of your personality. Simply recognizing this can defuse anxiety; otherwise, consider counseling, or try reading a book on relaxation technique. Your physician will probably only prescribe tranquillizers as a last resort.
* Sweating; nervy.
* Inability to concentrate.
* A fear of something unpleasant always being near.

POSSIBLE

■ HEART RHYTHM IRREGULARITY
The heart goes into either a very rapid or a very slow rhythm. It pumps less efficiently, giving a sensation of weakness or breathlessness or, at worst, collapse. These irregularities can stop as abruptly as they begin, making diagnosis difficult between attacks.
* Thumping in chest.
* Lightheadness, faintness.
* Abrupt disappearance of symptoms.
* Coffee, tea, alcohol may set off attacks.

■ LOW BLOOD SUGAR
The brain runs on sugar and a fall in blood sugar levels between meals is common.
* Light-headedness, difficulty in concentrating.
* Feeling cold.
* Symptoms rapidly relieved by a sweet drink or a snack.

■ PREGNANCY
Tiredness associated with early pregnancy can be a puzzle, since it can occur before the first missed menstrual period.
* Tender breasts.
* Desire to pass urine frequently.

RARE

■ HEMORRHAGE
Internal bleeding is worth considering in someone who has had a heavy blow to the belly, fractured a long bone or had severe abdominal pain; or has a history of peptic ulcers.
* Weakness, progressing to drowsiness, confusion.
* Swelling of the abdomen.
* Pale skin, sweating, clammy skin.
* Rapid pulse, rapid breathing.

■ DEHYDRATION
Excessive loss of body fluid from sweating, vomiting or diarrhea can cause acute weakness.

■ HEART ATTACK
Normally a dramatic event, but it can be quite mild, especially in the elderly, causing:
* Sudden general deterioration.
* Weakness, breathlessness.
* Swollen ankles, breathlessness at night.

"GENERAL" SYMPTOMS

■ INFECTIOUS HEPATITIS
Unexplained tiredness that precedes the appearance of the jaundice:
* Fever, sickness, nausea, loss of appetite.
* Possibly soreness under ribs on right.
* Jaundice appears after about seven days; then recovery is rapid.

■ GUILLAIN-BARRE SYNDROME
A neurological disorder of unknown cause, which leads to rapid development of muscle weakness. As it can affect the muscles involved in breathing, it needs hospital treatment. Recovery can take months.
* Typically accompanies a minor illness.
* Initial tingling of hands, feet, then numbness.
* Weakness rapidly involves the limbs.
* Muscles of breathing may be affected.

PROLONGED WEAKNESS

By its very nature, the cause of prolonged weakness is not likely to be clear from physical symptoms alone: investigation is needed. The following are a few of the commonest causes.

PROBABLE
POST-VIRAL WEAKNESS
ANEMIA
THYROID DISEASE

POSSIBLE
HEART FAILURE
LOW BLOOD PRESSURE
KIDNEY DISEASE
MALNUTRITION
MEDICATION

RARE
MUSCLE OR NERVE DISEASE
CANCER

PROBABLE

■ POST-VIRAL WEAKNESS
There is a major, continuing debate about whether this is a physical problem or a psychological disorder. It is probably both. In its most prolonged form it is known as chronic fatigue syndrome. Glandular fever (mono) (*see page 462*) is the best-known infection associated with prolonged weakness. The best treatment is simply to avoid overexertion.
* Tiredness on mild effort.
* No physical findings.
* Rarely lasts for more than a few months.

■ ANEMIA
See page 420. Mild anemia causes a feeling of being "below par". Those at most risk are:
– Women during the years of menstruation.
– Children during growth spurts.
– The elderly and the poor, with diets lacking iron.
– Alcoholics.

■ THYROID DISEASE
Weakness is a feature of both over- and underactivity, either of which are easily treated. An underactive thyroid gland gives:
* Progressive pallor, constipation, coarse features.
* Sensitivity to cold.
* Slowing of thought.

An overactive thyroid is more dramatic, causing:
* Sweating, weight loss, hunger.
* Tremor, nervousness and bulging eyes.

POSSIBLE

■ HEART FAILURE
Weakness can be a feature before other symptoms of heart failure become prominent. Usually there is some warning of heart trouble, such as angina, high blood pressure, previous heart attack or alcoholism. Eventually there will be:
* Breathlessness on mild activity.
* Ankle swelling, breathlessness at night.

■ LOW BLOOD PRESSURE
Usually results from blood loss, fluid loss, or certain medication side effects.

■ KIDNEY DISEASE
Very early symptoms are:
* Increased passage of urine, day and night.
* Vague weakness and tiredness.
* Later, anemia, nausea.

■ MALNUTRITION
This should not be a problem in developed countries, even so, it is still seen in the poor, in alcoholics or in other cases of self neglect. The weakness results from a combination of protein and vitamin deficiencies.
* Easy bruising, bleeding from gums (vitamin C deficiency).
* Tender calves (vitamin B1 deficiency); *see page 130.*
* In children, swollen wrists, stunted growth (vitamin D deficiency).

■ MEDICATION
Many medications such as diuretics (fluid pills), blood pressure pills, cause weakness. Your physician or pharmacist should help you clarify this problem.

RARE

■ MUSCLE OR NERVE DISEASE
Diagnosis is a matter for specialists, since early changes are subtle and non-specific.
Neurological disease might be suspected if there is:
* Progressive weakness of a group of muscles.
* Tingling, numbness or tremors of limbs.
* Unsteady gait.

Muscular disease in childhood affects boys:
* Thin thighs, but enlarged calves.
* Waddling gait, difficulty getting up from squatting position.
* In adults, twitching of muscles.

■ CANCER
It is unexplained why cancer can cause weakness before other, more obvious, symptoms.

"GENERAL" SYMPTOMS

Suspicion would be aroused by unusual weakness in:
* Smokers.
* Someone who has had recent indigestion, or noticed change of bowel habit.
* Someone with loss of appetite, weight loss.
* Unusual bleeding from chest, bowel or vagina, or blood in the urine.

For further details, see specific entries for the symptoms listed.

COLLAPSE

Sometimes called prostration, and characterized by overwhelming weakness, thready pulse, pale skin, sweating and confusion. Underlying most cases is low blood pressure, or toxic effects from serious infection or medications. While sudden collapse suggests a stroke or a heart attack (*see COLLAPSE WITH SHOCK OR COMA, page 471*), less abrupt collapse can mean a more general disruption of body function, for instance diabetes. However, there is no clear-cut distinction. In any case, get medical help fast.

Recovery position
Anyone who collapses should be laid on their side, leaning forwards. Make sure their airway — neck and throat — is not obstructed. If possible, keep their head lower than, or at the same level as, their heart.

Check for pulse and breathing. Start CPR if needed and you know how. Call out for assistance from persons nearby.

Always call for professional medical help immediately when anybody collapses.

PROBABLE
FAINT

POSSIBLE
SEVERE INFECTION
DRUG OVERDOSE
PULMONARY EMBOLUS
DEHYDRATION

RARE
PNEUMOTHORAX
SEPTICEMIA
HYPOADRENALISM
SEVERE HYPOTHYROIDISM

PROBABLE

■ FAINT
Short-lived unconsciousness, caused by temporary reduction in blood supply to the brain. Caused typically by standing upright in warm or hot conditions. Lying flat will lead quickly to recovery. *See page 418.*

POSSIBLE

■ SEVERE INFECTION
The possibilities are considered in detail in *FEVER, pages 440-51.*

■ DRUG OVERDOSE
Including alcohol. Suspected in someone who collapses and is confused or unconscious, especially a young, otherwise fit person.
* Smell of alcohol, empty pill containers.
* Neglected appearance.
* Inflamed veins.
* Pupils may be widely dilated or pin-point sized.
* Puncture marks on skin, made by a needle, usually at front of elbow or on back of hand.

Blood and urine tests will be necessary.

■ PULMONARY EMBOLUS
See page 218.

A blood clot settles in the lung, cutting off blood flow.

■ DEHYDRATION
See page 483.

RARE

■ PNEUMOTHORAX
Collapse of a section of lung.
* Sudden, knife-like chest pain, worse on breathing in.
* Slight breathlessness.
* Serious cases progress to faintness, collapse and cyanosis.

■ SEPTICEMIA
Infection in the blood, causing rigors and sweats. *See page 191.*

■ HYPOADRENALISM
Progressive, generalized weakness until some one-off stress causes collapse. *See page 488.*

■ SEVERE HYPOTHYROIDISM
An underactive thyroid gland is usually spotted well before the patient collapses. *See page 460.*

COLLAPSE WITH ABDOMINAL PAIN

Often hard to diagnose, because the reasons for abdominal pain differ with age. The following are the obvious, but not a complete list, of illnesses that can cause collapse in adults. Neglect at this stage will lead to shock and coma *– see page 471.*

PROBABLE
PEPTIC ULCER
PANCREATITIS
GALL BLADDER DISEASE
ECTOPIC PREGNANCY

POSSIBLE
SEVERE GASTROENTERITIS
INFLAMMATORY BOWEL DISEASE

RARE
INTESTINAL OBSTRUCTION
INTESTINAL ISCHEMIA

PROBABLE

The possibilities below all involve inflammation of internal organs, which can progress to rupture of the organ. It is frequently impossible to differentiate these

"GENERAL" SYMPTOMS

causes without tests or surgery.
All need urgent medical care.

■ PEPTIC ULCER
If a stomach or duodenal ulcer ruptures, acid, food and blood gush into the abdomen.
* Commonest in middleage.
* A history of upper abdominal discomfort or indigestion.
* Severe indigestion, often at night.
* Severe pain in the upper belly, apparently radiating into the back.
* Vomit containing blood or particles looking like coffee grounds.
* Stools may be black, tarry-looking or bloody.

■ PANCREATITIS
The pancreas lies at the back of the upper abdomen. There is usually existing gall bladder disease or a history of heavy drinking.
* Severe upper belly pain, worsening over a few hours.
* Pain in the back.
* Vomiting.
* Collapse.
Needs intensive treatment to prevent peritonitis, *page 149*.

■ GALL BLADDER DISEASE
Inflammation or obstruction of the gall bladder, usually connected with gall stones and commonest in middle-aged women.
* Pain felt in the upper right abdomen, under the ribs.
* Often a long history of discomfort on that side.
* Excruciating pain for hours at a time.
* Fever.

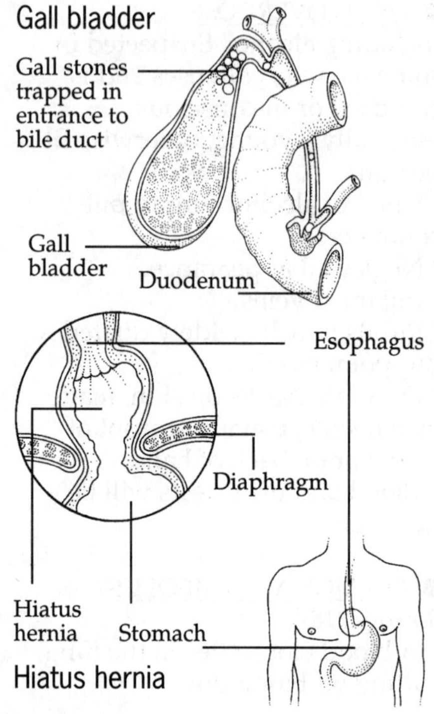

■ ECTOPIC PREGNANCY
If a fertilized egg lodges in a Fallopian tube, it can grow for a few weeks, eventually rupturing the tube, causing serious internal bleeding. This possibility should not be ignored in any fertile woman, even if there are no symptoms of pregnancy. Precise diagnosis is now relatively easy, thanks to ultrasound scanning.
* A missed menstrual period, tender breasts, nausea.
* Rapidly increasing lower belly pain, usually one-sided.
* Vaginal bleeding.

POSSIBLE

■ GASTROENTERITIS
An infection of the bowels which, if severe, causes rapid dehydration as well as toxic effects from the actual infection.
* Cramping abdominal pains.
* Vomiting.
* Diarrhea immediately, or after a few hours.

■ INFLAMMATORY BOWEL DISEASE
Typically ulcerative colitis or Crohn's disease. Associated with:
* A long history of recurrent abdominal pains, diarrhea.
* Bleeding or mucus in stools.

RARE

■ INTESTINAL OBSTRUCTION
Most often due to a trapped hernia or a growth in the intestine.
* A trapped hernia gives a tender swelling in the groin.
* At first, cramping abdominal pains.
* Vomiting, swelling of the abdomen.
* Within hours, fever, generalized abdominal pains.

■ INTESTINAL ISCHEMIA
A clot blocks blood supply to the intestines. Most likely in the elderly, with pre-existing heart disease.
* Sudden abdominal pain.
* Diarrhea, vomiting, blood in stools.
* Rapid progression to collapse.

Surgical removal of the clot can be successful, but must be done early.

COLLAPSE WITH SHOCK OR COMA

An emergency. Making a precise diagnosis is less important than resuscitating the individual. As an term, "shock" strictly means drastic reduction in blood flow around the tissues. Here the term is used in a less technical sense, so as to include a wider range of symptoms:
* Skin clammy, cold, pale.
* Thready, weak pulse.
* Blue lips, finger-nails.
* Individual reaction can vary from confusion to coma.

Coma may here be taken as unconsciousness. In trying to work out the cause of collapse with shock or coma, also consider the possibilities in the two preceding sections.

PROBABLE
STROKE
HEART ATTACK
HEART RHYTHM IRREGULARITY
BLOOD LOSS
OVERWHELMING INFECTION
SEVERE PAIN

"GENERAL" SYMPTOMS

POSSIBLE
DIABETIC COMA
ALCOHOL/DRUG OVERDOSE
LEAKING AORTIC ANEURYSM
BURNS

RARE
ALLERGIC SHOCK

PROBABLE

■ STROKE
Mainly affects the elderly. Caused by a blood clot or bleeding in the brain.
* Loss of consciousness for a few minutes.
* Vomiting at first.
* Paralysis of one side of the body.
* "Sighing", rough breathing.

The outlook depends on the reason for the stroke and the person's overall health.

■ HEART ATTACK
A risk in the middle-aged and elderly. Quick medical help is essential to maximize chances of survival.
* Sudden, crushing, central chest pain.
* Pain radiates up into jaws or down left arm.
* Breathlessness, sweating.

Not all heart attacks are so dramatic. In the elderly especially, they can occur without much pain.

■ HEART RHYTHM IRREGULARITY
Very rapid, very slow or very irregular heart rhythms reduce the blood output from the heart. You may notice:
* Abrupt onset of thumping or fluttering in chest.
* Breathlessness.
* Shock.

■ BLOOD LOSS
See also DEHYDRATION, page 483.
Not always obvious, but easy to recognize if the blood loss is visible, for example in vomit, stools, or from the vagina. A risk after injury, especially:
* Trauma to the abdomen, which can rupture the spleen.
* Fractured thigh bone with severe bleeding into muscle.

■ OVERWHELMING INFECTION
For complex reasons, a major infection, that gets into the blood stream, causes collapse via a drop in blood pressure. There will be the general symptoms of infection, such as:
* Fever, chills and shaking, headache.
* Spontaneous bleeding and bruising.

■ SEVERE PAIN
Severe pain from any source can cause collapse and coma as reflex actions.

POSSIBLE

■ DIABETIC COMA
Diabetics can have two types of coma. Collapse due to low blood sugar gives:
* Sweating, light-headedness, irritability.
* Rapid progression to confusion, then collapse.

If blood sugar remains high for

long, another, less sudden, form of collapse — ketoacidosis — can occur:
* Usually during another mild illness.
* Onset over a few hours or days.
* Dehydration (*page 483*), intense thirst.
* Sweet smell on breath.

Both these conditions respond rapidly to the appropriate treatment.

■ ALCOHOL/DRUG EXCESS
See DRUG OVERDOSE, page 469.

■ LEAKING AORTIC ANEURYSM
The aorta is the major artery leading from the heart, and carries its whole blood output. After years of service, its walls can swell out, weaken and then split, just like a car tire may bulge and blow out. A not uncommon cause of sudden death, but there are sometimes warning symptoms:
* Unusual pulsation in the belly, in time with the heart beat.
* A lump you can feel in the abdomen.
* Onset of backache as the aorta starts to leak.

Surgery is highly successful in early cases.

■ BURNS
Loss of body fluids invariably accompanies serious burns, with shock resulting both from this loss and from pain.

RARE

■ ALLERGIC SHOCK
This term describes the worst form of allergic reaction.

It is an unpredictable risk, to be borne in mind whenever someone is given an injection, but allergic shock can happen in response to foods and insect stings. Minor warning signs of allergic reaction are:
* Swelling of the lips.
* Itchy, raised skin wheals that come and go.

In allergic shock there is:
* Abrupt wheezing, progressing to cyanosis.
* Difficulty in swallowing, from swelling of the throat.
* Collapse.

People who know that they are at risk should carry the appropriate medication, or a warning bracelet.

NO APPETITE, OR VERY POOR APPETITE

Occasional loss of appetite accompanies our changing moods and minor infections. Indeed the regaining of appetite is among the earliest signs of recovery from these minor upsets, as is the disappearance of fever. If loss of appetite is accompanied by abdominal pain or weight loss (*see these symptoms*) then more serious disease is a possibility.

"GENERAL" SYMPTOMS

PROBABLE
MINOR FEVERISH ILLNESS
STRESS

POSSIBLE
DEPRESSION
ALCOHOLISM
INFECTIOUS HEPATITIS

RARE
CANCER OF THE STOMACH
HEART DISEASE

PROBABLE

■ MINOR FEVERISH ILLNESS
* Fever, muscle aches, sore throat or cough.
* Appetite disappears suddenly.
* The return of appetite lags a day or two behind the disappearance of fever.

■ STRESS
Stress may either stimulate or reduce appetite.
* Tense feelings in head, neck, shoulders.
* Irritability, mild depression.
Mood and appetite recover rapidly when the source of stress is absent.

POSSIBLE

■ DEPRESSION
See page 389. Suggested by prolonged loss of appetite as well as:
* Loss of interest in general.
* Expressions of despair, crying, poor self-image.
* Apathetic mood, neglect of self and others.
* Early morning waking (or disturbed sleep pattern).

■ ALCOHOLISM
The high carbohydrate content of alcohol satisfies hunger and causes loss of appetite for normal solid food. Of course, drink is not at all nutritious, and eventually symptoms of vitamin deficiency appear, as well as those of alcoholism. Symptoms such as:
* Self-neglect, smell of alcohol.
* Memory disturbance, swings of mood.
* Sore mouth, cracks at corners of lips, recurrent infections.
* Dilated veins over the face.

■ INFECTIOUS HEPATITIS
The combination of loss of appetite, fever for five to seven days, plus muscular aches and abdominal pains should arouse suspicion.
* Jaundice appears with yellowed eyes, dark urine.
* As the jaundice clears up, you begin to feel better.

RARE

■ CANCER OF THE STOMACH
For reasons not understood, early cancer, especially of the stomach, can cause loss of appetite before other features appear. However, it is rare for loss of appetite alone to continue for long without the other symptoms described under

NO APPETITE, LOSING WEIGHT, this page and NO APPETITE, LOSING WEIGHT AND CHEST PAIN, page 476.

Most common in the 45-plus age group.
* Persistent, otherwise unexplained, loss of appetite.
* Feeling of fullness very soon after eating a small amount.
* Otherwise unexplained symptoms, such as generally feeling unwell, tiredness, unusual bleeding, unusual pains.

■ HEART FAILURE

In certain forms of heart failure, loss of appetite is a noticeable symptom, probably related to congestion of blood in the liver. Among the many other symptoms which appear over days or weeks are:
* Breathlessness on activity; tiredness.
* Breathlessness when attempting to lie flat.
* Pre-existing chest disease, such as chronic bronchitis, bronchiectasis or heart disease, typically angina.
* An early feature is swollen ankles, and eventually a swollen abdomen.
* Tenderness over the liver; reduction in the volume of urine.

NO APPETITE, LOSING WEIGHT

In the under-40s, the cause is usually a prolonged feverish illness. In the middle-aged and elderly, more serious disease must be carefully considered. If you have noticed loss of appetite and weight loss, check whether you have any of the symptoms in the lists below. Then look them up elsewhere in the book, where they are featured under a heading of their own.

PROBABLE
PROLONGED FEVERISH ILLNESS
ANOREXIA NERVOSA

POSSIBLE
EMOTIONAL UPSET
CANCER

PROBABLE

■ PROLONGED FEVERISH ILLNESS

In children and young adults, loss of appetite and weight loss will accompany any moderately extended illness such as a bad chest infection or prolonged gastroenteritis. Both appetite and weight are rapidly regained after a couple of weeks. In adults, a wider range of causes can be found to account for them, plus other symptoms such as:
* Chills or night sweats.
* Recent abdominal surgery.
* Prolonged cough, diarrhea, abdominal pains.
* Unusual bleeding.
* Changes in amount of urine.

Follow up these symptoms individually, looking at other pages in this book where they are discussed in detail.

"GENERAL" SYMPTOMS

■ <u>ANOREXIA NERVOSA</u>
See page 423. Weight loss due to obsessional dieting.

POSSIBLE

■ <u>EMOTIONAL UPSET</u>
If severe enough, self-neglect may follow. Usually there is an obvious cause of stress.
* Other symptoms of emotional upset, such as swings of mood, irritability, crying, depression.

■ <u>CANCER</u>
In the 40-plus age range these symptoms also require a careful check for other features suggestive of cancer such as:
* Unusual pains.
* Unusual bleeding from mouth, vagina, bowel, in sputum, in urine.
* Swellings, lumps, enlarged lymph nodes.
* Feeling sick, tiredness.

NO APPETITE, LOSING WEIGHT AND CHEST PAIN

PROBABLE
PEPTIC ULCER
HIATUS HERNIA
ESOPHAGITIS

POSSIBLE
GALL BLADDER DISEASE
CANCER OF THE STOMACH

RARE
MALABSORPTION
LUNG CANCER
TUBERCULOSIS

PROBABLE

■ <u>PEPTIC ULCER</u>
The lining of the stomach and duodenum is washed by strong acid and salts. The digestive system has mechanisms to cope with this, but if the mechanisms break down, inflammation and eventually ulceration occurs. Smoking, drinking, stress, infection in the stomach, and most anti-rheumatic drugs can contribute to peptic ulcers.
* Burning pains behind the breastbone and in the upper abdomen.
* May have hunger pains.

* Food may help or worsen the pain.
* If it worsens pain, food is avoided, causing weight loss.
* You may be woken at night by the pain.
* Bleeding from ulcer may cause black stools and anemia.
* Simple antacids give temporary relief.

The treatment of peptic ulcers is one of the outstanding successes of modern medicine, making surgery, which used to be the only long-term cure, unnecessary.

Peptic ulcers: the two types
Two types of peptic ulcer exist. *Duodenal ulcers* are four times more common than *gastric ulcers*.

Duodenal ulcers do not turn into cancers; gastric ulcers may become cancerous. Twice as many men as women have ulcers. One in ten of all people will have some ulcer-related disease during their lifetime.

■ HIATUS HERNIA
A failure of the one-way valve mechanism that keeps stomach contents from regurgitating up into the esophagus. Often just a nuisance, but if long-standing, it can cause scarring which interferes with normal swallowing of food. Weight loss then results.

A condition of middle to later life, especially in the overweight.
* Burning pains.
* Belching, especially on bending over or lying flat.

Very commonly, the symptoms are worse during pregnancy.

Peptic ulcer

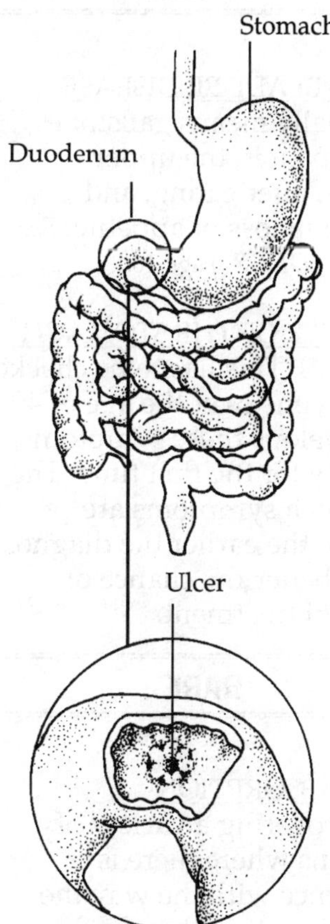

■ ESOPHAGITIS
Inflammation of the esophagus due to excess acid.
* Burning pain behind the breastbone (heartburn).
* Worse after hot or acid food.
* Pain may appear to spread across the chest, and up to the jaw.

Treatment is aimed at preventing scarring and narrowing of the esophagus .

"General" Symptoms

POSSIBLE

■ GALL BLADDER DISEASE
This usually means gallstones, causing pain in the upper abdomen after eating, and resulting in loss of appetite. *See GALL BLADDER, page 163.*

■ CANCER OF THE STOMACH
See page 474. This has to be checked for in anyone over the age of 40 who develops these symptoms, especially for the first time. The earlier such symptoms are reported, the earlier the diagnosis and the better the chance of successful treatment.

RARE

■ MALABSORPTION
A term covering a variety of conditions where there is interference with the way the digestive system absorbs food. Particularly a problem of children; symptoms include:
* Failure to grow.
* Loose, greasy, bulky, offensive stools.
* Frequent chest infections.
* Swollen belly with discomfort or pain.

■ LUNG CANCER
In addition to the three main symptoms there may also be:
* Breathlessness.
* Coughing of blood.
See details on page 223.

■ TUBERCULOSIS
Weight loss and loss of appetite, and sweating, are general features of this disease. Chest pain results from swelling of glands inside the chest. *See details on page 447.*

ABNORMAL HUNGER

PROBABLE
INDIGESTION
LOW BLOOD SUGAR

POSSIBLE
HYPERTHYROIDISM

RARE
INTESTINAL WORMS
BULIMIA
HYPOTHALAMIC DISEASE

PROBABLE

■ INDIGESTION
Food reduces the feelings of pain or emptiness caused by excess acid present in indigestion. You feel like taking frequent snacks to relieve the discomfort.
* Burning sensation behind the breastbone.
* Burping, belching or other signs of wind.

Persistent symptoms may signify a peptic ulcer.

■ LOW BLOOD SUGAR
Very common in a mild form if you miss a meal. Diabetics, especially those on insulin, must be alert to the early symptoms.
* At first, you feel light-headed and have difficulty concentrating; also, irritability, headache.
* As it worsens, sweating, confusion, drowsiness.
* Symptoms rapidly eased by taking sugar, candy or fruit juice.

POSSIBLE

■ HYPERTHYROIDISM
An over-active thyroid gland, developing over weeks or months.
* Weight loss, sweating, trembling of the hands.
* Often, bulging eyes.
* Hyperactivity, restlessness, nervousness.

RARE

■ INTESTINAL WORMS
The worm infects humans by way of under-cooked beef, pork or fish.
* Usually no other symptoms until segments of worm appear in stools.

■ BULIMIA
Bulimia is binge eating, associated with *ANOREXIA NERVOSA,* *page 423.*
* Typically in young women worried about their weight.
* Excess dieting, interrupted by bouts of excessive eating followed by vomiting.

"GENERAL" SYMPTOMS

■ HYPOTHALAMIC DISEASE
Disease of the hypothalamus gland in the brain can gradually cause excess appetite and:
* Passage of large amounts of urine.
* Drowsiness, narrowing of visual field.

PUTTING ON WEIGHT

PROBABLE
EATING TOO MUCH

POSSIBLE
HYPOTHYROIDISM
MEDICATION-RELATED

RARE
HORMONAL
HYPERADRENALISM

PROBABLE

■ EATING TOO MUCH
Some individuals really do eat very little, yet gain weight. The reason is unknown. Overweight is a major cause of ill health, including osteoarthritis, heart disease, diabetes and breathing problems.
* Worsens with age.
* Fat is generally spread around the body.
* Honest, purposeful dieting can achieve weight loss.

"GENERAL" SYMPTOMS

Most people who are overweight eat the wrong kinds of foods (too much fat and sugar) instead of a balanced diet, high in fiber, fruit and vegetables.

POSSIBLE

■ HYPOTHYROIDISM
* Slow, progressive weight gain. *See page 460.*

■ MEDICATION-RELATED
Commonest culprits are the contraceptive pill, anti-depressants and steroids which are widely used in inflammatory and rheumatic diseases, eventually causing:
* A "moon" face.
* Weight gain mainly in body, limbs remaining relatively thin.
* High blood pressure, diabetes.

RARE

■ HORMONAL
Several unusual hormonal disorders, mainly in boys, cause obesity.
* Obese child is unusually small or unusually tall.
* Delayed puberty.
* Under-development of penis and testicles.

■ HYPERADRENALISM
Results from overproduction of natural steroids by the body.
* Gross obesity of body, with prominent purple stretch marks.
* Thin, stick-like limbs.
* "Moon" face.
* Pronounced hump of fat on the back.
* Symptoms of diabetes (thirst, excess urine and so on, *see page 484).*
* Thin skin, easy bruising.

There are sophisticated treatments, depending on the cause.

TEMPERATURE, SUB-NORMAL

See ABNORMALLY LOW TEMPERATURE, page 451.

EXTREME THIRST

Read also CRAVING *FOR WATER, FEELING DEHYDRATED, page 483.*

PROBABLE
POOR FLUID INTAKE
SWEATING
DIARRHEA

POSSIBLE
EXCESS OF DIURETIC DRUG
INTERNAL BLEEDING

RARE
MEDICATION SIDE-EFFECT

PROBABLE

■ POOR FLUID INTAKE
Circumstances which could make this a possibility are:
– Prolonged vomiting.
– Disabled individual: for example, stroke victim, must rely on others for drinks.
– Obstruction of the esophagus.

The symptoms are:
* Dry mouth, low output of concentrated, dark urine.
* Skin becomes lax and loses its elasticity, eyes appear to sink.
* In babies, the soft spot on the skull becomes sunken.
* In extremes, apathy, confusion.

■ SWEATING
The fluid lost in sweat has to be replaced, otherwise thirst will follow. Fever, heavy exercise and hot weather might all cause profuse sweating. The symptoms are the same as for poor fluid intake.

■ DIARRHEA
The body can cope with brief episodes of diarrhea, but if it is prolonged, dehydration and thirst will follow. Babies are particularly susceptible to the effects of diarrhea, which is also often accompanied by vomiting at that age. A careful watch must be kept for signs of dehydration. Provide fluids after each bowel movement. If it is vomited back consistently, take child for medical evaluation.

POSSIBLE

■ EXCESS OF DIURETIC DRUGS
These medications are widely used to treat heart disease. They rid the body of fluid: even so, thirst is not often a problem, unless doses are excessive, when you may see:
* Passage of large quantities of urine for hours after taking the diuretic.
* Increasing weakness over several days or weeks.
* Constipation.

■ BLEEDING
This has to be heavy and sustained to cause thirst. External bleeding is usually obvious, but internal bleeding may be another matter:
* Pale skin, rapid pulse, collapse and thirst.

Suspect internal bleeding following:
* Recent abdominal injury (for example, a ruptured spleen).
* Recent severe abdominal pain (from, say, a perforated ulcer).
* Abdominal distension.
* Fractured thigh bone.

RARE

■ MEDICATION SIDE-EFFECT
Many medications cause a dry mouth; not, strictly speaking, true thirst —but the remedy is sips of fluid. Common medications with this side effect are anti-depressants and medications for urinary incontinence.

"GENERAL" SYMPTOMS

EXTREME THIRST, HIGH URINE OUTPUT

PROBABLE
DIABETES MELLITUS
PSYCHOLOGICAL

POSSIBLE
POTASSIUM DEFICIENCY
CHRONIC KIDNEY FAILURE

RARE
HYPER-PARATHYROIDISM
DIABETES INSIPIDUS

PROBABLE

■ DIABETES MELLITUS
See page 484. This combination of symptoms is the classical presentation of diabetes.

■ PSYCHOLOGICAL
A vicious cycle of high fluid intake followed by urinating to excess. Surprisingly common, especially in children, where consuming sodas becomes their main source of comfort. Other causes must be excluded first.

POSSIBLE

■ POTASSIUM DEFICIENCY
Nearly always secondary to the long-term use of diuretic medications. Suggested by:
* Elderly person on diuretics.
* Muscle weakness, tiredness, constipation.

(In very rare cases, caused by disease, such as chronic gastroenteritis.)

■ CHRONIC KIDNEY FAILURE
The passage of large quantities of dilute urine is an early sign of this problem, whose other symptoms are rather vague.
* Excessive urine day and night.
* Feeling sick.
* As it worsens, thirst, mild anemia, fatigue.

The outcome depends on the underlying cause.

RARE

■ HYPER-PARATHYROIDISM
The parathyroid glands lie next to the thyroid gland in the throat; they control calcium balance. Too much calcium in the blood gives:
* Excessive thirst and urine output.
* Pains in bones, constipation.
* Kidney stones that may be painful.
* Depression, sickness.

■ DIABETES INSIPIDUS
See page 485.

CRAVING FOR WATER, FEELING DEHYDRATED

Dehydration is the result of fluid loss exceeding fluid intake. Water is lost not just in urine but in feces (especially in diarrhea), sweat (especially in heat exhaustion), blood (especially in hemorrhage) and via breathing (especially in prolonged asthma). Thirst is frequently a symptom of dehydration; other signs, in order of severity, are:
* Dry tongue.
* Reduced output of urine, the urine being dark and strong-smelling.
* Dry, lax skin.
* Sunken eyes.
* In babies, a sunken soft spot in the skull.
* Eventually apathy, confusion, collapse.

Depending on the cause, dehydration can develop over any length of time, from days to weeks, unless there has been a large and sudden loss of fluid. It is important to realize that babies and elderly people can dehydrate in a matter of hours, typically from diarrhea and vomiting, and may not show any symptoms apart from restlessness until fluid loss is extreme.

PROBABLE
VOMITING
DIARRHEA
SWEATING
DECREASED FLUID INTAKE

POSSIBLE
OVER-USE OF DIURETICS
DIABETES MELLITUS (SUGAR DIABETES)

RARE
HIGH BLOOD CALCIUM
CHRONIC KIDNEY FAILURE
KIDNEY FAILURE
DIABETES INSIPIDUS

PROBABLE

■ VOMITING
Whatever the reason for the vomiting, eventually dehydration results simply because no water is being kept down. In both children and adults, the usual cause is gastroenteritis, known as gastric flu or stomach upset, with:
* Abrupt onset of vomiting.
* Chills, muscular aches.
* Diarrhea may accompany these, or begin a few hours later.

After two or three days, gastroenteritis can cause significant dehydration, but it is unusual for both the diarrhea and the vomiting together to last so long. So, dehydration is actually a remote risk except in babies, who should be carefully watched.

Babies and small children will often have vomiting and diarrhea as a symptom of ear and throat infections or meningitis.

"GENERAL" SYMPTOMS

■ DIARRHEA
A few episodes of diarrhea cause no harm. Profuse, watery diarrhea is a different matter because if that continues for more than a day or two dehydration becomes a real risk, especially in the very old and the very young.

■ SWEATING
In a hot, dry atmosphere it is possible to lose large amounts of fluid by sweating without noticing. Those who run for pleasure should also remember this and take fluids regularly, even when on the move. Early features would be:
* Muscle cramps.
* Thirst, but not as a prominent symptom.
* Weakness, vomiting.

■ DECREASED FLUID INTAKE
If disease interferes with swallowing, dehydration, and indeed starvation, are a risk unless arrangements are made to enable food to be taken some other way.

Similarly, with anyone unable to take sufficient fluid because of confusion, stroke or unconsciousness. The symptoms of dehydration can become confused with the symptoms of their disease. Look for:
* Low urine output.
* Increasingly lax skin.
* A tongue so dry it begins to crack.
* Increasing confusion.

POSSIBLE

■ OVER-USE OF DIURETICS
These invaluable and widely-used medications cause an increased output of urine. They are used to treat heart failure or high blood pressure; also to relieve fluid retention such as swollen ankles or swollen breasts. When they are used over long periods, they can cause a slow dehydration. You may come to accept as normal a dry mouth or increased thirst.

It is rare for diuretics to cause rapid dehydration except through deliberate overdose, for instance, if used as a slimming aid. The symptoms would be those of dehydration, as listed above, with:
* General weakness, also muscle weakness.
* If very severe, apathy and vomiting.

■ DIABETES MELLITUS (SUGAR DIABETES)
In this condition, excess sugar in the blood stream starts to "leak" into the kidneys, pulling large quantities of water with it. The result is a high volume of urine, day and night, giving the combination of thirst and dehydration. Other features might include:
* Vague feeling of ill-health.
* Weight loss.
* Frequent skin infections, especially thrush.
* A sweet smell on the breath.
* Visual changes.
* Eventually, confusion.

In teenagers and young adults, diabetes does tend to show itself in the above dramatic way, appearing over just a few days. In elderly people, the onset is usually less dramatic: the main symptoms are passing larger-than-usual amounts of urine, and very severe thirst.

RARE

■ HIGH BLOOD CALCIUM
Occurs mainly in association with diseases that affect the bones and tends to be part of a rather vague, gradually developing picture which might include:
* Weakness, drowsiness, nausea, vomiting.
* Pains in the abdomen, constipation.

■ CHRONIC KIDNEY FAILURE
Among the many functions of the kidneys is the job of concentrating the urine so that only enough is made as is needed to carry off waste products. One of the earliest features of kidney failure is loss of efficiency in this task resulting in increased flow of dilute urine, plus:
* Mild dehydration.
* Vague weakness, tiredness.

The disease is more likely in diabetics or those with high blood pressure.

■ KIDNEY FAILURE
In serious kidney failure, usually after months or years of illness, there comes a stage of many distressing symptoms including:
* Severe dehydration.
* Dry, brown tongue with the smell of urine on the breath.
* Weakness, anemia, hiccups, nausea.

■ DIABETES INSIPIDUS
This results from damage — typically as a result of head injury, tumors or meningitis — to the part of the brain that controls water balance (the pituitary gland).
* Output of gallons of urine a day.
* A huge compensating thirst.

This condition is now readily treatable.

HICCUPS

Hiccups result from a sudden contraction of the diaphragm, the sheet of muscle which separates the chest from the abdomen. It is an uncontrollable reflex action, like blinking. They are not associated with disease except for chronic kidney failure.

The diaphragm

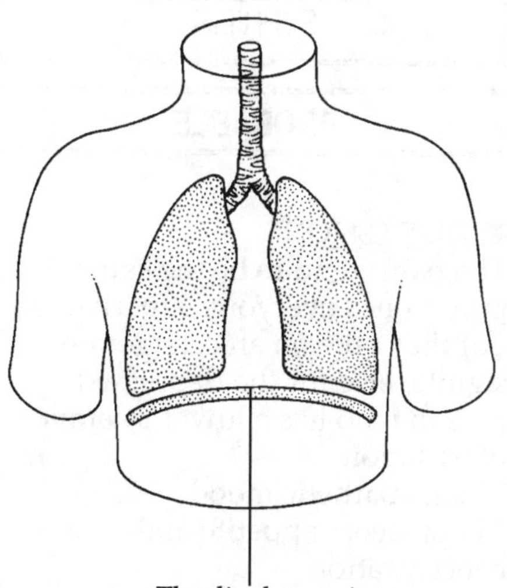

The diaphragm is a horizontal sheet of muscle

"GENERAL" SYMPTOMS

GENERALIZED PAIN

Considered here is *recurrent, generalized pain* as opposed to pain in a specific part of the body. Such generalized pains can include the vague aches and pains which plague most people from time to time, and which may have a psychological origin.

PROBABLE
DEPRESSION
HYPOCHONDRIA
FIBROMYALGIA

POSSIBLE
DIABETES MELLITUS
POLYMYALGIA RHEUMATICA
RHEUMATOID ARTHRITIS
SICKLE CELL DISEASE

RARE
SYPHILIS

PROBABLE

■ DEPRESSION
The pains tend to be the same minor ones everyone experiences, but they take on an exaggerated significance for the depressed person who has a lower tolerance of irritation.
* Flat, apathetic mood.
* Poor sleep, appetite and concentration.
* Crying, negative feelings.

■ HYPOCHONDRIA
Describes people who are constantly concerned, without good reason, that they have a serious medical illness. Persistent hypochondriacs — the ones who see their physicians as often as once a week — are characterized by:
* Lack of insight.
* Resistance to reasoned explanation or proof, after investigation, that they are healthy.
* Often, a long history of neurotic behavior.

■ FIBROMYALGIA
See page 271.

POSSIBLE

■ DIABETES MELLITUS
Sugar diabetes affects the working of nerves all over the body and can cause widespread nerve disturbance. This is usually a late complication: the disease should have been diagnosed long before.
* Pain, tingling of lower limbs.
* Pain worse at night.
* Muscle tenderness.

Unfortunately this complication is possible even in well controlled diabetes.

■ POLYMYALGIA RHEUMATICA
A not uncommon illness mainly affecting women in their 60s. It comes on over a period of a few weeks giving pains in any muscles, but particularly:
* Across the shoulders.
* Tenderness at the side of forehead.
* Vague sickness, occasional fever.

Easily and effectively treated, though treatment has to continue for a year or two.

■ RHEUMATOID ARTHRITIS
When arthritis affects many joints and muscles, pain can be widespread.
* Swollen joints.
* Wasted muscles.
* Stiffness.

■ SICKLE CELL DISEASE
In which hemoglobin, the blood's oxygen carrier, is abnormal. Found mostly in people of African origin.
* Normal, pain-free existence interrupted by bouts of pain in limbs, abdomen.
* Pains set off by infection, surgery under anesthetic, pregnancy.
* Screening is simple.

RARE

■ SYPHILIS
This sexually transmitted disease is now relatively rare in developed countries, but it is still worth considering if there is any odd or otherwise unexplained neurological disturbance. Years after the actual infection, syphilis can affect nerves in the spine, giving widespread nerve disorders such as:
* Severe, knife-like stabbing pains in the limbs.
* Pins and needles in hands or feet.
* Unsteady gait.
* Painless ulcers on limbs.
* Distorted but painless joints.

Though treatment will prevent any further disease, it will not reverse these symptoms.

PUFFINESS

See SWOLLEN BODY, page 429.

FEELING COLD

PROBABLE
NATURAL TENDENCY

POSSIBLE
RAYNAUD'S PHENOMENON AND DISEASE
HYPOTHYROIDISM

RARE
HYPOADRENALISM

PROBABLE

■ NATURAL TENDENCY
In the great majority of cases, sensitivity to cold is a natural feature of your constitution: you may have always suffered from numb and/or bluish fingers and toes *(see also BLUISH SKIN, page 424)*. The elderly often find that they "feel the cold". Similarly, babies have a reduced ability to compensate for low temperature, making adequate room temperature and warm clothing essential.

"GENERAL" SYMPTOMS

POSSIBLE

■ RAYNAUD'S PHENOMENON and RAYNAUD'S DISEASE
Common conditions in which the circulation of the fingers and toes over-reacts to changes in temperature.
* Fingers and toes always feel cold; go white or blue easily.
* Pain and redness are evident as they warm up.

Severe forms of Raynaud's can cause ulceration of fingers and toes. The problem may occasionally arise as a side-effect of taking beta-blockers for high blood pressure, or of working with vibrating equipment; it might also be a complication of a connective tissue disorder.

■ HYPOTHYROIDISM
Slowly increasing sensitivity to the cold is one of the specific features of this easily treated disorder. *See page 460.*

RARE

■ HYPOADRENALISM
A gradually developing hormone deficiency causing generalized weakness and lack of resistance to physical stress, including low temperature. People look strikingly pale.

SWOLLEN LYMPH NODES

The lymphatic system, consisting of the lymph nodes (glands), liver and spleen, is in the front line of defence against infection. It is the major part of the immune system of the body. Temporary swelling for a week or two is of little significance, being a feature of many minor viral illnesses and injuries. Benign problems account for 80 percent of lymph gland swelling in people under 30 years of age; 40 percent for people over 50 years.

However, prolonged swelling of lymph glands can be a sign of several serious conditions. Frequently, these conditions are treatable, especially at an early stage, making it essential to report persistently swollen glands. Blood tests and lymph node biopsy are usually needed to confirm the diagnosis.

PROBABLE
GLANDULAR FEVER (MONO)
TONSILLITIS
LOCAL INFECTION
CAT SCRATCH FEVER

POSSIBLE
HODGKIN'S DISEASE
LYMPHOMA
CANCER
TOXOPLASMOSIS
TUBERCULOSIS
LEUKEMIA
SARCOIDOSIS

RARE
SECONDARY SYPHILIS
YAWS
AIDS

"GENERAL" SYMPTOMS

Lymphatic system

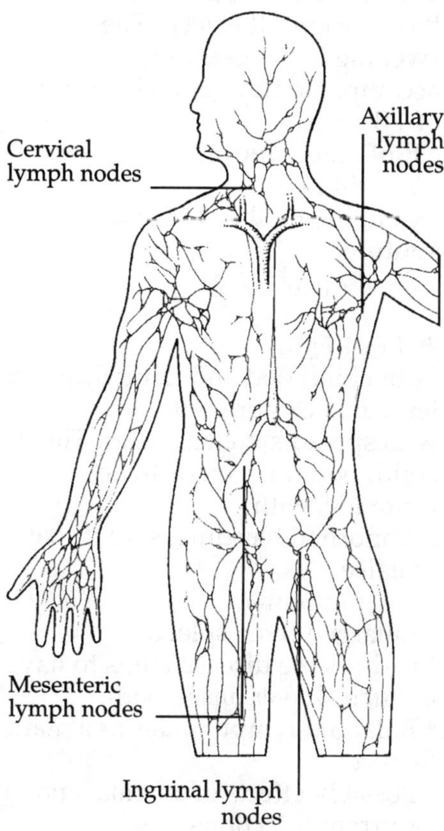

PROBABLE

■ <u>GLANDULAR FEVER (MONO)</u>
An extremely common infection, with a combination of severe sore throat, swollen glands and tiredness. No specific treatment; you will eventually make a full recovery. *See also page 462.*

■ <u>TONSILITIS</u>
A sore throat can cause massive swelling of lymph glands below the chin. This can be particularly dramatic in children; *see page 442.*

■ <u>LOCAL INFECTION</u>
Infection in a limb, like an infected toenail, can cause swelling of the nearest lymph glands, such as in the groin.

■ <u>CAT SCRATCH FEVER</u>
A probably under-recognized, reason for enlarged glands. Said to be one of the commonest causes of a single persistently swollen gland in the U.S.A. Over 4 percent of the population gets the disease.

* At first, just broken skin from the scratch.
* After a week or two, a small red lump appears.
* Swollen local glands, for example, underarm.
* Glands enlarge, and may discharge pus.
* Illness settles over a few weeks.

Sometimes there are also joint pains. The organism responsible has only recently been identified. Can be cured with antibiotics.

POSSIBLE

In most of the following, the lymph nodes gradually enlarge and remain enlarged:

■ <u>HODGKIN'S DISEASE</u>

* Painless.
* Rubbery feel to glands.
* Glands grow steadily over a few weeks.
* Tiredness, sweats at night.

Swelling of the neck glands is the most likely to be noticed. The feel of the glands in this disease is characteristic, but diagnosis requires biopsy of a gland.

"GENERAL" SYMPTOMS

■ LYMPHOMA
Another form of cancer of the lymphatic system, but in an older age group — 35-plus. Symptoms are similar to those in Hodgkin's disease, with:
* Widespread, painless swollen lymph nodes.
* Weight loss, sweats at night.

Treatment depends on the type of lymphoma — determined by blood test, plus bone marrow and lymph node biopsy.

■ CANCER
By the time it causes generalized swelling of glands, the cancer will be so advanced that it is bound to be obvious from other features. More important from the point of view of early diagnosis is enlargement of a single group of lymph nodes, which may signal the presence of an early cancer in such sites as the breast or the thyroid gland before there other obvious features.

The sites most noticeable are:
* Neck (cancers of lung, thyroid, nose and stomach).
* Groin (cancer of bowel, womb, prostate).
* Armpit (breast cancer).

■ TOXOPLASMOSIS
An infection acquired through eating infected meat, or sometimes from cat feces. If caught during pregnancy, it causes brain and eye damage in the baby.
* In mild cases, generalized, painless, swollen lymph nodes.
* Possibly fever, weakness as well.

■ TUBERCULOSIS
The usual glands involved are those around the neck. The swelling is painless and accompanied by general features of TB such as:
* Prolonged illness.
* Weight loss.
* Cough, possibly with blood in sputum.

See also page 447.

■ LEUKEMIA
Both childhood and adult forms of leukemia can present with widespread swollen nodes. The childhood form tends to be dramatic, with:
* Abnormal bleeding, sore throat, malaise.
* Fever, anemia.
* Enlarged liver, spleen.

In adults the disease tends to have a much slower onset, with:
* Enlarged lymph nodes as a main feature.
* Possibly effects of anemia, and recurrent infections.

Treatment of childhood leukemias is good and improving. Outlook in adults depends on the form of leukemia.

■ SARCOIDOSIS
A condition of unknown origin, often picked up by chance from seeing enlarged glands deep inside the chest on an X-ray. Usually benign, but may cause:
* Rashes, joint pains.
* Sickness.
* Large, painful red lumps on shin.
* Painful, red eye.

"GENERAL" SYMPTOMS

RARE

■ SECONDARY SYPHILIS
This remains globally a widespread disease.
* The initial sign is a painless sore on the genitals.
* General lymph node swelling after several months.
* Wart-like growths around genitalia.
* Vague malaise.

Diagnosis is by blood test; antibiotic treatment is effective and essential in order to prevent progression to serious nerve disorders, possibly years later.

■ YAWS
A syphilis look-alike found in the tropics. Unlike syphilis, it is spread by poor hygiene, rather than sexually transmitted.
* Ulcerating skin rash, mainly on palms and soles of feet.
* Widespread enlargement of the lymph nodes.

Treatment prevents disfiguring destruction of bone.

■ AIDS
An increasingly common problem, now affecting people with all types of sexual habits. The AIDS virus damages the immune system, leaving the person without resistance to infection by many unusual organisms.
* Fever.
* Night sweats.
* Widespread swollen lymph glands.
* Attacks of diarrhea.
* Itching of skin.
* Breathlessness.
* White patches inside cheeks.

INDEX

INDEX

INDEX